NUTRITION AND DIET RESEARCH PROGRESS SERIES

FLAVONOIDS: BIOSYNTHESIS, BIOLOGICAL EFFECTS AND DIETARY SOURCES

NUTRITION AND DIET RESEARCH PROGRESS SERIES

Diet Quality of Americans
Nancy Cole and Mary Kay Fox
2009. ISBN: 978-1-60692-777-9

School Nutrition and Children
Thomas J. Baxter
2009. ISBN: 978-1-60692-891-2

Appetite and Nutritional Assessment
Shane J. Ellsworth and Reece C. Schuster
2009. ISBN: 978-1-60741-085-0

Flavonoids: Biosynthesis, Biological Effects and Dietary Sources
Raymond B. Keller
2009. ISBN: 978-1-60741-622-7

NUTRITION AND DIET RESEARCH PROGRESS SERIES

FLAVONOIDS: BIOSYNTHESIS, BIOLOGICAL EFFECTS AND DIETARY SOURCES

RAYMOND B. KELLER
EDITOR

Nova Science Publishers, Inc.
New York

For permission to use material from this book please contact us:
Telephone 631-231-7269; Fax 631-231-8175
Web Site: http://www.novapublishers.com

LIBRARY OF CONGRESS CATALOGING-IN-PUBLICATION DATA

Flavonoids : biosynthesis, biological effects and dietary sources / [edited by] Raymond B. Keller.
p. ; cm.
Includes bibliographical references and index.
ISBN 978-1-60741-622-7 (hardcover)
1. Flavonoids. I. Keller, Raymond B.
[DNLM: 1. Flavonoids--biosynthesis. 2. Flavonoids--metabolism. QU 220 F58906 2009]
QP671.F52F527 2009
612'.0154--dc22

2009015647

Published by Nova Science Publishers, Inc. ✝ New York

CONTENTS

PREFACE

Flavonoids, also referred to as bioflavonoids, are polyphenol antioxidants found naturally in plants. They are secondary metabolites, meaning they are organic compounds that have no direct involvement with the growth or development of plants. Flavonoids are plant nutrients that when consumed in the form of fruits and vegetables are non-toxic as well as potentially beneficial to the human body. Flavonoids are widely disbursed throughout plants and are what give the flowers and fruits of many plants their vibrant colors. They also play a role in protecting the plants from microbe and insect attacks. More importantly, the consumption of foods containing flavonoids has been linked to numerous health benefits. Though research shows flavonoids alone provide minimal antioxidant benefit due to slow absorption by the body, there is indication that they biologically trigger the production of natural enzymes that fight disease.

Recent research indicates that flavonoids can be nutritionally helpful by triggering enzymes that reduce the risk of certain cancers, heart disease, and age-related degenerative diseases. Some research also indicates flavonoids may help prevent tooth decay and reduce the occurrence of common ailments such as the flu. These potential health benefits, many of which have been proven, have become of particular interest to consumers and food manufacturers.

Foods that contain high amounts of flavonoids include blueberries, red beans, cranberries, and blackberries. Many other foods, including red and yellow fruits and vegetables and some nuts, also contain flavonoids. Red wine and certain teas also are rich in flavonoids.

Chapter 1 - There have been many epidemiological studies linking flavonoid intake to health benefits and many *in vitro* studies demonstrating various biological effects of flavonoids that should be reflected by health benefits. It has been widely assumed that these observations are linked and dietary flavonoids are readily absorbed into the circulation and influence many regulatory and signalling pathways in tissues. More recently, it has become apparent that only a small proportion of dietary flavonoid intake is actually absorbed directly and measured relative absorption varies about 2 orders of magnitude between different compounds.

It is also apparent that most of the dietary load of flavonoids finds its way to the colon where the numerous and varied microflora metabolise them into simpler but much more bioavailable compounds. Further complications to the bioavailability of flavonoids are added by human Phase II conjugative metabolism, which is thought to convert most absorbed flavonoids into polar conjugates.

There is no doubt that some unconjugated flavonoids do get into the circulation at low concentrations, but they are quantitatively swamped by the bulk of flavonoid conjugates and colonic metabolites.

In contrast with the much-studied metabolism of flavonoids, relatively little is known about the biological activities of their conjugates and metabolites, although what is known comes from a predominance of *in vitro* studies and suggests that the metabolites do have numerous and significant biological activities. Hence very little is known about the real and mostly indirect benefits and mechanisms of action of dietary flavonoids.

In this review, the current state of knowledge in this area is discussed, with the aim of stimulating further research (especially by intervention studies) to aid greater understanding.

Chapter 2 - Flavonoids are widely distributed in fruit and vegetables and form part of the human diet. These compounds are thought to be a contributing factor to the health benefits of fruit and vegetables in part because of their antioxidant activities. Despite the extensive use of chemical antioxidant assays to assess the activity of flavonoids and other natural products that are safe to consume, their ability to predict an *in vivo* health benefit is debateable. Some are carried out at non-physiological pH and temperature, most take no account of partitioning between hydrophilic and lipophilic environments, and none of them takes into account bioavailability, uptake and metabolism of antioxidant compounds and the biological component that is targeted for protection. However, biological systems are far more complex and dietary antioxidants may function via multiple mechanisms. It is critical to consider moving from using ‘the test tube’ to employing cell-based assays for screening foods, phytochemicals and other consumed natural products for their potential biological activity. The question then remains as to which cell models to use. Human immortalized cell lines derived from many different cell types from a wide range of anatomical sites are available and are established well-characterized models.

The cytoprotection assay was developed to be a more biologically relevant measurement than the chemically defined antioxidant activity assay because it uses human cells as a substrate and therefore accounts for some aspects of uptake, metabolism and location of flavonoids within cells. Knowledge of structure activity relationships in the cytoprotection assay may be helpful in assessing potential *in vivo* cellular protective effects of flavonoids. This chapter will discuss the cytoprotective properties of flavonoids and focuses on the relationship between their cytoprotective activity, physicochemical properties such as lipophilicity (log P) and bond dissociation enthalpies (BDE), and their chemical structures. The factors influencing the ability of flavonoids to protect human gut cells are discussed, and these support the contention that the partition coefficients of flavonoids as well as their rate of reaction with the relevant radicals help define the protective abilities in cellular environments. By comparing the geometries of several flavonoids, its possible to explain the structural dependency of the antioxidant action of these flavonoids.

Chapter 3 - The determination by Matrix-Assisted Laser Desorption/Ionization time–of-flight (MALDI-TOF) mass spectroscopy of the oligomeric nature of the two major industrial polyflvonoid tannins which exist, namely mimosa and quebracho tannins, and some of their modified derivatives indicates that: (i) mimosa tannin is predominantly composed of prorobinetinidins while quebracho is predominantly composed of profisetinidins, that (ii) mimosa tannin is heavily branched due to the presence of considerable proportions of "angular" units in its structure while quebracho tannin is almost completely linear. These structural differences also contribute to the considerable differences in viscoity of water solutions of the two tannins. (iii) the interflavonoid link is more easily hydrolysable, and does appear to sometime hydrolyse in quebracho tannin and profisetinidins, partly due to the linear structure of this tannin, and confirming NMR findings that this tannin is subject to polymerisation/depolymerisation equilibria. This tannin hydrolysis does not appear to occur in mimosa tannin in which the interflavonoid link is completely stable to hydrolysis. (iv) Sulphitation has been shown to influence the detachment of catechol B-rings much more than pyrogallol-type B-rings. (vi) The distribution of tannin oligomers, and the tannins number average degree of polymerisation obtained by MALDI-TOF, up to nonamers and decamers, appear to compare well with the results obtained by other techniques. As regards procyanidin tannins, it has been possible to determine for mangrove polyflavonoid tannins that: (i) procyanidins oligomers formed by catechin/epicatechin, epigallocatechin and epicatechin gallate monomers are present in great proportions. (ii) oligomers, up to nonamers, in which the repeating unit at 528-529 Da is a catechin gallate dimer that has lost both the gallic acid residues and an hydroxy group are the predominant species. (iii) oligomers of the two types covalently linked to each other also occur.

Water solution of non-purified polyflavonoid extracts appear to be incolloidal state, this being due mainly to the hydrocolloid gums extracted with the tannin as well as to the tannin itself.

Commercial, industrially produced mimosa, quebracho, pine and pecan polyflavonoid tannin extracts water solutions of different concentrations behave mainly as viscous liquids at the concentrations which are generally used for their main industrial applications. Clear indications of viscoelastic response are also noticeable, among these the cross-over of the elastic and viscous moduli curves at the lower concentrations of the range investigated, with some differences being noticeable between each tannin and the others, pine and quebracho tannin extracts showing the more marked viscoelastic behaviour. Other than pH dependence (and related structural considerations), the parameters which were found to be of interest as regards the noticeable viscoelastic behaviour of the tannin extracts were the existence in the solutions of labile microstructures which can be broken by applied shear. This is supported by the well known thixotropic behaviour of concentrated, commercial polyflavonoid tannin extracts water solutions.

Such microstructures appear to be due or (i) to the known colloidal interactions of these materials, or (ii) to other types of secondary interactions between tannin oligomers and particularly between tannin and carbohydrate oligomers. The latter is supported by the dependence of this effect from both the average molecular masses of the tannin and of the carbohydrate oligomers.

The behaviour of polyflavonoid tannins as regards their antioxydant capacity and radical scavenging ability has been examined. Radical formation and radical decay reactions of some polyflavonoid and hydrolysable tannins has been followed, and comparative kinetics determined, for both light induced radicals and by radical transfer from a less stable chemical species to the tannin as part of an investigation of the role of tannin as antioxidants.

The five parameters which appear to have a bearing on the very complex pattern of the rates of tannin radical formation and radical decay were found to be (i) the extent of the colloidal state of the tannin in solution (ii) the stereochemical structure at the interflavonoid units linkage (iii) the ease of heterocyclic pyran ring opening, (iv) the relative numbers of A- and B-rings hydroxy groups and (v) solvation effects when the tannin is in solution. It is the combination of these five factors which appears to determine the behaviour as an antioxidant of a particular tannin under a set of application conditions.

The chapter ends with some recent results on the antiviral activity of polyflavonoid tannins for a great variety of viruses.

Chapter 4 - Naringin is the flavonoid compound found in grapefruit that gives grapefruit its characteristic bitter flavor. Grapefruit processors attempt to select fruits with a low naringin content, and often blend juices obtained from different grapefruit varieties to obtain the desired degree of bitterness. Naringin is believed to enhance our perception of taste by stimulating the taste buds; some people consume a small amount of grapefruit juice before a meal for this reason.

Naringin and its aglycone naringinin are commonly used health supplements; they exert a variety of biological actions. This article attempts to review their pharmacokinetics and pharmacological actions from scientific publications up to November 2008 including effects on the cardiovascular system, on the skeletal system, on smooth muscle, on the gastric intestinal system, on the endocrine system, also effects against tumours, protection against toxins in chemotherapy drugs and the environment, antioxidant effects, drug interactions, anti-inflammatory effects, and the newly discovered osteogenic and antibacterial actions.

Chapter 5 - Numerous epidemiological studies show that some nutrients may protect against vascular diseases, cancers and associated inflammatory effects. Consequently, the use of phytoconstituents, namely those from the human diet, as therapeutic drugs is relevant. Various studies report the efficiency of phyto-molecules which have cellular targets similar to those of the new drugs developed by pharmaceutical companies. Indeed, more than 1600 patents are currently reported concerning flavonoids and 3000 patents concerning polyphenols. Pleiotropic pharmaceutical activities are claimed in fields such as cancer, inflammation arthritis, eye diseases and many other domains. The increase of activities after combination with other natural compounds or therapeutic drugs is also patented. In addition, the aforementioned molecules, from natural origin, generally exhibit low toxicities and often a multipotency which allow them to be able to simultaneously interfere with several signalling pathways. However, several in vivo studies revealed that polyphenols / flavonoids are efficiently absorbed by the organism, but unfortunately have a low level of bioavailability, glucuronidation and sulphation being limiting factors. Therefore, many laboratories are developing elements to increase bioavailability and consequently the biological effects of these natural molecules. For example, the modifications in the lipophilicity of molecules increase the cellular uptake and consequently involve a best absorption without loss of their activities. Moreover isomerisation and methylation of hydroxyl groups of polyphenols (e.g. resveratrol) change the cell molecular targets and are crucial to improve the molecule efficiency in blocking cell proliferation. In this review, the focus is on the relevance of using flavonoid and polyphenol combinations or chemical modifications to enhance their biological effects. Innovative directions to develop a new type of drugs which may especially be used in combination with other natural components or pharmacological conventional drugs in order to obtain synergistic effects is discussed.

Chapter 6 - Cocoa has recently become an object of interest due to its high content of flavonoids, mainly the monomers epicatechin and catechin and various polymers derived from these monomers called procyanidins. Previous *in vitro* studies have shown the ability of cocoa flavonoids to down-regulate inflammatory mediators produced by stimulated macrophages, but there are no studies that consider the effects of *in vivo* cocoa intake on inflammatory response. The present article, reports the *in vivo* cocoa inhibitory effect on the acute inflammatory response. Female Wistar rats received Natural Forastero cocoa containing 21.2 mg flavonoids/g for 7 days (2.4 or 4.8 g per rat kg, p.o.). Then, acute inflammation was induced by means of carrageenin, histamine, serotonin, bradykinin or PGE_2 hind-paw injection. Rats fed 4.8 g/kg/day cocoa showed a significant reduction in the hind-paw edema induced by carrageenin from the first hour after induction ($P<0.05$). However, cocoa intake did not modify the edema induced by histamine, serotonin or PGE_2. Only a certain protective effect was observed at the lowest dose of cocoa in the bradykinin model. Moreover, peritoneal macrophages from rats that received 4.8 g/kg/day cocoa for 7 days showed a reduced ability to produce radical oxygen species (ROS), nitric oxide (NO), tumor necrosis factor α (TNFα) and interleukin 6 (IL-6). This fact could justify, at least partially, the beneficial effect of cocoa on carrageenin-induced inflammation. In summary, a diet rich in cocoa flavonoids was able to down-regulate the acute inflammatory response by decreasing the inflammatory potential of macrophages.

Chapter 7 - The biological activity of flavonoids was first recognized when the antiestrogenic principle present in red clover that caused infertility in sheep in Western Australia was discovered. These adverse effects of flavonoids placed these substances in the class of endocrine-disrupting chemicals. On the other hand, flavonoids are recently claimed to prevent several cancer types and to reduce incidence of cardiovascular diseases, osteoporosis, neurodegenerative diseases, as well as chronic and acute inflammation. Despite these controversial effects, a huge number of plant extracts or mixtures, containing varying amounts of isolated flavonoids, are commercially available on the market as dietary supplements and healthy products. The commercial success of these supplements is evident, even though the activity and mechanisms of flavonoid action are still unclear.

Owing to their chemical structure, the most obvious feature of flavonoids is their ability to quench free radicals. However, in the last few years many exciting new indication in elucidating the mechanisms of flavonoid actions have been published. Flavonoids inhibit several signal transduction-involved kinases and affect protein functions via competitive or allosteric interactions. Among others, flavonoids interact with and affect the cellular responses mediated by estrogen receptors (ERα and ERβ). In particular, our recent data indicate that some flavonoids (i.e., naringenin and quercetin) decouple specific ERα action mechanisms, important for cell proliferation, driving cells to the apoptosis. Therefore, distinct complex mechanisms of actions, possibly interacting one another, for nutritional molecules on cell signalling and response can be hypothesized.

Aim of this review is to provide an updating picture about mechanisms by which flavonoids play a role in cellular response and in preventing human pathologies such as cancer. In particular, their direct interaction with nuclear receptors and/or by their ability to modulate the activity of key enzymes involved in cell signaling and antioxidant responses will be presented and discussed.

Chapter 8 - Vegetal extracts usually have a large diversity of bioactive compounds showing several pharmacological activities, including antiophidian properties. In this study, both coumarin and tannic acid (100 μg/mL) showed no changes in the basal response of twitches in mouse nerve phrenic diaphragm preparations. In opposite, *Crotalus durissus terrificus* (Cdt 15 μg/mL) or *Bothrops jararacussu* (Bjssu 40 μg/mL) venoms caused irreversible neuromuscular blockade. Tannic acid (preincubated with the venoms), but not coumarin, was able to significantly inhibit ($p<0.05$) the impairment of the muscle strength induced by Cdt (88 ± 8%) and Bjssu (79 ± 7.5%), respectively. A remarkable precipitation was observed when the venoms were preincubated with tannic acid, but not with coumarin. *Plathymenia reticulata* is a good source of tannins and flavonoids whereas *Mikania laevigata* contain high amounts of coumarin. *P. reticulata* (PrHE, 0.06 mg/mL) and *M. laevigata* (MlHE, 1 mg/mL) hydroalcoholic extracts were assayed with or without Bjssu or Cdt venoms. Both PrHE and MlHE showed protection against Bjssu (79.3 ± 9.5% and 65 ± 8%, respectively) and Cdt (73.2 ± 6.7% and 95 ± 7%, respectively) neuromuscular blockade. In order to observe if the protective mechanism could be induced by protein precipitation, tannins were eliminated from both extracts and the assay was repeated. MlHE protected against the blockade induced by Bjssu (57.2 ± 6.7%), but not against Cdt. The conclusion is that plants containing tannins could induce the precipitation of venoms' proteins and plants containing coumarin showed activity against *Bothrops* venoms, but not against *Crotalus* venoms. Also concluded is that the use of isolated bioactive compounds could not represent the better strategy against ophidian venoms, since the purification may exclude some bioactive components resulting in a loss of antivenom activity. In addition, *M. laevigata* showed better antiophidian activity than *P. reticulata*.

Chapter 9 - There are serious concerns about the increasing global cancer incidence. As currently used chemotherapeutics agents often show severe toxicity in normal cells, anti-carcinogenic compounds included in the dietary intakes of natural foods are expected to be applicable to a novel approach to preventing certain types of cancer without side effects. Polyphenolic compounds, such as flavonoids, are ubiquitous in plants and are presently considered to be the most promising in terms of having anti-carcinogenic properties probably due to their antioxidant effect. To gain further insights into how flavonoids exert anti-carcinogenic actions on cancer cells at the molecular level, many intensive investigations have been performed. Currently, the common signaling pathways elicited by flavonoids are recognized as tumor suppressor p53 and survival factor AKT. These factors are potential effectors of flavonoid-induced apoptosis via activation of Bax and caspase family genes. The present chapter emphasizes pivotal molecular mechanisms underlying flavonoid-induced apoptosis in human cancer cells. In particular, this chapter focuses on representative flavonoids such as soy isoflavone, green tea catechin, quercetin, and anthocyanin.

Chapter 10 - Flavan-3-ols with the most well known members being catechin and epicatechin are a group of phenolic compounds widely distributed in nature. The oligomers and polymers of flavan-3-ols are known as condensed tannins which used to be considered as anti-nutritional components. In recent years, more and more evidences proved that these compounds were beneficial to human health as nutrition and lifestyle have fundamentally changed in modern society. These phenolic compounds showed great potential for the treatment of lifestyle related diseases, such as type 2 diabetes, obesity, and metabolic syndrome. They were also reported to have effects on slowing down the aging progress as well as on prevention of Alzheimer's disease, cardiovascular disease, and cancer. This chapter describes the structures, chemical properties, isolation and identification methods, bioactivity and distribution of flavan-3-ol monomers and condensed tannins in dietary sources and medicinal plants. Case studies such as the chemical and biological investigations of tannins in the stems of *Cynomorium songaricum* (a well known tonic in China) and in other plants are provided.

Chapter 11 - Accurate taxonomic groupings are important for many applications, especially for medicinal plants. For example, structural analogues of the antitumour agent, paclitaxel, found in common *Taxus* species have increased the availability of this life-saving medicine without relying on the slow growing and comparatively uncommon, *T. brevifolia* [1]. Flavonoids have a long history of use as chemotaxonomic markers and have assisted in resolving many taxonomic disputes that have arisen as a result of morphological classification. In recent times, there has been increased interest in using molecular systematics and bioinformatics as alternatives to traditional chemotaxonomic techniques, however the investigation of the types flavonoids present in plants is still a useful technique to rapidly assess plant taxonomy.

Planchonia careya is a medicinal plant that contains a range of antibacterial compounds. Species of this genus are morphologically related to *Barringtonia* and *Careya* species and there have been several changes of nomenclature to reflect the uncertainty of these relationships.

Our recent investigation of some of the comprising flavonoids from *Planchonia careya* has revealed similar distinctive compounds to those found in *Planchonia grandis* that are notably absent from *Barringtonia* and *Careya* taxa. Therefore the comparatively simple analysis of the flavonoid component of plant extracts can confirm or contest phenetic groupings to help resolve taxonomic discrepancies.

Chapter 12 - y ubiquitously occur in all parts of plants including the fruit, pollen, roots and heartwood. Plant extracts rich in flavonoids such as: Ginkgo biloba extract, soy bean extract and green tea extract are popular dietary supplements. Numerous physiological activities have been attributed to them and their potential roles in the prevention of hormone-dependent cancers have been investigated. Over 5000 different flavonoids have been described to date and they are classified into at least 10 chemical groups. Flavonoid compounds usually occur in plants as glycosides in which one or more of the phenolic hydroxyl groups are combined with sugar residues.

Quality control of these plant-extract products is problematic due to the many varying factors in herbal medicine. Unlike synthetic drugs (in which the concentration and activity of a single known bio-molecule is monitored), there are many uncertainties in terms of species variation, geographical source, cultivation, harvest, storage and processing techniques which may lead to a product of different quality and efficacy. To evaluate the quality of flavonoids contained within plant extracts it is therefore very important to develop an analytical method which can monitor the quantity and variety of flavonoids efficiently. Also the study of the absorption and retention of these compounds within individuals is more problematic as more than one active compound is ingested from the plant extracts.

The challenge presented by such extracts is therefore to determine the different flavonoid species present in any given extract and also to determine any modification or fortification of the extract. Furthermore, Administration, Distribution, Metabolism and Excretion (ADME) studies require the quantitative analysis of multiple components rather than a single drug compound. The increase in the number of new flavonoid reports is due to two main factors: the advances in methods of separation and the rapid development and application of modern mass spectrometry (MS). Mass spectrometry proved to be the most effective technique in flavonoids research both in plant extract and in biological samples. This expert commentary ll reviews the methods available for studying this wide-ranging class of compounds and also how modern techniques have been applied in order to "mine" the data obtained for flavonoid specific information from a complex metabolomic analysis.

Chapter 13 - *Afrofittonia silvestris* Lindau, commonly known as the hunter's weed, is a procumbent herb trailing on moist ground. The leaves of the plant are used to heal sore feet, skin infections and as laxative. The leaves were macerated in 50 % ethanol and the liquid extract concentrated to dryness. The dry extract was evaluated for antibacterial activity by adopting agar diffusion method. The extract was partitioned between water, ethyl acetate and butanol successively and further subjected to antibacterial testing. The most active extract, ethyl acetate extract, was purified through various chromatographic methods to obtain pure compounds identified by spectroscopic methods as kaempferide 3–O–β–D–glucopyranoside and kaempferol 5,4'-dimethoxy-3,7-O- α-L-dirhamnoside. These compounds produced significant antibacterial effects, while the minimum inhibitory concentrations of the fractions and the pure compounds ranged between 25 and 250 μg/mL. These flavonoids are reported for the first time in this plant, while kaempferol 5,4'-dimethoxy-3,7-O- α-L-dirhamnoside is a new compound.

Chapter 14 - Anthocyanins are water-soluble plant pigments conferring blue to pink colour to plant organs [1]. Nearly 600 different molecules have been identified so far, 97% of which occurs as glycosylated compounds. Their aglycone moiety is a flavonoid named anthocyanidin. The six most common anthocyanidins display various hydroxylation and methoxylation patterns. The repertoire of anthocyanins is so large, because various types of glycosyl moieties are bound to the aglycone core [1].

These pigments occur not only in petals, but also in fruits, vegetables and grains [2] and thus are constituents of the human diet. Their intake is highly variable, depending on the consumption of anthocyanin-rich food; data collected in the United States lead to estimate that anthocyanin daily individual intake may span from 12.5 [3] to 650 mg [4].

In: Flavonoids: Biosynthesis, Biological Effects...
Editor: Raymond B. Keller
ISBN: 978-1-60741-622-7

Chapter 1

BIOAVAILABILITY AND METABOLISM OF DIETARY FLAVONOIDS – MUCH KNOWN – MUCH MORE TO DISCOVER

David E. Stevenson*[1], Arjan Scheepens[2] and Roger D. Hurst[1]
[1]The New Zealand Institute for Plant and Food Research Limited,
Private Bag 3123, Waikato Mail Centre, Hamilton 3240, New Zealand
[2]The New Zealand Institute for Plant and Food Research Limited,
Private Bag 92-169, Mt Albert, Auckland, New Zealand

ABSTRACT

There have been many epidemiological studies linking flavonoid intake to health benefits and many *in vitro* studies demonstrating various biological effects of flavonoids that should be reflected by health benefits. It has been widely assumed that these observations are linked and dietary flavonoids are readily absorbed into the circulation and influence many regulatory and signalling pathways in tissues. More recently, it has become apparent that only a small proportion of dietary flavonoid intake is actually absorbed directly and measured relative absorption varies about 2 orders of magnitude between different compounds.

It is also apparent that most of the dietary load of flavonoids finds its way to the colon where the numerous and varied microflora metabolise them into simpler but much more bioavailable compounds. Further complications to the bioavailability of flavonoids are added by human Phase II conjugative metabolism, which is thought to convert most absorbed flavonoids into polar conjugates.

There is no doubt that some unconjugated flavonoids do get into the circulation at low concentrations, but they are quantitatively swamped by the bulk of flavonoid conjugates and colonic metabolites.

In contrast with the much-studied metabolism of flavonoids, relatively little is known about the biological activities of their conjugates and metabolites, although what is

* Correspondence: Dr. David E Stevenson. Tel: +64 7 959 4485. Fax: +64 7 959 4431, E-Mail: dstevenson@hortresearch.co.nz
* Correspondence: Dr. Jingli Zhang. Tel: ++64 9 9257100, Fax: ++64 9 9257001, Email jzhang@hort research.co.nz

known comes from a predominance of *in vitro* studies and suggests that the metabolites do have numerous and significant biological activities. Hence we actually know very little about the real and mostly indirect benefits and mechanisms of action of dietary flavonoids.

In this review, we discuss the current state of knowledge in this area, with the aim of stimulating further research (especially by intervention studies) to aid greater understanding.

INTRODUCTION

Numerous epidemiological trials have associated dietary flavonoid intake with health benefits, such as reductions in incidence of cardiovascular disease, stroke, diabetes and some types of cancer [1-12].

In addition, numerous *in vitro* studies have linked flavonoids to biological effects that could reasonably underlie the observed health benefits [13]. Although it is very tempting to assume a simple relationship between the two observations, decades of research into the absorption, distribution, metabolism and excretion (ADME) of flavonoids strongly contradicts this simplistic idea.

Research into this field started in the 1950s and was so prolific that in 1991, Scheline was able to include over 100 studies (mostly in animals) on flavonoid metabolism in his comprehensive "Handbook of mammalian metabolism of plant compounds" [14]. The main conclusion from all this work was that, unlike pharmaceutical compounds, which are mainly found relatively intact, as glucuronide derivatives in plasma or urine, flavonoids were much more extensively metabolised.

In addition to glucuronides, sulphates and methyl conjugates, the main urinary metabolites found were phenolic acids of the type also found to be produced by biotransformation using intestinal bacteria. A few studies using, ^{14}C-labelled flavonoids, found significant or even extensive degradation into simple compounds such as acetate, butyrate and carbon dioxide.

It appeared that the major part of the dietary flavonoid intake was not absorbed directly, but found its way into the colon where the extensive and varied microflora metabolised the flavonoids into simpler and apparently more bioavailable compounds. Examples of structures of the major compound classes discussed here are shown in Figure 1 (common flavonoids) and Figure 2 (common metabolites).

In recent years, much more detail has been added and we now have a relatively good understanding of flavonoid ADME. It appears that only a tiny proportion (approx 1-2%) of most dietary flavonoids is actually available to tissues and cells.

Most is metabolised by colonic microflora and most of the remainder that is absorbed through the gut is conjugated, mainly by glucuronidation, but also by sulphation and methylation.

The distribution of flavonoids is made more complex by factors like binding of flavonoids to serum proteins, such as albumin and the activities of cellular efflux pumps expressed by some cell types.

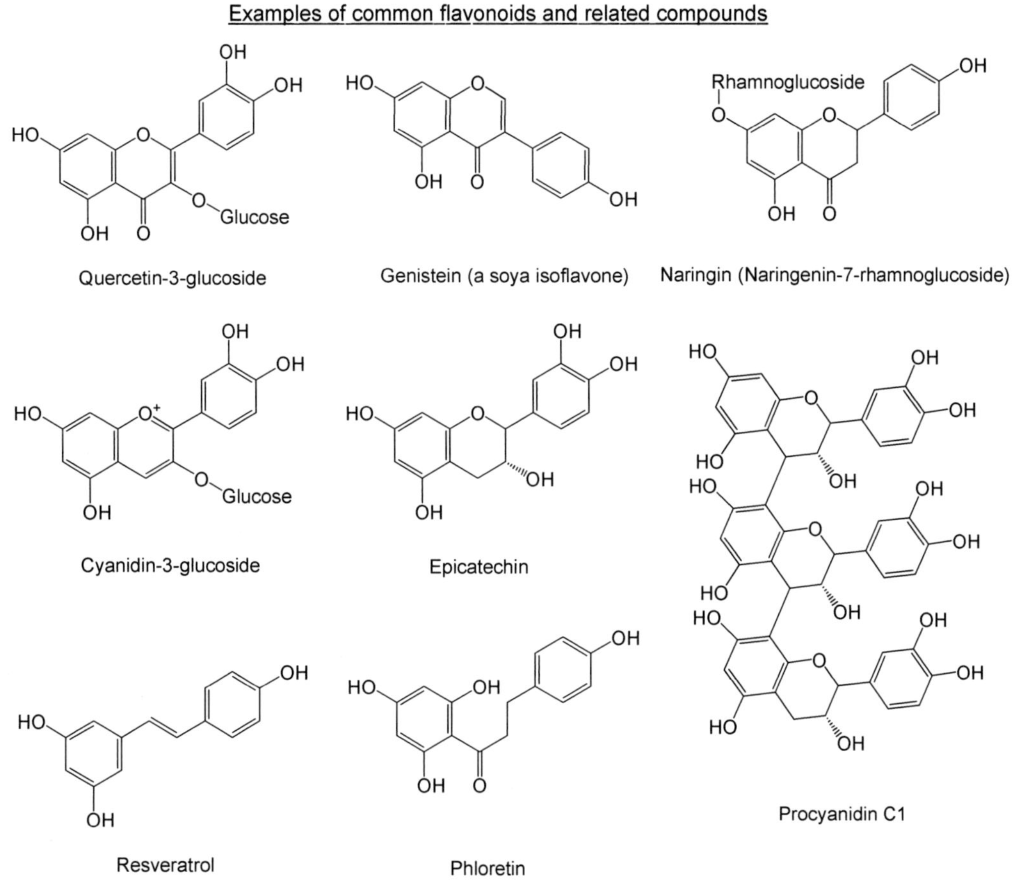

Figure 1. Structures of common flavonoids. Most flavonoids occur in plants predominantly as glycosides, with the exception of catechins and procyanidins. Resveratrol, a stilbene, is often found as its glucoside (piceid) and phloretin, a chalcone, as its glucoside (phloridzin).

There have been many excellent reviews discussing various aspects of these findings [15-30], but it is only relatively recently that serious attention has been given to determination of the biological activities of flavonoid metabolites and comparison with the parent compounds.

In contrast to the many hundreds of published studies on the biological effects of the quantitatively very minor species absorbed *in vivo*, i.e., flavonoid aglycones, published studies on metabolites only number around 50 at the time of writing.

We still, therefore, have little idea of the actual, as opposed to potential, relative contributions to health of flavonoid aglycones, flavonoid conjugates and colonic metabolites.

We have attempted to bring together all available information to date, to stimulate further research into the biology of flavonoid metabolites.

Our overall understanding of flavonoid ADME is summarised in Figure 3 and the chapter is organised to follow flavonoids through the various stages of digestion, absorption, distribution and metabolism and cover what is known about each stage.

The last section describes what we currently understand about the biological activities of the metabolites.

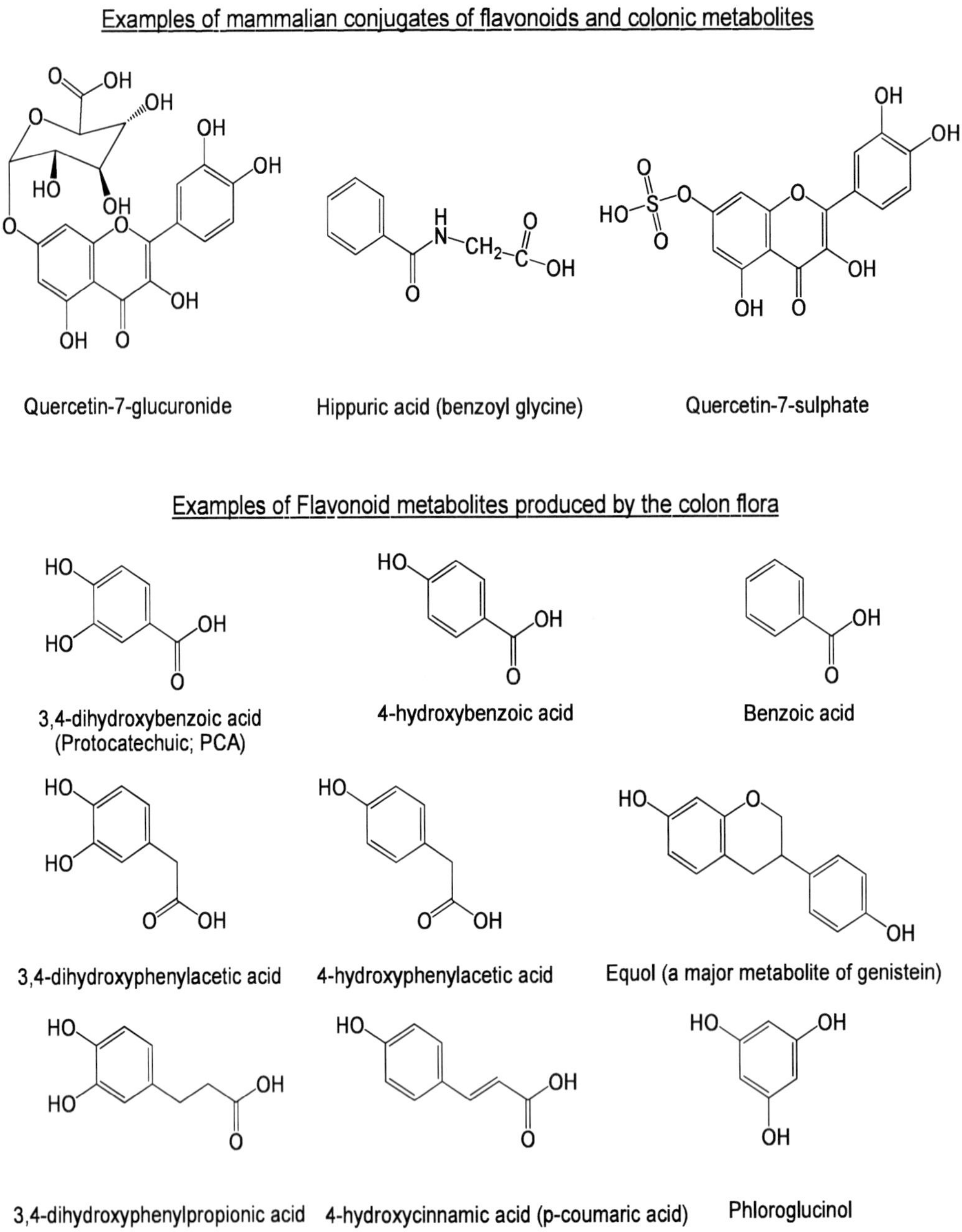

Figure 2. Structures of some flavonoid conjugates and colon flora-derived metabolites. Many other isomers of the phenolic acids have been detected, e.g., 2-, 3-, and 4-hydroxybenzoic acid and also O-methylated metabolites.

It is important to note that, although hundreds of different flavonoids are produced by plants, in thousands of differently glycosylated forms, only a small proportion occurs commonly in human foods.

The majority of scientific studies to date have focussed on the major human dietary flavonoids and the information obtained does not necessarily apply to the majority of flavonoids.

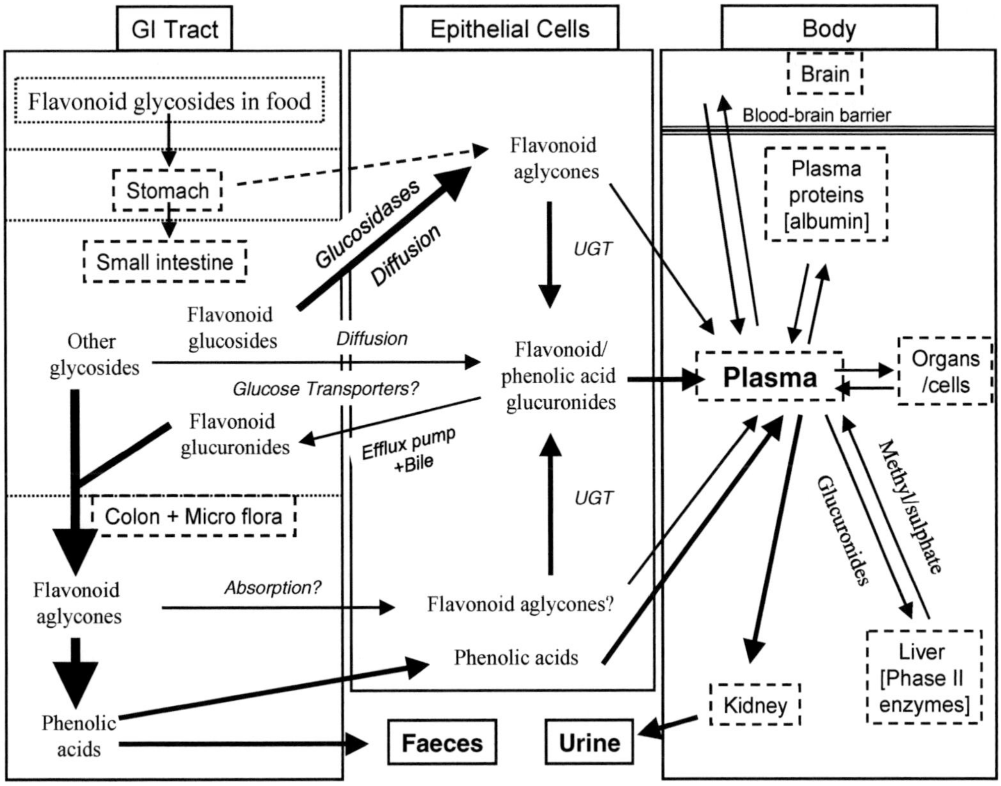

Figure 3. Summary of the great complexity of flavonoid metabolism, as currently understood. Thickness of arrows is an indication of relative quantitative significance of flows. UGT = Uridine diphosphoglucuronyl transferase. It has been estimated that dietary intake of flavonoids is ~100-200 mg/day [16, 31]; ~5% of this intake is absorbed via the intestine, ~95% passes into the colon [16].

Flavonoid Absorption and Metabolism in the Gastrointestinal Tract

The Oral Cavity

Human saliva was found to have significant, but highly variable hydrolytic activity [32], and hence hydrolysis of flavonoid glucosides may start in the oral cavity. It was not clear whether detached epithelial cells or bacteria, or both are the source of glucosidases. The resulting aglycones may be absorbed from the stomach, most likely by passive transport, whereas glycosides appear only to be absorbed by the intestine [33].

The Stomach

It is unclear whether procyanidins are metabolised in the stomach. In one study under simulated stomach acid conditions, procyanidins (epicatechin polymers, trimers to hexamers) have been found to be partially broken down, primarily to monomers and dimers [34]. This would be expected to enhance both bioavailability via intestinal absorption and colonic metabolism. In contrast, however, another study found that procyanidins were stable in the stomach [35], suggesting that they should be predominantly available to colonic flora.

Quercetin was absorbed in the rat stomach whereas its glycosides were not [33]. This suggests absorption by passive diffusion and the probable relative absence of suitable transporters or glycosidases. This result is the opposite of what is generally found in the intestine (see below). Anthocyanins at the very high concentration of 750 μM were absorbed directly from rat stomach to the extent of ~20% of the administered dose over 30 minutes [36]. The stomach is therefore clearly capable of anthocyanin absorption, but the physiological relevance of the high concentration used is questionable. Investigation of raspberry fruit extracts in an *in vitro* digestion model [37] suggested that anthocyanins and other flavonoids bind reversibly to other food components (protein, polysaccharides etc) and that this may increase their stability. This binding to polymers appears to modify the absorption and excretion of anthocyanins, but not their metabolism in rats [38], or pigs [39].

The Small Intestine

Manach *et al* [20] provided an excellent overview of the bioavailability of various flavonoids (aglycones and conjugates) and other relevant information obtained from a collection of human studies. Pharmacokinetic behaviour from these studies was very diverse, for example, the time to maximum plasma concentration ranged from 1-6 hours after dosing and elimination half-life from 1.5 hours to as long as nearly 20 hours. The percentage of dose excreted in the urine also varied from ~40% for isoflavone glycosides to under 1% for epigallocatechin gallate (EGCG), anthocyanins and rutin (quercetin rutinoside). Maximum reported plasma concentrations (C_{max}) also varied widely from 1-2 μM for isoflavones, quercetin glucosides and epigallocatechin (EGC), to 0.5 μM for naringin, 0.2 μM for rutin, 0.12 μM for EGCG and 0.03 μM for anthocyanins. Given that many studies have demonstrated that conjugates predominate in plasma, these results suggest that the concentrations of individual flavonoid aglycones are likely to be sub-micromolar [16, 18].

Table 1 summarises the main outcomes of human and animal studies, mostly carried out since the Manach *et al* review. In general, the results are very similar, but one recent development has been longer-term feeding studies to augment the more commonly studied single-dose trials. Resveratrol is a stilbene that has been relatively well-studied and its ADME appears similar to that of flavonoids, so some studies on resveratrol have also been included.

Table 2 summarises the main outcomes of *in vitro* cell-based studies, mostly using Caco-2 (human colon carcinoma) cell monolayers, a well-established system to measure parameters like permeability of the gut cell wall [40, 41]. The cells are grown to confluency on a semi-porous membrane, the upper or "apical" side corresponding to the intestinal lumen side and the lower or "basolateral" side corresponding to the "tissue" side of the intestinal wall. Samples are added to the apical medium and may or may not be detected in the basolateral medium, after passing through the cells. Caco-2 cells also express both functional Phase II conjugative enzymes and multi-drug resistance (MDR) efflux pumps, such as P-glycoprotein and breast cancer resistance protein (BCRP). Flavonoid conjugates have been detected in both the apical and basolateral medium, indicating that a compound has been taken up by the cells, conjugated and pumped back out [42]. This suggests that efflux pumps can limit bioavailability by returning flavonoid conjugates to the apical side/lumen, but cannot completely prevent some material from reaching the basolateral side/circulation.

The overall picture that emerges from the numerous bioavailability/metabolism studies is that there are essentially three groups of flavonoids with distinctively different behaviour, anthocyanins, procyanidins/catechins and "everything else". The aglycone forms of common flavonoids, such as quercetin, naringenin, or daidzein (and probably less common but structurally similar flavonoids) have been tested in many studies and are consistently the best-absorbed. These flavonoids are generally both more hydrophobic and more stable than anthocyanins or catechins and this may account for their higher observed plasma concentrations. Single doses routinely give plasma C_{max} values in the low micromolar range in humans (Table 1). Long-term dosing of pigs with quercetin gave similar results to single doses (~1 μM) [43], but in rats, plasma concentrations were over 20 μM, suggesting that pigs are probably a better model of human physiology [44]. Flavonoid aglycones, however, are rare in plant foods, glycosides usually being the only form found, with the exception of the relatively polar catechins, which are rarely glycosylated but, nevertheless, apparently much less bioavailable than hydrophobic compounds like quercetin. Where flavonoid aglycones are found in foods (specifically quercetin in onion skin), they appear to be more bioavailable than even glucoside derivatives [45].

The nature of glycosylation has an important influence on absorption. A number of studies have demonstrated the abundance of β-glucosidase, but the absence of other glycosidase activities in the GI tract and its tissues. Two β-glucosidases capable of hydrolysing flavonoid glycosides were found in human small intestinal mucosa. Lactase-phloridzin hydrolase (LPH) was localized in the apical membrane of gut epithelial cells while β-glucosidase was found in the cytosol [46]. This suggests that LPH can facilitate absorption by deglycosylating flavonoids and promoting passive diffusion, whereas the cytosolic enzyme can only act after absorption of the glucoside. Ovine lactase phloridzin hydrolase, a β-glucosidase found on the brush border of the mammalian small intestine, was readily able to hydrolyse glucosides of quercetin, genistein and daidzein [47]. Intestinal and liver β-glucosidases readily cleaved flavonoid glucosides, but not other glycosides [48]. There is some evidence from the studies in Table 2, that quercetin glucosides and maybe other flavonoid glucosides, can be transported intact by glucose transporters, but the main mechanism of glucoside absorption appears to be deglycosylation by membrane-bound β-glucosidase, followed by relatively rapid diffusion of the aglycone across the cell membrane [49-51]. Other glycosides may diffuse slowly across cell membranes [52-55], but the major proportion appears to pass into the colon, where microflora expressing various glycosidases can liberate the aglycones for absorption. It appears, for example, that a relatively high proportion of quercetin from the glucoside is absorbed from the intestine, as its plasma concentration peaks in 1-2 hours and it is predominantly cleared in 5-6 hours. In contrast, Rutin is absorbed much more slowly [56], to a much lower C_{max}, but most is deglycosylated in and absorbed from the colon as quercetin, giving a low but more sustained plasma level of quercetin conjugates that can last more than 24 hours.

Intestinal epithelial cells have high glucuronyl transferase activity and appear to glucuronidate ~95% of flavonoids before transfer into the bloodstream, or efflux back into the lumen [57-60].

Table 1. Summary of recent published studies involving determination of plasma/tissue bioavailability (C_{max}) from oral ingestion of flavonoids or flavonoid-rich foods and /or identification of major detected metabolites

Flavonoid/Source	Species	Bioavailability in plasma/tissues; Metabolites detected	Reference
Acylated anthocyanins from purple sweet potato	Human	Study on anthocyanins acylated with benzoic or cinnamic acids; plasma Cmax 2.5 µM after 1.5 hours; urinary excretion 0.01-0.03%; suggests absorption and plasma half-life much longer than non-acylated anthocyanins.	[76]
Anthocyanins from blackberry	Rat	Anthocyanins and methylated and/or glucuronidated metabolites detected in plasma, liver, kidney and brain (~0.25 µM); 0.2% of dose in urine.	[77]
Anthocyanins from Blood orange (fed 12 days)	Rat	~20% of dose absorbed from stomach, but only ~0.1% excreted in urine. Metabolites detected were methylated intact anthocyanins, plus un-metabolised anthocyanins.	[74]
Anthocyanins from grape	Rat/gastric intubation	~0.5 µM anthocyanins in plasma and brain after 10 min.	[78]
Apigenin, luteolin, oral/200 mg/kg	Rat	Peak plasma concentrations/% excreted in urine: Apigenin 50 µM/16%, Luteolin 15µM/6%; total recoveries ~40%, suggesting metabolism to simpler compounds in colon.	[79]
Apple juice	Ileostomised humans	Variable extent of metabolism of some unabsorbed flavonoids: Phloretin glycosides partially converted to phloretin and its 2-glucuronide; 90% of procyanidins recovered intact.	[60]
Apple juice, blueberries	Ileostomised humans	<33% of apple polyphenolics passed into collection bags, but up to 85% of those from blueberry. Suggests that berry phenolics are much more available for colonic metabolism.	[80]
Baicalein	Perfused rat intestine and Caco-2 monolayer	Extensive glucuronidation in both systems and efflux of glucuronide apically and basolaterallly. Glucuronidation reduced proportionally at higher loadings of flavonoid.	[57]
Baicalin (plant-derived glucuronide of the flavone baicalein.	Rat	Baicalein readily absorbed in small intestine, to yield plasma baicalin. Baicalin poorly absorbed, but apparently readily de-glucuronidated by colonic flora, absorbed and then re-glucuronidated.	[81]
Bilberry extract, oral/400 mg/kg	Rat	Plasma anthocyanin C_{max} 1.2 µM after 15 minutes, 30% of dose excreted in urine.	[82]
Blackcurrant juice or whole fruit	Human	0.05% of anthocyanins excreted intact with ~5% of dose excreted in the form of hippuric acid and its 3- and 4-hydroxyl derivatives.	[71]
Blueberries up to 4% of diet	Pig	No anthocyanins in plasma or urine, but traces detected in all tissues tested.	[83]
Blueberry extract, 2% of diet/10 weeks	Aged rat	Anthocyanins detected in brain of treatment but not control group.	[84]

Flavonoid/Source	Species	Bioavailability in plasma/tissues; Metabolites detected	Reference
Breviscapine (plant extract; 85% scutellarin)	Rat	11 glucuronides, methyl-glucuronides and sulpho-glucuronides.	[85]
Catechin epicatechin,	Isolated rat intestine	O-methylated (~30%), glucuronidated (~45%) conjugates (~20% with both) detected in the isolated jejunum after perfusion; 5 fold more flavanols overall, were detected in the isolated ileum after perfusion, predominantly unconjugated.	[86]
Catechins from tea	Human	Plasma C_{max} 1 μM catechins, after enzymic de-conjugation.	[87]
Catechins from tea	Rat foetal organs	Approx. 1 nM concentrations of catechins detected in foetal organs between 0.5-1 hour after dosing of mother	[88]
Cyanidin-3-glucoside (a common anthocyanin)	Isolated rat intestine	Cyanidin glucoside absorption was inhibited by quercetin glucoside, suggesting the involvement of active transport in absorption of anthocyanin glucosides	[89]
EGCG, Radio-labelled (^{3}H-aromatic protons)	Mouse	Widely distributed in mouse organs and tissues, indicating ability of EGCG or its metabolites to access all tissues. Excretion was 6% in urine and 35% in faeces. It appears likely that the remainder was lost as water vapour, following complete degradation by colon flora.	[90]
Chokeberry extract	Human	Peak of ~0.5 μM total anthocyanins in serum, Intact anthocyanins and conjugates, trace of protocatechuic acid (PCA) in plasma and urine.	[91]
Cyanidin glucoside orally; 400 mg/kg	Rat	Plasma C_{max} ~0.3 μM cyanidin glucoside and ~2.5μM protocatechuic acid (PCA).	[92]
Daidzein or daidzin (glucoside) 1mg/kg	Human (7 men)	C_{max}/T_{max} (intact and conjugated) 2.5 μM/10 hours from daidzin, 0.5 μM/8 hours from daidzein; main metabolites equol (one subject), dihydrodaidzein, *O*-desmethylangolensin.	[93]
Delphinidin glucoside	Rat	Main plasma metabolite 4'-O-methyl derivative; suggests that methylation is a major metabolic pathway for compounds with pyrogallol moiety (1, 2, 3-trihydroxyphenyl).	[94]
Dihydrocaffeic acid/18 mg/Kg (3,4-dihydroxypropionic acid; a putative colonic metabolite of flavonoids)	Rat	Rapid absorption, plasma T_{max} 30 min; 1% of dose excreted un metabolised in urine, along with methyl, glucuronide and sulphate conjugates.	[95]
Elderberry extract	Elderly women	Peak of ~0.16 μM total anthocyanins in serum, only intact anthocyanins observed in plasma and urine.	[96]
Genistein, hesperetin	Perfused rat intestine	Significant proportion of absorbed flavonoid glucuronidated and excreted back into lumen/perfusate.	[58]
Glabridin 10 mg/kg	Rat	Peak plasma concentration of ~0.1 μM; un-metabolised material, conjugates not detected: monocyte chemo-attractant protein-1 secretion reduced in dosed rats.	[97]

Table 1. (Continued)

Grapefruit extract	Dog	Plasma C_{max} 0.3-0.4 μM, primarily naringin, with small proportions of naringenin and its glucuronide.	[98]
Hesperetin, naringenin (aglycones) 135 mg each	Human	Plasma Max concentrations 3 and 7 μM respectively, mostly as conjugated forms. Phenolic acid metabolites also detected.	[99]
Isoflavones (glucosides of genistein and daidzein)	Human	Intact isoflavones are absorbed in 2 "peaks"; apparently the first from direct intestinal absorption and the second from the colon after microbial metabolism.	[100]
Kaempferol (a flavonol, like quercetin)	Human	Even a low dose (9 mg) resulted in a peak plasma concentration of 0.1 μM and urinary excretion of 2% of dose. Suggests that bioavailability higher than quercetin.	[101]
Luteolin and related permethylated flavone, Nobiletin	Rat	Nobiletin much better absorbed and widely distributed in tissues. Major metabolites were 3 mono-demethylated and 2 di-demethylated forms.	[64]
Naringenin and its glucoside	Rat	Orally, ~10% of both compounds absorbed and mainly recovered as glucuronide. Intravenously, glucoside recovered largely unchanged. Glucoside readily cleaved and glucuronidated during intestinal absorption.	[102]
Naringenin, hesperetin glycosides from Blood orange juice	Human	Peak plasma concentrations reached after 5 hours of ~0.1-0.2 μM, 95% detected as conjugates.	[103]
Normal diet	Human	Thirteen polyphenols and metabolites were found suitable as biomarkers of polyphenol intake; cinnamic acids: chlorogenic acid, caffeic acid, m-coumaric acid, gallic acid, 4-O-methylgallic acid; flavonoids: quercetin, isorhamnetin, kaempferol, hesperetin, naringenin, phloretin; lignans: enterolactone, enterodiol. Suggests that cinnamic acids, hydrophobic flavonoids and lignans are the most bioavailable phenolics.	[104]
Pelargonidin aglycone by oral gavage	Rat	18% of dose absorbed after 2 hours and detected in liver, kidney, brain, lung but not heart, spleen. Main metabolites glucuronide and 4-hydroxybenzoic acid.	[73]
Phloretin, quercetin and their glucosides	Rat intestine *in situ*	Perfusion of glucosides or aglycones generated same mixture of conjugates in blood. Glucosylation increased quercetin absorption, but reduced phloretin absorption.	[105]
Polymethoxylated flavone mixture isolated from Chinese herb	Rat	Plasma metabolites all glucuronides of parent compound or demethylated forms.	[106]
Procyanidin dimers	Isolated rat intestine	95% absorbed as unconjugated epicatechin, i.e., the dimers were cleaved into monomers by the intestinal cells.	[107]
Procyanidin-rich chocolate	Human	Plasma C_{max} of epicatechin range from 0.13-0.35 μM.	[108]

Flavonoid/Source	Species	Bioavailability in plasma/tissues; Metabolites detected	Reference
Procyanidins and catechins from oral grape seed extract	Rat	Conjugates of catechins only, no evidence of absorption or degradation of procyanidins.	[109]
Procyanidins and catechins from oral grape seed extract	Rat	No evidence of procyanidin absorption, only gallic acid and catechin monomers detected.	[110]
Puerarin (daidzein-8-C-glucoside)	Rat	Un-metabolised puerarin plasma conc 6 μM after 4 hours, detected in brain extracts. Metabolites detected: hydroxylated and reduced forms including equol.	[111]
Quercetin	Rat intestine	Quercetin rapidly absorbed, but ~ half glucuronidated and excreted back in to lumen.	[59]
Quercetin	Rat	Quercetin conjugates (no aglycone) appeared in lymphatic fluid, with the maximum concentration at 30 minutes.	[112]
Quercetin aglycone from Shallot skin, quercetin glucosides (shallot flesh/1.4 mg/kg total quercetin	Human	C_{max} 1μM from flesh and 4μM from skin; suggests that food matrix increases aglycone solubility/absorption compared with pure compound.	[45]
Quercetin and its glucoside	Isolated rat intestine	Glucoside absorbed faster than aglycone, via hexose transporter, but deglycosylated during or after absorption. Only aglycone and glucuronides found in mucosal tissue.	[49]
Quercetin glycosides	Rat intestine	Deglycosylation and absorption of quercetin aglycone was much higher from glucosides than other glycosides.	[50]
Quercetin glycosides from onions	Human	Quercetin-3-glucuronide, 3'-methyl-quercetin-3-glucuronide and quercetin-3'-sulfate, no source glycosides detected.	[113, 114]
Quercetin glycosides from onions	Human	Five isomeric quercetin glucuronides.	[115]
Quercetin in diet	Pig	Single dose of 25 mg/kg (50 mg/kg/day/4 weeks) resulted in μM concentrations of: plasma 1.6 (0.8), liver 0.03 (0.15), muscle 0.3 nM (both), brain (0.07 nM).	[43]
Quercetin mono- and di-glucoside from fried onions	Human	Sub-micromolar maximum concentrations of intestinal conjugates (glucuronide, sulphate) after~40 min and peak of liver metabolite (sulpho-glucuronide) after 2.5 hours. Considerable differences between plasma and urinary conjugate profiles. Total urinary excretion 4.7%.	[116]
Quercetin, catechin, red wine polyphenols, orally	Rat	Only quercetin could be detected in plasma, as conjugates. None of the supplements reduced lipid peroxidation markers.	[117]
Quercetin, long-term dietary supplementation	Rat, Pig	Rats, 0.1% quercetin in diet/11 weeks resulted in ~20 μM total quercetin (inc. conjugates) in plasma and 0-4 μM in organs; pigs, 500mg/kg in diet/3 days resulted in 1.25 μM in plasma, 6 μM in liver and 2.5 μM in kidney.	[44]
Quercetin, oral/6 weeks	Rat	11 different conjugates after absorption, major one a methyl, sulpho, glucuronide.	[70]

Table 1. (Continued)

Flavonoid/Source	Species	Bioavailability in plasma/tissues; Metabolites detected	Reference
Quercetin-3- and -4'-glucosides	Isolated rat intestine	Quercetin from 3–glucoside was only absorbed after hydrolysis by lactase phloridzin hydrolase in lumen; 4-glucoside was absorbed both after hydrolysis and directly by SGLT1. (Note contrast with [51], this table, below)]).	[118]
Quercetin glycosides from apple or onion	Human	Bioavailability of quercetin from apples and of pure quercetin rutinoside both 30% relative to onions. Plasma C_{max} at~40 min after ingestion of onions, 2.5 h after apples and 9 h after the rutinoside. Half-lives of elimination were 28 h for onions and 23 h for apples.	[56]
Quercetin supplement, 500 mg/3 times daily/7 days	Human	Plasma concentration >0.6 μM for 8 hours after last dose, C_{max} 1.1 μM, 94.5% present as conjugates.	[119]
Red wine whole/de-alcoholised	Rat intestinal preparation	Absorption of quercetin (3-fold) and its 3-glucoside (1.5-fold) was increased in the presence of alcohol, compared with de-alcoholised wine.	[120]
Resveratrol	Isolated rat intestine	Predominantly glucuronide found in mucosal tissue.	[121]
Resveratrol, catechin, quercetin	Human	Proportion of compound present in plasma as conjugates/proportion of dose excreted in urine/: Resveratrol – 98%/17%, catechin – 97%/2%, quercetin – 80%/5%.	[122]
Resveratrol; radio-labelled (^{14}C)	Rat	Apparently predominantly intact resveratrol conjugates predominated and were distributed throughout tissues.	[123]
Scutellarin (plant-derived 7-glucuronide of flavone scutellarein)	Human	Peak plasma concentration ~0.3 μM, urinary metabolites were 6-glucuronide, 2 sulpho-glucuronides and methyl scutellarin, scutellarein.	[124]
Semi-synthetic diet	Rat	Numerous flavonoid conjugates and colonic metabolites detected in intestinal mucosa, plasma and caecal contents.	[125]
Various flavonoids and glucosides	Isolated rat intestine	Glucosides except quercetin-3-glucoside (absorbed directly) deglycosylated during absorption and extensively glucuronidated.	[51]
Vitexin-rhamnoside (flavone derivative)	Isolated rat intestine	Good permeability by passive diffusion, increased by P-glycoprotein inhibitors; suggests P-glycoprotein involved in luminal efflux.	[62]

Table 2. Summary of recent published studies involving determination of absorption/bioavailability using Caco-2 and/or other gut epithelial cell cultures

Test compound	Outcome	Reference
Apigenin	At low apical concentrations main conjugate formed is sulphate, which is mainly effluxed apically. At higher concentrations, glucuronidation predominates and is mostly effluxed basolaterallly. Enteric recycling apparently limited by low efflux pump capacity.	[42]
Benzoic acid, p-coumaric acid, gallic acid, mono-hydroxybenzoic acids	Indication that observed rapid transport is mediated by a mono-carboxylic acid-specific carrier.	[126-129]
Blackcurrant anthocyanins	~11% apparently absorbed by cells, no basolateral efflux.	[130]
Catechins from tea	Catechins inhibit drug efflux by multidrug resistance P-glycoprotein . This effect may potentially enhance absorption of other flavonoids by inhibiting efflux.	[131]
Catechins from tea	Catechins inhibit mono-carboxylic acid transporter (MCT) but are absorbed by paracellular diffusion and also effluxed apically.	[132, 133]
Diosmin, hesperidin, naringin (rutinosides of flavones) and algycones	Aglycones had measurable permeabilities, rutinosides did not. Supports low absorption of glycosides other than glucosides.	[52]
Flavonoid aglycones	The human organic anion transporter OAT1 is inhibited by flavonoids and may be involved in their cellular absorption.	[134]
Galangin (5,7-dimethoxy flavone), mono- and di-methyl derivatives.	Methylated forms 5-8 times more permeable and more resistant to metabolism in Caco-2 cells and hepatocytes. Suggests that methylation should greatly increase oral bioavailability of flavonoids.	[135, 136]
Genistein, apigenin with siRNA treatment	Determination of which glucuronyl transferase (UGT) iso-forms expressed by Caco-2 cells.	[137]
Glabridin (isoflavan from liquorice)	Extensive glucuronidation observed and apical efflux appears to be meditated by P-glycoprotein and MDR1.	[61]
Hesperetin	Apically applied hesperetin slowly diffused basolaterallly, but most conjugates formed were transported back to the apical medium; addition of efflux pump inhibitors suggested the main pump operating was breast cancer resistance protein (BCRP).	[53]
Hesperetin, hesperidin (hesperetin-7-rutinoside)	Hesperidin absorbed by proton-coupled active transport, apparently by MCT transporter; hesperidin is not and is likely only bioavailable after deglycosylation by micro flora.	[54, 55]
Hydroxy tyrosol (3,4-dihydroxyphenylethanol)	Absorption is by passive diffusion and a methylated metabolite was detected.	[138]
Luteolin and its permethylated derivative, Nobiletin	Nobiletin, but not luteolin, preferentially accumulated in the Caco-2 cell monolayer, suggesting much higher bioavailability.	[139]
Quercetin and 3-glucoside	Glucoside absorbed unchanged and as aglycone, aglycone absorbed better.	[140]
Quercetin-3-glucoside	Absorption by Caco-2 and Chinese hamster ovary cells facilitated by sodium-dependent glucose co-transporter (SGLT1).	[141]
Quercetin-3-glucoside	Basolateral efflux from cells appears to be mediated by GLUT2 glucose transporter.	[142]

Various efflux pumps have been implicated in the return of glucuronidated flavonoids to the lumen [61, 62]. The material returned to the lumen is thought to pass into the colon and to subsequently become available for microbial metabolism. The positional isomer distribution of absorbed glucuronides may be influenced not only by the positional selectivity of intestinal epithelial cell glucuronyl transferase iso-forms, but also by selective efflux back into the lumen. The MRP2 efflux pump shows selectivity between quercetin glucuronide isomers [63] and this may contribute to the observed isomer distribution in the circulation. Some flavonoids, primarily from citrus fruits (e.g., Nobiletin, Sinensetin, Tangeretin) are permethylated, i.e., they have O-methyl groups in place of phenolic hydroxyl groups. Other flavonoids can also be easily methylated chemically and permethylated flavonoids have considerably different ADME properties from other flavonoids [64-68]. Methylation increases hydrophobicity and therefore intestinal absorption. Blocking of all potential conjugation sites (i.e., phenols) by methylation inhibits Phase II conjugative metabolism, requiring Phase I, cytochrome P_{450}-mediated demethylation before conjugation is possible [66]. These findings suggest an approach to counteract the issue of low flavonoid bioavailability for health studies (assuming that it is desirable), and also highlight the effectiveness of mammalian cell metabolism at limiting the absorption of flavonoids.

The array of flavonoid conjugates from gut cell metabolism appears to be further expanded by the liver, which appears to accumulate higher concentrations of flavonoids than any other organ [44]. Liver β-glucuronidase can apparently remove glucuronidation added by the intestinal cells and sulpho-transferase and catechol O-methyl transferase (COMT) can substitute (or add) sulphation and/or methylation. For example, quercetin is primarily glucuronidated by intestinal cells, before passage into the bloodstream. When cultured hepatocytes were treated with purified quercetin glucuronides to investigate potential further metabolism in the liver, three major processes were observed. Firstly, methylation of the quercetin moiety of the glucuronides by COMT was noted before removal of glucuronyl residues by β-glucuronidase, followed by sulphation [69]. The potential for a complex conjugate mixture resulting from conjugation by both intestine and liver was highlighted by a rat study with quercetin [70]. Eleven conjugates were detected, the most abundant having all 3 conjugate groups, i.e., methyl, glucuronide and sulphate, in the same molecule.

Anthocyanins are very unstable compared with other flavonoids, particularly at neutral or alkaline pH. The anthocyanin content of a wide variety of processed blackcurrant products was only 0.05-10% of that in fresh fruit. Although they should be relatively stable in the acidic environment of the stomach, degradation in the neutral small intestine may be very rapid [71]. Bioavailability studies on anthocyanins consistently find barely detectable concentrations in plasma (<0.05 μM) with only a tiny proportion of the dose (often <0.1%) excreted in urine (Tables 1, 4). This low urinary excretion compares with up to ~20% for some other flavonoids (see below). Elevated levels of phenolic acid metabolites can account for only a low percentage of intake (Tables 1, 4). It is becoming clear from the numerous bioavailability studies on anthocyanins that 60-90% of the dietary load disappears from the GI tract within 4 hours of a meal [72]. It is not clear, however, what happens to them. Possibilities are that they are degraded/structurally rearranged into as-yet unidentified derivatives, or covalently bound to proteins or other polymers (i.e., resistant to extraction/detection), either in the intestinal lumen, plasma, or inside cells. Anthocyanin detection is commonly achieved using very sensitive techniques such as liquid chromatography-mass spectroscopy (LC-MS). However, recoveries from anthocyanin extraction procedures performed from plasma are often very low (less than 20%) and hence it is possible that the apparently low bioavailability of anthocyanins is partly due to a lack of robust techniques to enable complete extraction and detection.

Anthocyanins are unusual in that, unlike other flavonoids, the predominant forms detected in plasma and urine are intact, un-metabolised glycosides, rather than aglycones or conjugates. They may be very unstable under physiological conditions after deglycosylation, because, apart from the strawberry anthocyanin, pelargonidin [73], there is very little evidence of significant deglycosylation or conjugation of anthocyanins. Although it may appear that anthocyanins probably do not have significant biological activities because of their apparently low bioavailability, there is some evidence that absorption from the stomach [74] and the jejunum [75], may be both rapid and relatively high. Particularly rapid degradation after absorption, however, appears to severely limit the duration of significant anthocyanin plasma concentrations, in normal circumstances. Only traces survive long enough to be detected in the urine. Localised biological effects of anthocyanins immediately after absorption, or direct effects on the gastrointestinal tract or its microflora are possible, however.

The Colon and Microflora

Colonic microflora display an extensive capability to metabolise flavonoids that reach the colon either directly, or after intestinal epithelial cell metabolism and apical efflux of glucuronides, biliary excretion etc. Numerous studies (Table 3) have demonstrated the ability of isolated cultures, faecal slurries, etc, to remove glycosylation that is resistant to endogenous mammalian β-glucosidases and cleave flavonoids into simpler compounds. As with the published bioavailability studies, quercetin is the most studied and best understood. It appears that quercetin glucosides, for example, are relatively well absorbed in the small intestine (see above discussion), whereas the glucosidase-resistant rutin reaches the colon mostly intact where it can be deglycosylated by microflora making it potentially available for both absorption by colonic epithelial cells and degradation into simpler compounds. One report proposed a mechanism to explain the observed degradation of quercetin by pig caecum microflora, predominantly into phloroglucinol and 3,4-dihydroxyphenylacetic acid [143]. These degradation products appear to accumulate in the colon to concentrations 1-2 orders of magnitude higher than the flavonoid aglycones [144]. There is evidence from urinary studies [145-148], that the phenolic acid degradation products, particularly benzoic acid, a likely final product of these degradation pathways, are well absorbed and increased urinary excretion correlates with consumption of flavonoid-rich foods. Hippuric acid (benzoylglycine) is regularly detected at high concentrations in urine, following consumption of flavonoid-rich foods and is known to be the major human conjugate of benzoic acid [146]. Studies *in vitro* using Caco-2 and other gut epithelial cells (Table 2) have demonstrated that these low molecular weight acids are efficiently transported, possibly by a mono-carboxylic acid transporter present in the colonic epithelia and so rapid absorption through the gut wall is not unexpected. One recent study found various small aromatic compounds in urine resulting from quercetin consumption and in addition reported for the first time, mercapturic acid conjugates of phenolic acids in the urine, apparently derived from colonic breakdown of glutathione conjugates of quercetin that had been detected in the plasma [149].

Table 3. Summary of published studies of the biotransformation of flavonoids using microbial cultures

Flavonoid	Culture	Metabolites Found	Reference
Anthocyanins	Human faecal flora	Rapid conversion into phenolic acids; major products were: protocatechuic acid from cyanidin; syringic acid from malvidin; vanillic acid from peonidin; 4-hydroxybenzoic acid from pelargonidin.	[165]
Biochanin A, formononetin, glycitein (methylated isoflavones	Eubacterium limosum (human intestinal strict anaerobe	Demethylated isoflavones.	[166]
Catechin, epicatechin	Human faecal flora	Main metabolites from both catechins were 3-hydroxyphenyl-propionic acid and phenylpropionic acid; 3,4-dihydroxyphenylacetic acid and 3-hydroxyphenylacetic acid were not detected.	[167]
Catechins from tea (EGCG etc)	Human, rat faecal flora	15 compounds to be confirmed.	[168]
Catechins from tea (EGCG etc)	Eubacterium sp. strain SDG-2	Removal of esterified gallate and cleavage of flavanols to 1,3-diphenylpropan-2-ol derivatives.	[169]
Daidzein	Rat faecal flora	Daidzein, dihydrodaidzein, but no equol detected.	[170]
Flavonoid aglycones	Pig caecum micro flora	Major metabolites: 3-(4-hydroxyphenyl)-propionic acid, 3-phenylpropionic acid from naringenin; phloroglucinol, 3,4-dihydroxyphenylacetic acid, 3,4-dihydroxytoluene from quercetin; 3-(3-hydroxyphenyl)-propionic acid, phloroglucinol from hesperetin.	[171]
Flavonoids from tea, citrus and soy	*In vitro* colon model	3-methoxy-4-hydroxyphenylacetic acid, 4-hydroxyphenyl acetic acid, 3,4-dihydroxyphenylacetic acid, 3-(3-hydroxyphenyl) propionic acid, 2,4,6-trihydroxybenzoic acid, 3-(4-hydroxy-3-methoxyphenyl) propionic acid, 3-hydroxyphenyl acetic acid, hippuric acid.	[172]
Genistein, daidzein	Mouse intestinal isolate	Equol, 5-hydroxyequol.	[173]
Genistein, daidzein and their glycosides	Eubacterium ramulus	6'-hydroxy-O-desmethylangolensin, 2-(4-hydroxyphenyl)-propionic acid.	[174]
Procyanidins (epicatechin polymers)	Human colonic flora	Mainly mono-hydroxylated phenylacetic, phenylpropionic and phenylvaleric acids.	[175]
Quercetin glucoside	2 human isolates	Removal and metabolism of glucoside group by Enterococcus casseliflavus, degradation of flavonol moiety to 3,4-dihydroxyphenylacetic acid, acetate and butyrate by Eubacterium ramulus.	[176]

Flavonoid	Culture	Metabolites Found	Reference
Quercetin glycosides	Human faecal flora	3,4-dihydroxyphenylacetic acid, 3-hydroxyphenylacetic acid.	[177]
Quercetin, hesperetin, naringenin and their rutinosides	Human faecal flora	Rutinosides readily deglycosylated, accumulating hesperetin, naringenin, but not quercetin. Aglycones metabolised to phenolic acids.	[178]
Quercetin, luteolin	Eubacterium ramulus	Intermediate formation of taxifolin (quercetin) and eriodyctiol (luteolin), final conversion to 3,4-dihydroxyphenylacetic acid and 3-(3,4-dihydroxyphenyl)propionic acid.	[179]
Quercetin, Rutin	Pig caecum micro flora	3,4-dihydroxyphenylacetic acid, phloroglucinol.	[143]
Quercetin, taxifolin; luteolin, eriodictyol, apigenin, naringenin, phloretin and glycosides	Clostridium orbiscindens	No glycoside cleavage, but conversion of aglycones to 3,4-dihydroxyphenylacetic acid, 3-(3,4-dihydroxyphenyl)propionic acid, 3-(4-hydroxyphenyl)propionic acid.	[180]
Quercetin-3-glucoside	Germ free rats with/without, Enterococcus casseliflavus	Germ-free, urine, faeces contained quercetin and isorhamnetin (methylated quercetin). Colonised with bacteria, main metabolite found was 3,4-dihydroxyphenylacetic acid.	[181]
Unrestricted diet	Human faecal water	Compounds detected (micromolar concentrations): Naringenin (1.20); quercetin (0.63); other flavonoids (<= 0.17); phenylacetic acid (479); 3-phenylpropionic acid (166); 3-(4-hydroxy)-phenylpropionic acid (68); 3,4-dihydroxycinnamic (caffeic) acid (52); benzoic acid (51); 3-hydroxylphenylacetic acid (46); 4-hydroxyphenylacetic acid (19).	[144]
Various flavonoid aglycones and glycosides	Eubacterium ramulus	Luteolin-7-glucoside, rutin, quercetin, kaempferol, luteolin, eriodictyol, naringenin, taxifolin (dihydroquercetin), phloretin, were degraded to phenolic acids. Luteolin-5-glucoside, diosmetin-7-rutinoside, naringenin-7-neohesperidoside, (+)-catechin, (–)-epicatechin were not degraded.	[182]
Various flavonoid glycosides	Pig caecum micro flora	Deglycosylation was fastest for mono-glycosides, slower for di- or tri-saccharide glycosides; aglycones degraded to primarily 3,4-dihydroxyphenylacetic acid, 4-hydroxyphenylacetic acid, phloroglucinol.	[183]

It was proposed that the glutathione conjugates arose from a reaction between a quinone form of quercetin (resulting from oxidation) and glutathione. This is thought to occur both spontaneously and catalysed by glutathione-S-transferase.

Although it is clear that flavonoids can be degraded into phenolic acids, there are alternative dietary sources which make the picture more complicated. Blueberry fruits in particular (and presumably plant foods in general), contain large amounts of phenolic acid compounds bound to insoluble polymeric plant cell wall material, i.e., “fibre”. Simple esters between phenolic acids and other compounds, including, for example, caffeic-quinic acid esters (chlorogenic acid) are common in apples and coffee. *p*-Coumaric-tartaric acid esters (coutaric acid) are found at reasonable levels in grapes. Unbound acids are a relatively small proportion of the total phenolic acids present in the edible parts of plants. The bound or conjugated acids are predominantly hydroxy-benzoic and hydroxy-cinnamic acids and 12 were detected in hydrolysed blueberry fruit fibre [150]. When this insoluble fraction of blueberry was incubated with human faecal slurry, over 20 phenolic acids were detected, some clearly liberated unchanged from the fruit fibre, others, (phenylacetic acids in particular), apparently transformed by the faecal bacteria. An alternative source of phenolic acids may have been transformation of residual flavonoids. A widely occurring hydroxycinnamic acid, caffeic acid, can be metabolised by human faecal flora into similar compounds to those derived from flavonoids, i.e., 4-hydroxyphenylpropionic acid and benzoic acid [151]. Gut microbe-derived cinnamoyl esterases have been shown to be primarily responsible for the liberation of free phenolic acids from phenolic acid esters in the colon [152], whilst endogenous mammalian esterase activity can be found throughout the gastro-intestinal tract [153]. Since there are apparently three potential source materials for the phenolic acids generated by the colon flora, flavonoids, fibre and cinnamic acids, care must be taken linking particular phenolic acid metabolites and flavonoids, using animal or human studies, unless pure flavonoids are administered.

The occurrence of small phenolic acids in plants is also a complicating factor. It has been claimed that protocatechuic acid (PCA) is the major metabolite of cyanidin glycosides in humans, based on a trial involving the consumption of blood orange juice (BOJ). PCA was the main plasma and urinary metabolite detected and a relatively high (compared with other anthocyanin studies) proportion of anthocyanins (1.2%) were detected in urine [154]. It was claimed that the PCA came primarily from intestinal microbial metabolism of cyanidin. This assumption was based on the finding of PCA as a major metabolite of purified anthocyanins in rats [73, 92]. The former finding is not conclusive, however, because the T_{max} (time after dosing at which C_{max} is attained) of PCA was relatively short, at 2 hours (suggesting direct absorption). BOJ contains a small amount of PCA and its flavanone content (which may also be metabolised to PCA) is similar to its anthocyanin content [155]. BOJ consumption clearly results in significant amounts of absorbed PCA, but it does not necessarily derive from cyanidin.

Beer, unsurprisingly for a fermented product, is a good direct dietary source of small phenolic acids. Phenolic acids from beer (some of which are the same compounds as colonic metabolite acids) were readily absorbed in human subjects and the degree of conjugation varied considerably [156]. 4-Hydroxyphenylacetic acid reached much higher plasma concentrations (~1 μM) than cinnamic acids, such as ferulic or caffeic acids and was predominantly non-conjugated. This suggests that simple phenolic acids, both as produced by colonic microflora and in the diet, would be readily absorbed and may be conjugated to a much lesser extent than flavonoids. Similarly, consumed free *p*-coumaric acid is rapidly and extensively absorbed through the stomach wall and upper intestine using both passive diffusion and the mono-carboxylic transporter, reaching plasma levels of 165 μM, albeit with a very short plasma half-life of 10 minutes [157]. *In vitro* studies using these acids would have more physiological relevance than those on unconjugated flavonoids because of their higher bioavailability in relatively unaltered states.

It also appears that most of the flavonoids studied so far are not absorbed directly by the small intestine, based on total urinary excretion of conjugates of the intact flavonoid. The highest reported proportion of a dose of flavonoid excreted in urine was 20%, for phloridzin-derived phloretin [158].

Another study reported 10% from phloridzin or phloretin itself [159]. This implies that at least 80-90% would have passed on to the colon and been available for microfloral breakdown (or direct absorption contributing to percentage excreted in urine). Commonly reported percentages of urinary excretion of intact flavonoids are in single figures and those for anthocyanins rarely exceed 0.1% (Tables 1, 4).

There is some evidence that anthocyanins may be rapidly and relatively well absorbed from large doses, but their (presumed) instability under physiological conditions results in very little surviving to be excreted in the urine. It seems unlikely that the absorbed proportion could often exceed that for phloretin, so the major proportion of dietary anthocyanins would be potentially able to reach the colon. As discussed above, however, losses to as-yet unknown destinations or forms, appear to be extensive although a study in rats shows that at least part of the dietary intake of intact anthocyanins can reach the colon and undergo metabolism by faecal flora [160].

High-anthocyanin berryfruit extracts (2.5-5% of diet) were fed for 14 weeks. Recoveries of different individual anthocyanins from faeces were very variable (6-25%). Interestingly, it was noted that anthocyanin degradation in faecal samples stored at -18°C was rapid unless these were pasteurised before storage, suggesting that faecal bacteria were still active during storage.

An exception to the extensive degradation of flavonoids to phenolic acids are the soy isoflavones, which are metabolised to modified, but intact flavonoids such as equol or angolensin [161]. The isoflavones, (as discussed below), are also the best example of alternative flavonoid metabolism end products produced by individuals with different populations of gut microflora, where some individual's flora can produce equol, whereas others cannot [162].

Limited evidence suggests that the consumption of flavonoids in the diet can modify the composition of the colonic flora. This can in turn, modify the metabolism of the flavonoids by the microflora. Soy isoflavone metabolism was compared in children, who had been, or were being fed either soy- or cows-milk based infant formula. Those currently or recently consuming infant formula showed differences in metabolism depending on the type of formula consumed, but there was no difference in older children [163]. This suggests that dietary flavonoids can influence the composition of the colonic microflora that metabolise them, but the effect is not long-lasting.

Tea polyphenolics and their colonic metabolites were recently tested for their effects on the growth of human colonic microfloral cultures [164]. The phenolics and metabolites generally inhibited bacterial growth, and pathogenic strains were much more severely affected than commensal strains. This also suggests that dietary flavonoids can beneficially influence the composition of the colonic microflora.

Table 4. Summary of published studies on urinary metabolites of flavonoids

Flavonoid/source	Species	Excretion Level/Metabolites Found	Reference
Apple cider (phloretin, quercetin epicatechin and glycosides)	Human	Only phloretin (20% of dose) detected in urine directly, but 3-fold increase in hippuric acid.	[158]
Berry anthocyanins	Human, rat	Only un-metabolised anthocyanins detected in urine.	[184]
Biochanin A, quercetin, EGCG	Rat	Biochanin A absorption increased and clearance decreased, when co-administered with quercetin and EGCG; may be due to inhibition of efflux pumps.	[185]
Black tea	Human	Hippuric acid was the major excretion product and accounted for nearly all of the polyphenolic intake from the tea.	[146, 147]
Blackcurrant juice	Human	Essentially similar to above study.	[186]
Boysemberry extract	Human	Intact anthocyanins and glucuronides detected.	[187]
Chocolate	Human	Increased urinary extraction of 3-hydroxyphenylpropionic acid, ferulic acid, 3,4-dihydroxyphenylacetic acid, 3-hydroxyphenylacetic acid, vanillic acid, and 3-hydroxybenzoic acid.	[148]
Chokeberry, blackcurrant, elderberry, marionberry	Weanling pigs	0.1-0.2% urinary excretion of intact anthocyanins, glucuronides and methyl derivatives; colonic metabolites not analysed.	[188, 189]
Cocoa powder or epicatechin	Rat	Similar composition and concentration of urinary metabolites from cocoa procyanidins and epicatechin administration.	[190]
Cocoa procyanidins	Human	Epicatechin conjugate excretion increased relative to controls. Milk had no effect on apparent bioavailability.	[191, 192]
Daidzein, genistein	Human	Tetrahydrodaidzein, dihydrogenistein, 6'-hydroxy-O-demethylangolensin, 2-dehydro-O-demethylangolensin, equol, dehydrodaidzein, O-demethyl-angolensin, daidzein, genistein, glycitein, enterolactone.	[161]
Dried cranberry juice	Human	Main metabolites hippuric and 2-hydroxy hippuric acids, PCA, gentisic acid (methylated PCA) and quercetin conjugates. The juice contained PCA and other phenolic acids, so not all were necessarily flavonoid metabolites.	[193]
EGCG	Human, rat, mouse	0.1% of dose as EGCG, dimethylated EGCG, up to 16% as hydroxyphenyl-γ-valerolactone derivatives	[194]
Elderberry juice 400 ml	Human	~0.04% of anthocyanin dose excreted unchanged.	[195]
Epicatechin	Human, rat	Glucuronides and methyl glucuronides.	[196]
Flavonoid-rich meal	Human	Traces (<1 mg) of flavonoid and hydroxycinnamic acid conjugates, moderate amounts (1-20 mg) of glucuronides of 3-hydroxyphenylacetic, homovanillic, vanillic, isoferulic acids, 3-(3-methoxy-4-hydroxyphenyl)-propionic, 3-(3-hydroxyphenyl)-propionic acid, and 3-hydroxyhippuric acid, very large amounts (3-400 mg) of hippuric acid.	[145]
Genistein	Rat	Genistein glucuronide, dihydrogenistein glucuronide, genistein sulphate, dihydrogenistein, 4-hydroxyphenyl-2-propionic acid .	[197]
Green Tea	Human	(-)-5-(3',4',5'-Trihydroxyphenyl)-γ-valerolactone, (-)-5-(3',4'-dihydroxyphenyl)-γ-valerolactone.	[198]
Naringenin	Rat	Glucuronides and 3-(4-hydroxyphenyl) propionic acid.	[199]

Flavonoid/source	Species	Excretion Level/Metabolites Found	Reference
Normal diet	Human	Flavonoids sufficiently measurable to act as biomarkers for polyphenol-rich food intake were quercetin, isorhamnetin, kaempferol, hesperetin, naringenin, phloretin (all relatively hydrophobic) suggesting they are more bioavailable than more polar flavonoids, e.g. catechins.	[200]
Oral blackberry anthocyanins	Rat	Unchanged anthocyanidin glycosides (<1% of dose) detected in urine, no aglycones or conjugates.	[201]
Oral elderberry anthocyanins	Human	Unchanged anthocyanidin glycosides detected in urine (~0.1% of dose), no aglycones, but traces of conjugates.	[202, 203]
Phloretin, phloridzin	Rat	Both compounds led to ~10% urinary excretion of phloretin metabolites (glucuronides, sulphates). Phloridzin appears to be deglycosylated completely during absorption.	[159]
Procyanidins from apple, 1000mg/kg, oral	Rat	Plasma T_{max} 2 hours, C_{max} ~40 μM catechin equivalents; still present after 24 hours. The physiological relevance of this extreme dose is uncertain.	[204]
Quercetin	Human	3,4-Dihydroxyphenylacetic acid, 3-hydroxyphenylacetic acid, and homovanillic acid.	[205]
Quercetin/cooked onions	Human	First report of glutathione conjugates, in addition to glucuronides, sulphates. Also colonic metabolites, dihydroxytoluene, dihydroxybenzaldehyde, dihydroxyphenylacetic acid, dihydroxycinnamic acid, dihydroxyphenylpropionic acid and mercapturic acid conjugates of the colonic metabolites, presumably from microbial degradation of quercetin glutathione conjugates.	[149]
Radio labelled (^3H) catechin, epicatechin	Rat	Intravenous administration led to ~1/3 urinary and 2/3 faecal excretion. Oral administration led to ~5% urinary excretion and exchange of label with plasma water, suggesting that most radiolabel was transferred to water during metabolism by colon flora.	[206]
Radiolabelled EGCG	Rat	Plasma radioactivity peaked at 24 hours post dosing and 32% appeared in urine. Antibiotic-treated rats excreted <1% of radioactivity in urine. Implies that only EGCG colonic metabolites are bioavailable. Major identified metabolites; 5-(5'-hydroxyphenyl)-γ-valerolactone 3'-O-glucuronide (urine), 5-(3',5'-dihydroxyphenyl)-γ-valerolactone (faeces).	[207]
Red clover extract (methylated isoflavones)	Human	Demethylated, hydroxylated and reduced intact isoflavones.	[208, 209]
Red wine, grape juice, 400 ml	Human	~0.2% of anthocyanin dose excreted in urine.	[210]
Strawberries (pelargonidin-3-glucoside, a relatively non-polar anthocyanin)	Human	Relatively high proportion of anthocyanidin (~1.8%) detected in urine, as glucoside, aglycone, 3 glucuronides and one sulpho-glucuronide.	[211]
Strawberries, 200g (source of pelargonidin-3-glucoside)	Human	C_{max} 0.27 μM at T_{max} of 1.1 hours for main metabolite pelargonidin-glucuronide. Total urinary excretion of pelargonidin 1%.	[212]
Tea polyphenolics	Human, normal or with colostomy	Normal subjects produced large amounts of hippuric acid and ~20 other phenolic acids. (primarily phenylacetic and benzoic acid derivatives) Colostomy subjects produced almost no phenolic acids.	[213]

Distribution of Flavonoid Metabolites Round the Body

Blood proteins and lipoproteins appear to have a potentially major influence on the plasma transport, stability and biological activity of flavonoids. The main role of the major blood protein, serum albumin, appears to be regulation of the binding of lipophilic hormones to their receptors [214]. It has been proposed that one of many functions of flavonoids in plants is endocrine disruption of herbivores [215, 216]. Baker [214] has also suggested that albumin has evolved in mammals to inhibit the endocrine-disrupting effects of flavonoids, phytoestrogens in particular, by holding them in the plasma and reducing availability to cellular receptors. This system is complementary to conjugative metabolism, which probably evolved for similar reasons. A number of studies on albumin have produced evidence consistent with this hypothesis.

Considerable differences were found when quercetin and its metabolites were compared for their capacity to inhibit Copper(II)-induced LDL oxidation and their binding strength to serum albumin [217]. Quercetin and its glucuronides were much better inhibitors of LDL oxidation than its sulphate or methyl/glucuronide conjugates. Albumin binding was strongest for quercetin and its sulphate and up to 5-fold weaker for glucuronides. Furthermore, different isomers of quercetin glucuronides showed differences in albumin binding behaviour. A spectroscopic study of quercetin binding to bovine serum albumin in equimolar mixtures of the two found maximal binding at 10 μM and that bound quercetin was much more resistant to oxygen-dependent degradation [218]. Given that the human serum concentration of albumin is ~350-500 μM, ~100-fold higher than observed for any flavonoid, it was estimated that plasma flavonoids are probably predominantly albumin bound. A similar study found a relative binding affinity order of quercetin>rutin=(epi)catechin [219]. Flavonoid aglycones showed moderate affinity for bovine albumin, with binding constants of 1-15 x 10^4 M^{-1}, whereas conjugates had binding constants ~10 times lower. It was again estimated that, given realistic plasma concentrations, even conjugates of flavonoids like quercetin would be predominantly bound to albumin *in vivo* [220]. Resveratrol uptake by liver hepatocytes appears to be a combination of passive diffusion and carrier-mediated transport and is inhibited by competitive binding to serum albumin [221]. It is well known that human serum albumin has a major influence on drug pharmacokinetics [222], and hence the influence of serum albumin on flavonoid distribution and biological activity in the body could be similarly important.

Multi-drug resistance (MDR) efflux transporters/pumps in cells other than intestinal cells may also significantly modulate flavonoid distribution in the body. Absorption of EGCG by cultured cells expressing high levels of drug efflux pump proteins was increased around 10-fold in the presence of specific synthetic pump inhibitors [223]. Flavonoids have been demonstrated to inhibit transport of model substrates by p-Glycoprotein and organic anion transporters [131, 134]. It was not clear whether the flavonoids were inhibitors of the pumps, or competitive substrates. This suggests that MDR efflux pumps may significantly reduce net cellular absorption of flavonoids or their metabolites and that flavonoids may influence each other's transport. These findings also raise the interesting notion that pharmaceutical drug absorption into tissues for therapeutic activity and efficacy may be improved by a diet rich in isoflavones.

FLAVONOID BIOAVAILABILITY TO THE CENTRAL NERVOUS SYSTEM

It appears to be difficult for flavonoid metabolites to get into organs and tissues in general, but the central nervous system is a particular challenge. This is because of the relative impermeability of the interface between blood and brain – the blood-brain barrier (BBB), which is comprised of highly specialised cerebral endothelial cells which express a complex array of tight junction proteins and numerous MDR efflux transporters. Paradoxically, flavonoids have about the right hydrophobicity to cross the BBB, but glucuronidation and or sulphation greatly reduces their permeability, by greatly reducing their hydrophobicity. Flavonoid permeability into the brain has not been well investigated.

When evaluating *in vivo* organ bioavailability studies, it is important to consider whether the tissues were thoroughly perfused in order to remove circulating blood prior to tissue collection and analysis. This is especially important in studies evaluating brain bioavailability as there is generally a much larger difference between brain and blood content of specific compounds, than there is between the blood and other organs, because of the presence of the BBB. Practically, this is usually achieved by transcardial perfusion with saline or a similar physiological buffer at the time of euthanasia, but it can be technically difficult to remove all the blood, especially from brain blood vessels. Many variables can affect the quality of perfusion, including; the pressure applied to the perfusion apparatus, placement of the infusion needles, temperature and formulation of the perfusate, time taken and volume of perfusate used. It is generally recommended to fine-tune these procedures for any given study and a measure of haemoglobin content in the resulting organ homogenates can be used an indication of the quality of the perfusion. Given the extremely limited ability of any polyphenolic compound to enter the brain, if even 1-2% of the blood circulating in the brain (or other target organs) at the time of death is not washed away then spurious, variable and inaccurate measures will result. Some authors have used a correction method, where the amount of blood contamination is estimated in organ homogenates and the resulting blood-borne phytochemical content is then subtracted from the total found in organ homogenates [44]. This method may be especially useful if the compounds of interest are easily degraded and consequently the time between death and compound analysis is crucial.

In a study using an *in vitro* BBB cell monolayer model [224], hesperetin and naringenin aglycones had high permeabilities and were detected basolaterally (i.e., having crossed the cell monolayer) within 30 minutes, but their glycosides and glucuronide metabolites had much lower permeabilities, as did anthocyanins and these findings correlate well with their respective hydrophobicity. The latter were detected basolaterally only after incubation for 18 hours. Epicatechin, its glucuronides and 3 typical phenolic acid colonic metabolites had no detectable basolateral permeability, but accumulated within the cell monolayer [225]. In another study, however, when epicatechin was fed to rats at the extreme dose of 100 mg/kg, (equating to over 10 L of green tea in a single consumption in humans), epicatechin glucuronide and 3'-O-methyl epicatechin glucuronide were detected in the brain at 0.4 nmol/g brain tissue whilst plasma levels approximately 100-fold higher at 40 μM were detected [226].

The central nervous system also effectively limits anthocyanin access. In a study by Kalt *et al* [83], pigs which were fed a 1,2 or 4% blueberry fruit diet for 4 weeks and then fasted for a day before sacrifice and analysis had 11 anthocyanin moieties at detectable levels within the cerebral cortex and cerebellum, whereas none were detected in plasma. The total amount of anthocyanins detected was in the order of 0.7 to 0.9 pmol/g brain tissue and included the un-metabolised compounds: arabinose, galactose and glucose glycosides of cyanidin, delphinidin, malvidin and peonidin. This experimental method, where the phytochemical-containing diet is removed from the animals for 24 hours prior to euthanasia, thus allowing phytochemical clearance from blood, is a convenient way to prevent blood-borne phytochemical contamination of organs. Similar low levels of anthocyanins (0.25nmol/g brain tissue) were found in the brains of rats after 14 days of a blackberry fruit supplemented diet [77]. In this study the anthocyanins consisted primarily of un-metabolised anthocyanins, except for a methylated peonidin 3-glucoside. In another study where rats were administered red grape anthocyanins directly into the stomach, the authors found brain levels of intact anthocyanins of up to 192 ng/g (~0.6 μM) after only 10 minutes, unfortunately the tissues were not perfused and the unusually high levels of anthocyanins measured were therefore likely of both brain and blood origin [78].

The BBB has an extensive expression of MDR efflux transporter pumps which remove many xenobiotics, phytochemicals and drugs from the BBB endothelial cell layer and thereby prevent access to the brain proper. The most well characterised and possibly most relevant to the export of phytochemicals from the brain is P-glycoprotein (P-gp), an ATP-driven efflux pump which has a preference for lipophilic compounds (reviewed in detail in [225]). *In vitro* BBB models can be used to elucidate which of the efflux pumps might be responsible for the export of specific compounds, for example, Youdim *et al* [227] showed that both quercetin and naringenin have some level of central nervous system access which is limited by the activity of BBB efflux pumps. Pre-treatment with a specific P-gp inhibitor demonstrated some specificity, inhibiting the efflux of naringenin but not quercetin. When their system was pre-treated with a P-gp inhibitor which also blocks the action of the breast cancer resistance protein (BCRP) efflux pump, quercetin efflux was also severely limited. These results indicate that the naringenin is primarily exported by P-gp whereas quercetin is preferentially exported by the BCRP efflux pump [227].

It is not clear whether the primary mode by which flavonoids cross the BBB is diffusion or carrier-mediated transport, but whatever the process, they are apparently very susceptible to export via efflux pumps with some specificity for individual compounds. This efflux system is, however, not completely effective, as indicated by *in vivo* studies showing the retention of flavonoids within brain tissue at the picomolar to low nanomolar range. It is, therefore, important that *in vitro* studies evaluating the action of phytochemicals on brain cell cultures make use of physiologically relevant doses within this low concentration range.

Biological Activity of Flavonoid Metabolites

The majority of *in vitro* studies of flavonoid biological activity have been carried out on aglycones, so their physiological relevance is questionable. Recently, however, increasing attention has been paid to determining the biological activity of known conjugates or putative colonic metabolites (Table 5).

Table 5. Summary of *in vitro* studies of biological activity of flavonoid metabolites

Compounds tested	Assay	Outcome	Reference
Quercetin (a flavonol), catechin (a flavanol) and their glucuronides, sulphates and methyl ethers, extracted from plasma of rats fed the algycones	Blood monocyte adhesion to cultured human aortic endothelial cells, or reactive oxygen species (ROS) formation stimulated by interleukin-1β (IL-1β) or hydrogen peroxide (H_2O_2).	Quercetin aglycone or catechin conjugates inhibited monocyte adhesion. Catechin or its conjugates inhibited H_2O_2-induced ROS and only catechin conjugates inhibited IL-1β-induced ROS.	[228]
Quercetin and several likely colonic microbial metabolites	Chemical and cell-based antioxidant assays, inhibition of cholesterol biosynthesis in hepatocytes	Quercetin was active in all three assays and other *ortho* diphenols were equally effective in the chemical antioxidant assay. Of the metabolites, only 3,4-diydroxy toluene was active in the cell-based antioxidant assays.	[229]
Quercetin glucuronide	Lipid peroxidation	Effective inhibitor.	[230]
Quercetin and its 3-glucuronide	Generation of H_2O_2-induced ROS in mouse 3T3 fibroblasts	Only glucuronide inhibited ROS generation, after 4 hours pre-treatment, apparently because quercetin was methylated to isorhamnetin. When applied simultaneously with H_2O_2, both were active, but quercetin was better.	[231]
Quercetin and its 3-glucuronide	Inhibition of angiotensin II-induced vascular smooth-muscle cell hypertrophy in a cell culture model	Both were effective, possibly by inhibition of c-Jun N-terminal kinase activation.	[232]
Quercetin conjugates (glucuronide, sulphate, O-methyl)	COX-2 gene expression	Reduced expression *in vitro* by Caco-2 gut epithelial cells.	[233]
Quercetin, isorhamnetin quercetin-3-glucuronide and quercetin-3-sulphate	Superoxide generation in aqueous buffer and inhibition of blood vessel vasodilatory activity of nitric oxide (NO)	Glucuronide inactive in all assays; quercetin active against NO; quercetin isorhamnetin and sulphate generated superoxide.	[234]
Quercetin	Neutrophil-mediated LDL oxidation	Inhibited LDL oxidation at 1 μM apparently by inhibiting myeloperoxidase (IC_{50} 1μM) and radical-induced LDL oxidation (IC_{50} 1.5 μM). 3'-methylation and 3-glucuronidation moderately weakened this activity, but both together, or 3-sulphation greatly reduced it.	[235]

Table 5. (Continued)

Compounds tested	Assay	Outcome	Reference
Quercetin, Isorhamnetin	Neurotoxicity in cell culture	Active, apparently through inhibition of survival signalling/induction of apoptosis but only at supra-physiological levels not attained in the brain *in vivo*. Isorhamnetin had lower toxicity; quercetin glucuronide was non-toxic.	[236]
Quercetin glucuronide isomers	Xanthine oxidase and lipoxygenase inhibition	All isomers active.	[237]
Quercetin glucuronide isomers	Inhibition of acetylation of carcinogen 2-amino fluorene by HL-60 leukaemia cells	All isomers were inhibitors and all exhibited cytotoxicity..	[238]
Quercetin and conjugates	Chromosomal damage in cultured lymphoblastoid cells	Quercetin caused damage, apparently through generation of H_2O_2, 3-sulphate and isorhamnetin did not. All reduced damage by added H_2O_2, in the order quercetin>isorhamnetin>3-sulphate.	[239]
Quercetin disulphate (potential but un-reported human metabolite)	Pig platelet aggregation; prevention may be of value in CVD	Effective inhibitor.	[240]
Morin (another flavonol)	Macrophage function	Conjugates modulated macrophage function.	[241, 242]
Quercetin	Inhibition of MDR efflux pumps	Quercetin conjugates as good as or better than quercetin.	[243]
Protocatechuic acid (PCA)	Oxidative stress in rat hepatocytes	PCA had cytoprotective effects, but only at very high concentrations.	[244]
PCA	Human leukaemia cells	Promoted apoptosis at 2 mM concentration.	[245]
PCA	Cultured hepatocytes treated with t-butylhydroperoxide (t-BH)	Reduced oxidative stress markers in hepatocytes and administered orally, protected rats from liver damage by oral t-BH, according to several biochemical parameters.	[246]
PCA and other isolated colonic metabolites	Antiproliferative activity on prostate and colon cancer cells	Only PCA showed activity.	[172]

Compounds tested	Assay	Outcome	Reference
PCA, cyanidin, cyanidin glucoside	Protection of cultured neuronal cells from H2O2-induced oxidative stress	All 3 compounds were effective at the membrane level, but only PCA and cyanidin operated at the cytosolic (i.e., intracellular) level, suggesting ability to enter cells.	[247]
Tea catechins and synthetic glucuronides	Scavenging of free radicals and inhibition of arachidonic acid release from HT-29 gut epithelial cells	Some synthetic tea catechin glucuronides retained similar activity to their aglycones.	[248]
Epicatechin and metabolites	Protection of cultured cells from H2O2-induced cytotoxicity	Epicatechin and a methylated metabolite had high protective capacity; glucuronides had almost none. The protection appears to arise from inhibition of the apoptotic associated enzyme, caspase-3.	[249, 250]
Mono- and di-demethylated metabolites of Nobiletin (hexamethoxyflavone)	Inhibition of bacterial lipopolysaccharide (LPS)-induced NO production and inducible nitric oxide synthase (iNOS), (COX-2) protein expression in RAW264.7 macrophages	The metabolites had stronger anti-inflammatory effects than nobiletin itself.	[251]
Quercetin, catechin, epicatechin, phloretin, phloridzin and corresponding mixtures of isomeric mono-glucuronides	Cytoprotection capacity for Jurkat T cells stressed with H2O2	All compounds reduced cell death, but glucuronide mixtures were less potent (IC50 1-16 μM) than aglycones (IC50 <0.5 μM).	[252]
Polyphenolic aglycones, glycosides and mammalian conjugates	Superoxide scavenging capacity	Flavonoid sophoroside, rhamnoglucoside and glucuronide derivatives had the highest capacity; sulphates and aglycones had much lower capacity. Cinnamic acids (caffeic and ferulic acids) were ineffective.	[253]
Hesperetin and glucuronides	UV-A-induced necrotic cell death	Hesperetin glucuronides were protective against cell death; the aglycone was not.	[254]

In addition to the numerous *in vitro* studies listed in Table 5, there have been a number of studies, often *in vivo,* combining investigation of metabolism and determination of biological activities of the metabolites.

Quercetin/Flavonols

Spencer *et al* investigated the uptake, metabolism and protection from oxidative stress of quercetin and its major metabolites (3'-O-methyl quercetin, 4'-O-methyl quercetin and quercetin 7-O-beta-D-glucuronide) in dermal fibroblasts [255]. Uptake and oxidative stress protection was highest with quercetin itself and lower with methyl derivatives. The glucuronide was not taken up by the cells and conferred no protection. In that study, quercetin appeared to be metabolised by the cells to a glutathione conjugate and a quinine derivative. Quercetin conjugates (glucuronide, sulphate, O-methyl) reduced COX-2 gene expression in *ex vivo* human lymphocytes, but a single feeding of human subjects with onions (containing 163.9 mg quercetin 3, 4'-diglucoside, 140.6 mg quercetin 4'-glucoside, and 2.4 mg quercetin aglycone) had no effect. Plasma quercetin metabolites attained a C_{max} of 4 μM [256].

Quercetin has been implicated in the anti-depressant effects of St John's Wort (SJW). When tested on rats using a forced swimming test, SJW extract, rutin and the quercetin metabolite isorhamnetin (3'-methyl quercetin) all exhibited anti-depressant activity after administration for 9 days; Isorhamnetin being most effective [257]. After eight days administration of SJW extract, concentrations in plasma and the central nervous system were 9.6 and 1.3 μM for quercetin and conjugates and 7.4 and 2 μM for methylated quercetin and conjugates.

High acute doses of quercetin glucopyranoside (Isoquercitrin; 100 mg/kg) achieved quercetin C_{max} in the plasma and central nervous system of 16.5 and 2.9 μM, respectively. Unfortunately, in this study the brains were not perfused prior to analysis and the brain levels of these compounds are likely overstated due to contamination from blood circulating in the brain at the time of death. The corresponding C_{max} values for methylated quercetin and conjugates were 10.7 and 2.7 μM. Human subjects fed a soup high in quercetin exhibited higher plasma quercetin conjugate concentrations and reduced collagen-stimulated platelet aggregation than controls on low quercetin soup [258].

Antibody staining of quercetin-3-glucuronide showed that it preferentially accumulated in macrophage-derived foam cells, abundant in human aortic atherosclerotic lesions, but not normal aorta, where foam cells are rare.

In addition, the glucuronide was taken up by murine macrophages and de-conjugated to quercetin aglycone. The aglycone suppressed expression of genes involved in foam cell formation, suggesting that quercetin conjugates may inhibit atherosclerosis [259]. Conjugation, therefore, appears to have the potential to considerably modify the *in vivo* biological activity of absorbed flavonoids.

The picture that emerges from the many studies on quercetin is that the aglycone and its conjugates share many activities, although often with considerably different efficacy. In addition, some conjugates lose activities or exhibit activities that the aglycone does not. It is clearly not valid to assume any relationship between *in vitro* activities of flavonoid aglycones and *in vivo* effects from that compound in the diet. In addition, positive results *in vitro*, even from verified conjugates, do not necessarily translate into *in vivo* effects following an acute dose.

Isoflavones

Some individuals produce equol, as a major metabolite of daidzein, whereas others do not produce detectable equol [162], presumably because of differences in colonic microflora composition and isoflavone metabolism. Equol has well characterised cardiovascular benefits [260]. It also inhibits neoplastic cell transformation *in vitro*, a potential mechanism for the anti-cancer effect attributed to daidzein [261]. With regard to cancer therapy genistein and daidzein glucuronides were oestrogenic, but ~10-fold weaker than their aglycones and weakly activated natural killer (NK) cells against cancer cells [262]. Microarray analysis of the effects of soy isoflavones on gene expression uncovered a relationship between the ability to produce equol and a greater expression in oestrogen-responsive genes [263]. Equol appears to affect gene expression more than daidzein. Dietary equol attenuated weight gain in ovariectomised rats, but did not prevent bone-loss and had an undesirable uterotrophic effect [264, 265]. In contrast, a similar study found that equol did prevent bone loss, but the other major daidzein metabolite, O-desmethylangolensin, did not [266]. In a study on menopausal women, 135 mg/day for one week of soy isoflavones only improved menopausal symptoms in individuals who were equol producers. Equol appears to be primarily responsible for the health benefits of dietary soy isoflavones. High-dose oral equol (400 mg/kg) in ovariectomised rats produced a mammotropic (stimulatory) effect, suggesting that equol is weakly oestrogenic [267].

Catechins

A human intervention trial suggested that the increase in flow-mediated arterial dilation resulting from tea consumption is inversely related to an individual's ability to methylate tea flavonoids [6], i.e., methylation decreases biological activity.

Other Flavonoids

Anthocyanins and their suspected colonic phenolic acid metabolites were tested for their ability to inhibit platelet activation *in vitro* [268], an ability thought to be beneficial in the prevention of coronary vascular disease (CVD). Significant inhibition was observed with 1 μM anthocyanins or 10 μM of most of the phenolic acids tested. Notable exceptions, showing no activity, were hippuric acid and homovanillic acid. A mixture of all the tested compounds, (probably more representative of the *in vivo* situation), was the most effective, even at 1 μM total concentration. Although the phenolic acids required a higher concentration, they are likely to be present individually at much higher concentrations than anthocyanins in the body. The "simulated metabolite mixture" of both individually active and inactive compounds exhibited a strong synergy, although which of the components were synergistic was not determined.

Some flavonoid conjugates demonstrate anti-inflammatory activity. Myricetin glucuronide had an anti-inflammatory effect in a carrageenan-induced rat model of inflammation and showed inhibitory activity for 5-lipoxygenase and cyclo-oxygenase (COX)-

1 and COX-2 and [269]. Oral administration to rats of 100 mg/Kg of astilbin (a flavanone rhamnoside) resulted in low micromolar concentrations in plasma of astilbin and a methylated metabolite, plus a glucuronide in bile only [270]. The methylated metabolite and astilbin had similar anti-inflammatory effects when injected intra-peritoneally into mice, i.e., ~halving picryl chloride-induced ear swelling and nearly normalising elevated levels of tumour necrosis factor α (TNF) and Interferon-γ (IFN-γ).

Apple juice phenolic extracts, fermented anaerobically by human faecal flora, had 30-50% of the Trolox equivalent antioxidant capacity (TEAC) of the unfermented extracts, but in Caco-2 cell-based antioxidant assays, the fermented extract was significantly better at inhibiting ROS formation induced by t-BH [271]. The main identified constituent of the fermented extract were 3,4-dihydroxy- and 4-hydroxy-phenylpropionic acid, phloroglucinol and 3,4-dihydroxyphenylacetic acid. These data indicate that inhibition of ROS formation by phenolics is not likely the result of their chemical antioxidant activity but rather, induction of endogenous cytoprotective mechanisms.

The plant-derived glucuronide baicalin (bicalein-7-glucuronide) is both the major natural form and the major human conjugate of the flavonoid baicalein [81]. The glucuronide was able to induce apoptosis in cultured prostate cancer cells [272] and Jurkat leukemic T lymphocytes [273]. In the latter case, it appeared to act by caspase activation via the mitochondrial pathway but cytotoxicity for normal peripheral blood mononuclear cells was much lower. The intestinal absorption of this compound is much lower than its aglycone [81] but these results demonstrate the biological activity of a flavonoid glucuronide.

Conclusion

Although there is considerable quantitative variation between different studies, even of the same compound, as to the proportions absorbed, excreted, degraded, or metabolised by different means, some generalisations can be made. It is clear that net intestinal absorption of a few individual flavonoids may be as high as 10-20% of intake, under experimental conditions, but under normal circumstances, figures of 1-2% appear more likely and some compounds may be lower still. The more hydrophobic flavonoids, when consumed as glucosides, appear to be the best absorbed, usually via enzymic deglycosylation, followed by diffusion of the aglycone across intestinal cell membranes. More polar compounds, such as catechins, are relatively poorly absorbed and glycosides other than glucosides are resistant to deglycosylation and are slowly absorbed, by diffusion or possibly sugar transporters. Anthocyanins appear to be hardly absorbed at all, based on urinary excretion measurements, but newer evidence suggests that their absorption may be both relatively extensive and rapid, but counterbalanced by very rapid degradation and a consequent very short plasma half-life. The plasma typically appears to contain only traces of most flavonoid aglycones or their original glycosidic forms; a very high, but somewhat variable, percentage is in the form of the polar conjugates, glucuronides and sulphates. The flavonoids in plasma appear to be predominantly bound to serum albumin and maybe other proteins and this, combined with cellular MDR efflux pumps, limits organ bioavailability, particularly to the brain. The only apparent exception is the liver, which may actively take up flavonoid glucuronides, to relatively high concentrations and appears to modify their conjugation. The intestine appears to predominantly glucuronidate flavonoids, whereas the liver may de-glucuronidate them and/or add sulphate and/or methyl groups.

It appears that ~90% of the dietary intake of most flavonoids passes into the colon, either directly, after absorption and MDR-mediated efflux by intestinal cells, or biliary excretion. The colonic microflora can deglycosylate most flavonoid glycosides, thus potentially increasing bioavailability, but can also further degrade the aglycones into phenolic acids and further into simple compounds like benzoic acid, acetic acid and carbon dioxide. The phenolic acids appear to be generally very well absorbed and may make a significant indirect contribution to any health benefits attributed to the flavonoid they were derived from.

Hence, although bioavailability and metabolism studies of flavonoids have discovered a great deal, the information is very fragmented and contradictory. We still have minimal ability to predict or model the expected intracellular concentrations of the numerous metabolites of even one flavonoid. The complex metabolite mixture arising from the numerous flavonoids in a typical diet may not be amenable to modelling in the foreseeable future.

Although the quantitative significance of the biological activities of flavonoid aglycones *in vivo* is doubtful, there are many examples of similarly potent *in vitro* activities of their metabolites, in many different biological aspects. The critical observation, however, is that the activity of the metabolites is, more often than not, considerably different in type of response or magnitude of biological effect, from the original flavonoid. There is one example (see above) in which a combination of weakly active phenolic acid metabolites showed a strong synergy [268], suggesting that a combination of *in vivo* metabolites may have greater health benefits than any of the individual compounds.

Theoretically, a detailed knowledge of flavonoid metabolism, combined with extensive *in vitro* testing of the metabolites, individually and in combination, could elucidate their specific health benefits, to the extent that health benefits could be attributed to individual compounds. However, the permutations of many metabolites and assays may be too numerous and complex for this to ever be a practical proposition. There is also at least one example of the failure of this approach [256]. In this study, an *in vitro* bioassay of identified metabolites of quercetin reduced COX-2 gene-expression but a human trial of quercetin failed to replicate the result.

An alternative approach has recently been proposed [274] that has potential to evaluate real *in vivo* activities of flavonoids, without the necessity to gather huge amounts of ADME data. This involves human subjects consuming the compound or food of interest and the application of their serum to cell cultures. The cells should thus be treated with a truly representative mixture of flavonoid metabolites, at physiologically relevant concentrations, along with any endogenous signalling molecules that they induce. In this particular study, it was found that endothelial cell cultures produced completely different responses in expression of CVD biomarker genes when treated with serum from red-wine drinkers or red wine itself. It is likely that better results could have been obtained from treating the cells with a simulated red-wine polyphenol metabolite mixture, but determining the composition of such a mixture would be a huge undertaking and probably impractical for the hundreds of foods that need to be tested. Another recent study detected anti-inflammatory effects from pomegranate phenolic extract using this approach on rabbits [275]. More work is needed to confirm the validity of this novel approach, but if it is proved successful, it would be a major step towards simplifying the whole area of flavonoid biological activity determination. This approach may be very useful to assist with interpretation of complex ADME data.

REFERENCES

[1] Heiss, C.; Finis, D.; Kleinbongard, P.; Hoffmann, A.; Rassaf, T.; Kelm, M.; and Sies, H. (2007). Sustained increase in flow-mediated dilation after daily intake of high-flavanol cocoa drink over 1 week. *Journal of Cardiovascular Pharmacology and Therapeutics*, *49*, 74-80.

[2] Tavani, A.; Spertini, L.; Bosetti, C.; Parpinel, M.; Gnagnarella, P.; Bravi, F.; Peterson, J.; Dwyer, J.; Lagiou, P.; Negri, E.; and La Vecchia, C. (2006). Intake of specific flavonoids and risk of acute myocardial infarction in Italy. *Public Health Nutrition*, *9*, 369-374.

[3] Mink, P. J.; Scrafford, C. G.; Barraj, L. M.; Harnack, L.; Hong, C.-P.; Nettleton, J. A.; and Jacobs, D. R., Jr. (2007). Flavonoid intake and cardiovascular disease mortality: a prospective study in postmenopausal women. *American Journal of Clinical Nutrition*, *85*, 895-909.

[4] Naissides, M.; Pal, S.; Mamo, J. C. L.; James, A. P.; and Dhaliwal, S. (2006). The effect of chronic consumption of red wine polyphenols on vascular function in postmenopausal women. *European Journal of Clinical Nutrition*, *60*, 740-745.

[5] Bayard, V.; Chamorro, F.; Motta, J.; and Hollenberg, N. K. (2007). Does flavanol intake influence mortality from nitric oxide-dependent processes? Ischemic heart disease, stroke, diabetes mellitus, and cancer in Panama. *International Journal of Medical Sciences*, *4*, 53-58.

[6] Hodgson, J. M.; Puddey, I. B.; Burke, V.; and Croft, K. D. (2006). Is reversal of endothelial dysfunction by tea related to flavonoid metabolism? *British Journal of Nutrition*, *95*, 14-17.

[7] Neuhouser, M. L. (2004). Dietary flavonoids and cancer risk: Evidence from human population studies. *Nutrition and Cancer*, *50*, 1-7.

[8] Hertog, M. G. L.; Feskens, E. J. M.; Hollman, P. C. H.; Katan, M. B.; and Kromhout, D. (1994). Dietary flavonoids and cancer risk in the Zutphen Elderly Study. *Nutrition and Cancer-an International Journal*, *22*, 175.

[9] Hertog, M. G. L.; Feskens, E. J. M.; Hollman, P. C. H.; Katan, M. B.; and Kromhout, D. (1993). Dietary antioxidant Ffonoids and risk of coronary heart-disease - the Zutphen Elderly Study. *Lancet*, *342*, 1007.

[10] Bosetti, C.; Rossi, M.; McLaughlin, J. K.; Negri, E.; Talamini, R.; Lagiou, P.; Montella, M.; Ramazzotti, V.; Franceschi, S.; and LaVecchia, C. (2007). Flavonoids and the risk of renal cell carcinoma. *Cancer Epidemiology Biomarkers and Prevention*, *16*, 98-101.

[11] Cui, Y.; Morgenstern, H.; Greenland, S.; Tashkin, D. P.; Mao, J. T.; Cai, L.; Cozen, W.; Mack, T. M.; Lu, Q.-Y.; and Zhang, Z.-F. (2008). Dietary flavonoid intake and lung cancer - A population-based case-control study. *Cancer*, *112*, 2241-2248.

[12] Hooper, L.; Kroon, P. A.; Rimm, E. B.; Cohn, J. S.; Harvey, I.; Le Cornu, K. A.; Ryder, J. J.; Hall, W. L.; and Cassidy, A. (2008). Flavonoids, flavonoid-rich foods, and

cardiovascular risk: a meta-analysis of randomized controlled trials. *American Journal of Clinical Nutrition, 88*, 38-50.

[13] Stevenson, D. E.; and Hurst, R. D. (2007). Polyphenolic phytochemicals - just antioxidants or much more? *Cellular and Molecular Life Sciences, 64*, 2900-2916.

[14] Scheline, R. R. (1991). *Handbook of mammalian metabolism of plant compounds*. Boca Raton: CRC Press.

[15] Aura, A.-M. (2008). Microbial metabolism of dietary phenolic compounds in the colon. *Phytochemistry Reviews, 7*, 407-429.

[16] Clifford, M. N. (2004). Diet-derived Phenols in plasma and tissues and their implications for health. *Planta Medica, 70*, 1103-1114.

[17] Kroon, P.; and Williamson, G. (2005). Polyphenols: dietary components with established benefits to health? *Journal of the Science of Food and Agriculture, 85*, 1239-1240.

[18] Kroon, P. A.; Clifford, M. N.; Crozier, A.; Day, A. J.; Donovan, J. L.; Manach, C.; and Williamson, G. (2004). How should we assess the effects of exposure to dietary polyphenols in vitro? *American Journal of Clinical Nutrition, 80*, 15-21.

[19] Manach, C.; and Donovan, J. L. (2004). Pharmacokinetics and metabolism of dietary flavonoids in humans. *Free Radical Research, 38*, 771-785.

[20] Manach, C.; Williamson, G.; Morand, C.; Scalbert, A.; and Remesy, C. (2005). Bioavailability and bioefficacy of polyphenols in humans. I. Review of 97 bioavailability studies. *American Journal of Clinical Nutrition, 81*, 230S-242S.

[21] Walle, T. (2004). Absorption and metabolism of flavonoids. *Free Radical Biology and Medicine, 36*, 829-837.

[22] Williamson, G. (2002). The use of flavonoid aglycones in in vitro systems to test biological activities: based on bioavailability data, is this a valid approach? *Phytochemistry Reviews, V1*, 215-222.

[23] Williamson, G.; and Manach, C. (2005). Bioavailability and bioefficacy of polyphenols in humans. II. Review of 93 intervention studies. *American Journal of Clinical Nutrition, 81*, 243S-255S.

[24] Scalbert, A.; Morand, C.; Manach, C.; and Remesy, C. (2002). Absorption and metabolism of polyphenols in the gut and impact on health. *Biomedicine and Pharmacotherapy, 56*, 276-282.

[25] Karakaya, S. (2004). Bioavailability of phenolic compounds. *Critical Reviews in Food Science and Nutrition, 44*, 453-464.

[26] Clifford, M. N.; and Brown, J. E. (2006). Dietary flavonoids and health - broadening the perspective. In O. M. Andersen; and K. R. Markham (Eds.), *Flavonoids: Chemistry, Biochemistry and Applications* (pp. 319-370). Boca Raton: CRC Press.

[27] Kay, C. D. (2006). Aspects of anthocyanin absorption, metabolism and pharmacokinetics in humans. *Nutrition Research Reviews, 19*, 137-146.

[28] McGhie, T. K.; and Walton, M. C. (2007). The bioavailability and absorption of anthocyanins: Towards a better understanding. *Molecular Nutrition and Food Research, 51*, 702-713.

[29] Zhang, L.; Zuo, Z.; and Lin, G. (2007). Intestinal and hepatic glucuronidation of flavonoids. *Molecular Pharmaceutics*, *4*, 833-845.

[30] Larkin, T.; Price, W. E.; and Astheimer, L. (2008). The key importance of soy isoflavone bioavailability to understanding health benefits. *Critical Reviews in Food Science and Nutrition*, *48*, 538-552.

[31] Mullie, P.; Clarys, P.; Deriemaeker, P.; and Hebbelinck, M. (2008). Estimation of daily human intake of food flavonoids. *International Journal of Food Sciences and Nutrition*, *59*, 291-298.

[32] Walle, T.; Browning, A. M.; Steed, L. L.; Reed, S. G.; and Walle, U. K. (2005). Flavonoid glucosides are hydrolyzed and thus activated in the oral cavity in humans. *Journal of Nutrition*, *135*, 48-52.

[33] Crespy, V.; Morand, C.; Besson, C.; Manach, C.; Demigne, C.; and Remesy, C. (2002). Quercetin, but not its glycosides, is absorbed from the rat stomach. *Journal of Agricultural and Food Chemistry*, *50*, 618-621.

[34] Spencer, J. P. E.; Chaudry, F.; Pannala, A. S.; Srai, S. K.; Debnam, E.; and Rice-Evans, C. (2000). Decomposition of cocoa procyanidins in the gastric milieu. *Biochemical and Biophysical Research Communications*, *272*, 236-241.

[35] Rios, L. Y.; Bennett, R. N.; Lazarus, S. A.; Remesy, C.; Scalbert, A.; and Williamson, G. (2002). Cocoa procyanidins are stable during gastric transit in humans'. *American Journal of Clinical Nutrition*, *76*, 1106-1110.

[36] Talavera, S.; Felgines, C.; Texier, O.; Besson, C.; Lamaison, J. L.; and Remesy, C. (2003). Anthocyanins are efficiently absorbed from the stomach in anesthetized rats. *Journal of Nutrition*, *133*, 4178-4182.

[37] McDougall, G. J.; Dobson, P.; Smith, P.; Blake, A.; and Stewart, D. (2005). Assessing potential bioavailability of raspberry anthocyanins using an in vitro digestion system. *Journal of Agricultural and Food Chemistry*, *53*, 5896-5904.

[38] Walton, M. C.; Hendriks, W. H.; Broomfield, A. M.; and McGhie, T. (2009). A viscous food matrix influences absorption and excretion but not metabolism of blackcurrant anthocyanins in rats. *Journal of Food Science*, *74, H22-H29*.

[39] Walton, M. C.; Lentle, R. G.; Reynolds, G. W.; Kruger, M. C.; and McGhie, T. K. (2006). Anthocyanin absorption and antioxidant status in pigs. *Journal of Agricultural and Food Chemistry*, *54*, 7940-7946.

[40] Sergent, T.; Ribonnet, L.; Kolosova, A.; Garsou, S.; Schaut, A.; De Saeger, S.; Van Peteghem, C.; Larondelle, Y.; Pussemier, L.; and Schneider, Y. J. (2008). Molecular and cellular effects of food contaminants and secondary plant components and their plausible interactions at the intestinal level. *Food and Chemical Toxicology*, *46*, 813-841.

[41] Shah, P.; Jogani, V.; Bagchi, T.; and Misra, A. (2006). Role of Caco-2 cell monolayers in prediction of intestinal drug absorption. *Biotechnology Progress*, *22*, 186-198.

[42] Hu, M.; Chen, J.; and Lin, H. M. (2003). Metabolism of flavonoids via enteric recycling: Mechanistic studies of disposition of apigenin in the Caco-2 cell culture model. *Journal of Pharmacology and Experimental Therapeutics*, *307*, 314-321.

[43] Bieger, J.; Cermak, R.; Blank, R.; de Boer, V. C. J.; Hollman, P. C. H.; Kamphues, J.; and Wolffram, S. (2008). Tissue distribution of quercetin in pigs after long-term dietary supplementation. *Journal of Nutrition*, *138*, 1417-1420.

[44] de Boer, V. C. J.; Dihal, A. A.; van der Woude, H.; Arts, I. C. W.; Wolffram, S.; Alink, G. M.; Rietjens, I. M. C. M.; Keijer, J.; and Hollman, P. C. H. (2005). Tissue distribution of quercetin in rats and pigs. *Journal of Nutrition, 135*, 1718-1725.

[45] Wiczkowski, W.; Romaszko, J.; Bucinski, A.; Szawara-Nowak, D.; Honke, J.; Zielinski, H.; and Piskula, M. K. (2008). Quercetin from shallots (Allium cepa L. var. aggregatum) is more bioavailable than its glucosides. *Journal of Nutrition, 138*, 885-888.

[46] Nemeth, K.; Plumb, G. W.; Berrin, J.-G.; Juge, N.; Jacob, R.; Naim, H. Y.; Williamson, G.; Swallow, D. M.; and Kroon, P. A. (2003). Deglycosylation by small intestinal epithelial cell beta-glucosidases is a critical step in the absorption and metabolism of dietary flavonoid glycosides in humans. *European Journal of Nutrition, 42*, 29-42.

[47] Day, A. J.; Canada, F. J.; Diaz, J. C.; Kroon, P. A.; McLauchlan, R.; Faulds, C. B.; Plumb, G. W.; Morgan, M. R. A.; and Williamson, G. (2000). Dietary flavonoid and isoflavone glycosides are hydrolysed by the lactase site of lactase phlorizin hydrolase. *FEBS Letters, 468*, 166-170.

[48] Day, A. J.; DuPont, M. S.; Ridley, S.; Rhodes, M.; Rhodes, M. J. C.; Morgan, M. R. A.; and Williamson, G. (1998). Deglycosylation of flavonoid and isoflavonoid glycosides by human small intestine and liver beta-glucosidase activity. *FEBS Letters, 436*, 71-75.

[49] Gee, J. M.; DuPont, M. S.; Day, A. J.; Plumb, G. W.; Williamson, G.; and Johnson, I. T. (2000). Intestinal transport of quercetin glycosides in rats involves both deglycosylation and interaction with the hexose transport pathway. *Journal of Nutrition, 130*, 2765-2771.

[50] Arts, I. C. W.; Sesink, A. L. A.; Faassen-Peters, M.; and Hollman, P. C. H. (2004). The type of sugar moiety is a major determinant of the small intestinal uptake and subsequent biliary excretion of dietary quercetin glycosides. *British Journal of Nutrition, 91*, 841-847.

[51] Spencer, J. P. E.; Chowrimootoo, G.; Choudhury, R.; Debnam, E. S.; Srai, S. K.; and Rice-Evans, C. (1999). The small intestine can both absorb and glucuronidate luminal flavonoids. *FEBS Letters, 458*, 224-230.

[52] Serra, H.; Mendes, T.; Bronze, M. R.; and Simplicio, A. L. (2008). Prediction of intestinal absorption and metabolism of pharmacologically active flavones and flavanones. *Bioorganic and Medicinal Chemistry, 16*, 4009-4018.

[53] Brand, W.; van der Wel, P. A. I.; Rein, M. J.; Barron, D.; Williamson, G.; van Bladeren, P. J.; and Rietjens, I. (2008). Metabolism and transport of the citrus flavonoid hesperetin in Caco-2 cell monolayers. *Drug Metabolism and Disposition, 36*, 1794-1802.

[54] Kobayashi, S.; and Konishi, Y. (2008). Transepithelial transport of flavanone in intestinal Caco-2 cell monolayers. *Biochemical and Biophysical Research Communications, 368*, 23-29.

[55] Kobayashi, S.; Tanabe, S.; Sugiyama, M.; and Konishi, Y. (2008). Transepithelial transport of hesperetin and hesperidin in intestinal Caco-2 cell monolayers. *Biochimica et Biophysica Acta-Biomembranes, 1778*, 33-41.

[56] Hollman, P. C. H.; Van Trijp, J. M. P.; Buysman, M. N. C. P.; V.d. Gaag, M. S.; Mengelers, M. J. B.; De Vries, J. H. M.; and Katan, M. B. (1997). Relative bioavailability of the antioxidant flavonoid quercetin from various foods in man. *FEBS Letters, 418*, 152-156.

[57] Zhang, L.; Lin, G.; Chang, Q.; and Zuo, Z. (2005). Role of intestinal first-pass metabolism of baicalein in its absorption process. *Pharmaceutical Research*, *22*, 1050-1058.

[58] Silberberg, M.; Morand, C.; Mathevon, T.; Besson, C.; Manach, C.; Scalbert, A.; and Remesy, C. (2005). The bioavailability of polyphenols is highly governed by the capacity of the intestine and of the liver to secrete conjugated metabolites. *European Journal of Nutrition*, *45*, 88-96.

[59] Crespy, V.; Morand, C.; Manach, C.; Besson, C.; Demigne, C.; and Remesy, C. (1999). Part of quercetin absorbed in the small intestine is conjugated and further secreted in the intestinal lumen. *American Journal of Physiology-Gastrointestinal and Liver Physiology*, *277*, G120-G126.

[60] Kahle, K.; Huemmer, W.; Kempf, M.; Scheppach, W.; Erk, T.; and Richling, E. (2007). Polyphenols are intensively metabolized in the human gastrointestinal tract after apple juice consumption. *Journal of Agricultural and Food Chemistry*, *55*, 10605-10614.

[61] Cao, J.; Chen, X.; Liang, J.; Yu, X. Q.; Xu, A. L.; Chan, E.; Duan, W.; Huang, M.; Wen, J. Y.; Yu, X. Y.; Li, X. T.; Sheu, F. S.; and Zhou, S. F. (2007). Role of P-glycoprotein in the intestinal absorption of glabridin, an active flavonoid from the root of Glycyrrhiza glabra. *Drug Metabolism and Disposition*, *35*, 539-553.

[62] Xu, Y. A.; Fan, G. R.; Gao, S.; and Hong, Z. Y. (2008). Assessment of intestinal absorption of vitexin-2"-O-rhamnoside in hawthorn leaves flavonoids in rat using in situ and in vitro absorption models. *Drug Development and Industrial Pharmacy*, *34*, 164-170.

[63] Williamson, G.; Aeberli, I.; Miguet, L.; Zhang, Z.; Sanchez, M. B.; Crespy, V.; Barron, D.; Needs, P.; Kroon, P. A.; Glavinas, H.; Krajcsi, P.; and Grigorov, M. (2007). Interaction of positional isomers of quercetin glucuronides with the transporter ABCC2 (cMOAT, MRP2). *Drug Metabolism and Disposition*, *35*, 1262-1268.

[64] Murakami, A.; Ohigashi, H.; Koshimizu, K.; Kawahara, S.; Matsuoka, Y.; Kuwahara, S.; Kuki, W.; Takahashi, Y.; and Hosotani, K. (2002). Characteristic rat tissue accumulation of nobiletin, a chemopreventive polymethoxyflavonoid, in comparison with luteolin. *BioFactors*, *16*, 73-82.

[65] Walle, T. (2007). Methylation of dietary flavones greatly improves their hepatic metabolic stability and intestinal absorption. *Molecular Pharmaceutics*, *4*, 826-832.

[66] Walle, T. (2007). Methoxylated flavones, a superior cancer chemopreventive flavonoid subclass? *Seminars in Cancer Biology*, *17*, 354-362.

[67] Walle, T.; Wen, X.; and Walle, U. K. (2007). Improving metabolic stability of cancer chemoprotective polyphenols. *Expert Opinion on Drug Metabolism and Toxicology*, *3*, 379-388.

[68] Walle, U. K.; and Walle, T. (2007). Bioavailable flavonoids: Cytochrome P450-mediated metabolism of methoxyflavones. *Drug Metabolism and Disposition*, *35*, 1985-1989.

[69] O'Leary, K. A.; Day, A. J.; Needs, P. W.; Mellon, F. A.; O'Brien, N. M.; and Williamson, G. (2003). Metabolism of quercetin-7-and quercetin-3-glucuronides by an in vitro hepatic model: the role of human beta-glucuronidase, sulfotransferase, catechol-O-methyltransferase and multi-resistant protein 2 (MRP2) in flavonoid metabolism. *Biochemical Pharmacology*, *65*, 479-491.

[70] Graf, B. A.; Ameho, C.; Dolnikowski, G. G.; Milbury, P. E.; Chen, C.-Y.; and Blumberg, J. B. (2006). Rat gastrointestinal tissues metabolize quercetin. *Journal of Nutrition, 136*, 39-44.

[71] Hollands, W.; Brett, G. M.; Radreau, P.; Saha, S.; Teucher, B.; Bennett, R. N.; and Kroon, P. A. (2008). Processing blackcurrants dramatically reduces the content and does not enhance the urinary yield of anthocyanins in human subjects. *Food Chemistry, 108*, 869-878.

[72] Prior, R. L.; and Wu, X. L. (2006). Anthocyanins: Structural characteristics that result in unique metabolic patterns and biological activities. *Free Radical Research*, *40*, 1014-1028.

[73] El Mohsen, M. A.; Marks, J.; Kuhnle, G.; Moore, K.; Debnam, E.; Srai, S. K.; Rice-Evans, C.; and Spencer, J. P. E. (2006). Absorption, tissue distribution and excretion of pelargonidin and its metabolites following oral administration to rats. *British Journal of Nutrition, 95*.

[74] Felgines, C.; Talavera, S.; Texier, O.; Besson, C.; Fogliano, V.; Lamaison, J.-L.; Fauci, L. l.; Galvano, G.; Remesy, C.; and Galvano, F. (2006). Absorption and metabolism of red orange juice anthocyanins in rats. . *British Journal of Nutrition, 95*, 898-904.

[75] Matuschek, M. C.; Hendriks, W. H.; McGhie, T. K.; and Reynolds, G. W. (2006). The jejunum is the main site of absorption for anthocyanins in mice. *Journal of Nutritional Biochemistry, 17*, 31-36.

[76] Harada, K.; Kano, M.; Takayanagi, T.; Yamakawa, O.; and Ishikawa, F. (2004). Absorption of acylated anthocyanins in rats and humans after ingesting an extract of Ipomoea batatas purple sweet potato tuber. *Bioscience Biotechnology and Biochemistry, 68*, 1500-1507.

[77] Talavéra, S.; Felgines, C.; Texier, O.; Lamaison, J.-L.; Besson, C.; Gil-Izquierdo, A.; and Réme?sy, C. (2005). Anthocyanin metabolism in rats and their distribution to digestive area, kidney, and brain. *Journal of Agricultural and Food Chemistry, 53*, 3902-3908.

[78] Passamonti, S.; Vrhovsek, U.; Vanzo, A.; and Mattivi, F. (2005). Fast access of some grape pigments to the brain. *Journal of Agricultural and Food Chemistry*, *53*, 7029-7034.

[79] Chen, T.; Li, L. P.; Lu, X. Y.; Jiang, H. D.; and Zeng, S. (2007). Absorption and excretion of luteolin and apigenin in rats after oral administration of Chrysanthemum morifolium extract. *Journal of Agricultural and Food Chemistry, 55*, 273-277.

[80] Kahle, K.; Kraus, M.; Scheppach, W.; Ackermann, M.; Ridder, F.; and Richling, E. (2006). Studies on apple and blueberry fruit constituents: Do the polyphenols reach the colon after ingestion? *Molecular Nutrition and Food Research, 50*, 418-423.

[81] Akao, T.; Kawabata, K.; Yanagisawa, E.; Ishihara, K.; Mizuhara, Y.; Wakui, Y.; Sakashita, Y.; and Kobashi, K. (2000). Balicalin, the predominant flavone glucuronide of scutellariae radix, is absorbed from the rat gastrointestinal tract as the aglycone and restored to its original form. *Journal of Pharmacy and Pharmacology, 52*, 1563.

[82] Ichiyanagi, T.; Shida, Y.; Rahman, M. M.; Hatano, Y.; and Konishi, T. (2006). Bioavailability and Tissue Distribution of Anthocyanins in Bilberry (Vaccinium myrtillus L.) Extract in Rats. *Journal of Agricultural and Food Chemistry, 54*, 6578-6587.

[83] Kalt, W.; Blumberg, J. B.; McDonald, J. E.; Vinqvist-Tymchuk, M. R.; Fillmore, S. A. E.; Graf, B. A.; O'Leary, J. M.; and Milbury, P. E. (2008). Identification of anthocyanins in the liver, eye, and brain of blueberry-fed pigs. *Journal of Agricultural and Food Chemistry*, *56*, 705-712.

[84] Andres-Lacueva, C.; Shukitt-Hale, B.; Galli, R. L.; Jauregui, O.; Lamuela-Raventos, R. M.; and Joseph, J. A. (2005). Anthocyanins in aged blueberry-fed rats are found centrally and may enhance memory. *Nutritional Neuroscience*, *8*, 111 - 120.

[85] Xia, H. J.; Qiu, F.; Zhu, S.; Zhang, T. Y.; Qu, G. X.; and Yao, X. S. (2007). Isolation and identification of ten metabolites of breviscapine in rat urine. *Biological and Pharmaceutical Bulletin*, *30*, 1308-1316.

[86] Kuhnle, G.; Spencer, J. P. E.; Schroeter, H.; Shenoy, B.; Debnam, E. S.; Srai, S. K. S.; Rice-Evans, C.; and Hahn, U. (2000). Epicatechin and catechin are O-methylated and glucuronidated in the small intestine. *Biochemical and Biophysical Research Communications*, *277*, 507-512.

[87] Yang, C. S.; Chen, L. S.; Lee, M. J.; Balentine, D.; Kuo, M. C.; and Schantz, S. P. (1998). Blood and urine levels of tea catechins after ingestion of different amounts of green tea by human volunteers. *Cancer Epidemiology Biomarkers and Prevention*, *7*, 351-354.

[88] Chu, K. O.; Wang, C. C.; Chu, C. Y.; Choy, K. W.; Pang, C. P.; and Rogers, M. S. (2006). Uptake and distribution of catechins in fetal organs following in utero exposure in rats. *Human Reproduction*, *22*, 280-287.

[89] Walton, M. C.; McGhie, T. K.; Reynolds, G. W.; and Hendriks, W. H. (2006). The flavonol quercetin-3-glucoside inhibits cyanidin-3-glucoside absorption in vitro. *Journal of Agricultural and Food Chemistry*, *54*, 4913-4920.

[90] Suganuma, M.; Okabe, S.; Oniyama, M.; Tada, Y.; Ito, H.; and Fujiki, H. (1998). Wide distribution of H-3 (-)-epigallocatechin gallate, a cancer preventive tea polyphenol, in mouse tissue. *Carcinogenesis*, *19*, 1771-1776.

[91] Kay, C. D.; Mazza, G.; Holub, B. J.; and Wang, J. (2004). Anthocyanin metabolites in human urine and serum. *British Journal of Nutrition*, *91*, 933-942.

[92] Tsuda, T.; Horio, F.; and Osawa, T. (1999). Absorption and metabolism of cyanidin 3-O-[beta]-glucoside in rats. *FEBS Letters*, *449*, 179-182.

[93] Ruefer, C. E.; Bub, A.; Moeseneder, J.; Winterhalter, P.; Stuertz, M.; and Kulling, S. E. (2008). Pharmacokinetics of the soybean isoflavone daidzein in its aglycone and glucoside form: a randomized, double-blind, crossover study. *American Journal of Clinical Nutrition*, *87*, 1314-1323.

[94] Ichiyanagi, T.; Rahman, M. M.; Kashiwada, Y.; Ikeshiro, Y.; Shida, Y.; Hatano, Y.; Matsumoto, H.; Hirayama, M.; Tsuda, T.; and Konishi, T. (2004). Absorption and metabolism of delphinidin 3-O-[beta]-glucopyranoside in rats. *Free Radical Biology and Medicine*, *36*, 930-937.

[95] Poquet, L.; Clifford, M. N.; and Williamson, G. (2008). Investigation of the metabolic fate of dihydrocaffeic acid. *Biochemical Pharmacology*, *75*, 1218-1229.

[96] Cao, G.; Muccitelli, H. U.; Sanchez-Moreno, C.; and Prior, R. L. (2001). Anthocyanins are absorbed in glycated forms in elderly women: a pharmacokinetic study. *American Journal of Clinical Nutrition*, *73*, 920-926.

[97] Ito, C.; Oi, N.; Hashimoto, T.; Nakabayashi, H.; Aoki, F.; Tominaga, Y.; Yokota, S.; Hosoe, K.; and Kanazawa, K. (2007). Absorption of dietary licorice isoflavan glabridin to blood circulation in rats. *Journal of Nutritional Science and Vitaminology, 53*, 358-365.

[98] Mata-Bilbao, M. D.; Andres-Lacueva, C.; Roura, E.; Jaduregui, O.; Escriban, E.; Torre, C.; and Lamuela-Raventos, R. M. (2007). Absorption and pharmacokinetics of grapefruit flavanones in beagles. *British Journal of Nutrition, 98*, 86-92.

[99] Kanaze, F. I.; Bounartzi, M. I.; Georgarakis, M.; and Niopas, I. (2007). Pharmacokinetics of the citrus flavanone aglycones hesperetin and naringenin after single oral administration in human subjects. *European Journal of Clinical Nutrition, 61*, 472-477.

[100] Franke, A. A.; Custer, L. J.; and Hundahl, S. A. (2004). Determinants for urinary and plasma isoflavones in humans after soy intake. *Nutrition and Cancer, 50*, 141-154.

[101] DuPont, M. S.; Day, A. J.; Bennett, R. N.; Mellon, F. A.; and Kroon, P. A. (2004). Absorption of kaempferol from endive, a source of kaempferol-3-glucuronide, in humans. *European Journal of Clinical Nutrition, 58*, 947.

[102] Choudhury, R.; Chowrimootoo, G.; Srai, K.; Debnam, E.; and Rice-Evans, C. A. (1999). Interactions of the flavonoid naringenin in the gastrointestinal tract and the influence of glycosylation. *Biochemical and Biophysical Research Communications, 265*, 410-415.

[103] Gardana, C.; Guarnieri, S.; Riso, P.; Simonetti, P.; and Porrini, M. (2007). Flavanone plasma pharmacokinetics from blood orange juice in human subjects. *British Journal of Nutrition, 98*, 165-172.

[104] Mennen, L. I.; Sapinho, D.; Ito, H.; Galan, P.; Hercberg, S.; and Scalbert, A. (2008). Urinary excretion of 13 dietary flavonoids and phenolic acids in free-living healthy subjects variability and possible use as biomarkers of polyphenol intake. *European Journal of Clinical Nutrition, 62*, 519-525.

[105] Crespy, V.; Morand, C.; Besson, C.; Manach, C.; Demigne, C.; and Remesy, C. (2001). Comparison of the intestinal absorption of quercetin, phloretin and their glucosides in rats. *Journal of Nutrition, 131*, 2109-2114.

[106] Zhou, D. Y.; Xing, R.; Xu, Q.; Xue, X. Y.; Zhang, F. F.; and Liang, X. M. (2008). Polymethoxylated flavones metabolites in rat plasma after the consumption of Fructus aurantii extract: Analysis by liquid chromatography/electrospray ion trap mass spectrometry. *Journal of Pharmaceutical and Biomedical Analysis, 46*, 543-549.

[107] Spencer, J. P. E.; Schroeter, H.; Shenoy, B.; Srai, S. K. S.; Debnam, E. S.; and Rice-Evans, C. (2001). Epicatechin is the primary bioavailable form of the procyanidin dimers B2 and B5 after transfer across the small intestine. *Biochemical and Biophysical Research Communications, 285*, 588-593.

[108] Wang, J. F.; Schramm, D. D.; Holt, R. R.; Ensunsa, J. L.; Fraga, C. G.; Schmitz, H. H.; and Keen, C. L. (2000). A dose-response effect from chocolate consumption on plasma epicatechin and oxidative damage. *Journal of Nutrition, 130*, 2115S-2119S.

[109] Donovan, J. L.; Manach, C.; Rios, L.; Morand, C.; Scalbert, A.; and Remesy, C. (2002). Procyanidins are not bioavailable in rats fed a single meal containing a grapeseed extract or the procyanidin dimer B-3. *British Journal of Nutrition, 87*, 299-306.

[110] Nakamura, Y.; and Tonogai, Y. (2003). Metabolism of grape seed polyphenol in the rat. *Journal of Agricultural and Food Chemistry, 51*, 7215 -7225.

[111] Prasain, J. K.; Jones, K.; Brissie, N.; Moore, R.; Wyss, J. M.; and Barnes, S. (2004). Identification of Puerarin and Its Metabolites in Rats by Liquid Chromatography-Tandem Mass Spectrometry. *Journal of Agricultural and Food Chemistry, 52*, 3708-3712.

[112] Murota, K.; and Terao, J. (2005). Quercetin appears in the lymph of unanesthetized rats as its phase II metabolites after administered into the stomach. *FEBS Letters, 579*, 5343-5346.

[113] Day, A. J.; Mellon, F.; Barron, D.; Sarrazin, G.; Morgan, M. R. A.; and Williamson, G. (2001). Human metabolism of dietary flavonoids: Identification of plasma metabolites of quercetin. *Free Radical Research, 35*, 941-952.

[114] Graefe, E. U.; Wittig, J.; Mueller, S.; Riethling, A. K.; Uehleke, B.; Drewelow, B.; Pforte, H.; Jacobasch, G.; Derendorf, H.; and Veit, M. (2001). Pharmacokinetics and bioavailability of quercetin glycosides in humans. *Journal of Clinical Pharmacology, 41*, 492-499.

[115] Wittig, J.; Herderich, M.; Graefe, E. U.; and Veit, M. (2001). Identification of quercetin glucuronides in human plasma by high-performance liquid chromatography-tandem mass spectrometry. *Journal of Chromatography B, 753*, 237-243.

[116] Mullen, W.; Edwards, C. A.; and Crozier, A. (2006). Absorption, excretion and metabolite profiling of methyl-, glucuronyl-, glucosyl- and sulpho-conjugates of quercetin in human plasma and urine after ingestion of onions. *British Journal of Nutrition, 96*, 107-116.

[117] Benito, S.; Mitjavila, M. T.; and Buxaderas, S. (2004). Flavonoid metabolites and susceptibility of rat lipoproteins to oxidation. *American Journal of Physiology - Heart and Circulatory Physiology, 287*.

[118] Day, A. J.; Gee, J. M.; DuPont, M. S.; Johnson, I. T.; and Williamson, G. (2003). Absorption of quercetin-3-glucoside and quercetin-4 '-glucoside in the rat small intestine: the role of lactase phlorizin hydrolase and the sodium-dependent glucose transporter. *Biochemical Pharmacology, 65*, 1199-1206.

[119] Moon, Y. J.; Wang, L.; DiCenzo, R.; and Morris, M. E. (2008). Quercetin pharmacokinetics in humans. *Biopharmaceutics and Drug Disposition, 29*, 205-217.

[120] Dragoni, S.; Gee, J.; Bennett, R.; Valoti, M.; and Sgaragli, G. (2006). Red wine alcohol promotes quercetin absorption and directs its metabolism towards isorhamnetin and tamarixetin in rat intestine in vitro. *British Journal of Pharmacology, 147*, 765-771.

[121] Kuhnle, G.; Spencer, J. P. E.; Chowrimootoo, G.; Schroeter, H.; Debnam, E. S.; Srai, S. K. S.; Rice-Evans, C.; and Hahn, U. (2000). Resveratrol is absorbed in the small intestine as resveratrol glucuronide. *Biochemical and Biophysical Research Communications, 272*, 212-217.

[122] Goldberg, D. A.; Yan, J.; and Soleas, G. J. (2003). Absorption of three wine-related polyphenols in three different matrices by healthy subjects. *Clinical Biochemistry, 36*, 79-87.

[123] Vitrac, X.; Desmouliere, A.; Brouillaud, B.; Krisa, S.; Deffieux, G.; Barthe, N.; Rosenbaum, J.; and Merillon, J. M. (2003). Distribution of C-14 -trans-resveratrol, a cancer chemopreventive polyphenol, in mouse tissues after oral administration. *Life Sciences, 72*, 2219-2233.

[124] Chen, X. Y.; Cui, L.; Duan, X. T.; Ma, B.; and Zhong, D. F. (2006). Pharmacokinetics and metabolism of the flavonoid scutellarin in humans after a single oral administration. *Drug Metabolism and Disposition, 34*, 1345.

[125] Gee, J. M.; Wroblewska, M. A.; Bennett, R. N.; Mellon, F. A.; and Johnson, I. T. (2004). Absorption and twenty-four-hour metabolism time-course of quercetin-3-O-glucoside in rats, in vivo. *Journal of the Science of Food and Agriculture, 84*, 1341-1348.

[126] Tsuji, A.; Takanaga, H.; Tamai, I.; and Terasaki, T. (1994). Transcellular Transport of Benzoic Acid Across Caco-2 Cells by a pH-Dependent and Carrier-Mediated Transport Mechanism. *Pharmaceutical Research, 11*, 30-37.

[127] Tamai, I.; Takanaga, H.; Maeda, H.; Yabuuchi, H.; Sai, Y.; Suzuki, Y.; and Tsuji, A. (1997). Intestinal brush-border membrane transport of monocarboxylic acids mediated by proton-coupled transport and anion antiport mechanisms. *Journal of Pharmacy and Pharmacology, 49*, 108-112.

[128] Konishi, Y.; Kobayashi, S.; and Shimizu, M. (2003). Transepithelial transport of p-coumaric acid and gallic acid in caco-2 cell monolayers. *Bioscience Biotechnology and Biochemistry, 67*, 2317-2324.

[129] Haughton, E.; Clifford, M. N.; and Sharp, P. (2007). Monocarboxylate transporter expression is associated with the absorption of benzoic acid in human intestinal epithelial cells. *Journal of the Science of Food and Agriculture, 87*, 239-244.

[130] Steinert, R. E.; Ditscheid, B.; Netzel, M.; and Jahreis, G. (2008). Absorption of black currant anthocyanins by monolayers of human intestinal epithelial Caco-2 cells mounted in using type chambers. *Journal of Agricultural and Food Chemistry, 56*, 4995-5001.

[131] Jodoin, J.; Demeule, M.; and Beliveau, R. (2002). Inhibition of the multidrug resistance P-glycoprotein activity by green tea polyphenols. *Biochimica et Biophysica Acta-Molecular Cell Research, 1542*, 149-159.

[132] Konishi, Y.; Kobayashi, S.; and Shimizu, M. (2003). Tea polyphenols inhibit the transport of dietary phenolic acids mediated by the monocarboxylic acid transporter (MCT) in intestinal Caco-2 cell monolayers. *Journal of Agricultural and Food Chemistry, 51*, 7296-7302.

[133] Konishi, Y.; Kubo, K.; and Shimizu, M. (2003). Structural effects of phenolic acids on the transepithelial transport of fluorescein in Caco-2 cell monolayers. *Bioscience Biotechnology and Biochemistry, 67*, 2014-2017.

[134] Hong, S. S.; Seo, K.; Lim, S. C.; and Han, H. K. (2007). Interaction characteristics of flavonoids with human organic anion transporter 1 (hOAT1) and 3 (hOAT3). *Pharmacological Research, 56*, 468-473.

[135] Wen, X.; and Walle, T. (2006). Methylation protects dietary flavonoids from rapid hepatic metabolism. *Xenobiotica, 36*, 387-397.

[136] Wen, X.; and Walle, T. (2006). Methylated flavonoids have greatly improved intestinal absorption and metabolic stability. *Drug Metabolism and Disposition, 34*, 1786-1792.

[137] Liu, X.; Tam, V. H.; and Hu, M. (2007). Disposition of flavonoids via enteric recycling: Determination of the UDP-Glucuronosyltransferase Isoforms responsible for the metabolism of flavonoids in intact caco-2 TC7 cells using siRNA. *Molecular Pharmaceutics, 4*, 873-882.

[138] Manna, C.; Galletti, P.; Maisto, G.; Cucciolla, V.; D'Angelo, S.; and Zappia, V. (2000). Transport mechanism and metabolism of olive oil hydroxytyrosol in Caco-2 cells. *FEBS Letters*, *470*, 341-344.

[139] Murakami, A.; Koshimizu, K.; Kuwahara, S.; Takahashi, Y.; Ito, C.; Furukawa, H.; Ju-Ichi, M.; and Ohigashi, H. (2001). In vitro absorption and metabolism of nobiletin, a chemopreventive polymethoxyflavonoid in citrus fruits. *Bioscience, Biotechnology and Biochemistry*, *65*, 194-197.

[140] Boyer, J.; Brown, D.; and Rui, H. L. (2004). Uptake of quercetin and quercetin 3-glucoside from whole onion and apple peel extracts by Caco-2 cell monolayers. *Journal of Agricultural and Food Chemistry*, *52*, 7172-7179.

[141] Walgren, R. A.; Lin, J.-T.; Kinne, R. K. H.; and Walle, T. (2000). Cellular uptake of dietary flavonoid quercetin 4'-beta -glucoside by sodium-dependent glucose transporter SGLT1. *Journal of Pharmacology and Experimental Therapeutics*, *294*, 837-843.

[142] Chen, C. H.; Hsu, H. J.; Huang, Y. J.; and Lin, C. J. (2007). Interaction of flavonoids and intestinal facilitated glucose transporters. *Planta Medica*, *73*, 348-354.

[143] Keppler, K.; Hein, E. M.; and Humpf, H. U. (2006). Metabolism of quercetin and rutin by the pig caecal microflora prepared by freeze-preservation. *Molecular Nutrition and Food Research*, *50*, 686-695.

[144] Jenner, A. M.; Rafter, J.; and Halliwell, B. (2005). Human fecal water content of phenolics: The extent of colonic exposure to aromatic compounds. *Free Radical Biology and Medicine*, *38*, 763-772.

[145] Rechner, A. R.; Kuhnle, G.; Bremner, P.; Hubbard, G. P.; Moore, K. P.; and Rice-Evans, C. A. (2002). The metabolic fate of dietary polyphenols in humans. *Free Radical Biology and Medicine*, *33*, 220-235.

[146] Clifford, M. N.; Copeland, E. L.; Bloxsidge, J. P.; and Mitchell, L. A. (2000). Hippuric acid as a major excretion product associated with black tea consumption. *Xenobiotica*, *30*, 317-326.

[147] Mulder, T. P.; Rietveld, A. G.; and van Amelsvoort, J. M. (2005). Consumption of both black tea and green tea results in an increase in the excretion of hippuric acid into urine. *American Journal of Clinical Nutrition*, *81*, 256S-260S.

[148] Rios, L. Y.; Gonthier, M. P.; Remesy, C.; Mila, L.; Lapierre, C.; Lazarus, S. A.; Williamson, G.; and Scalbert, A. (2003). Chocolate intake increases urinary excretion of polyphenol-derived phenolic acids in healthy human subjects. *American Journal of Clinical Nutrition*, *77*, 912-918.

[149] Hong, Y. J.; and Mitchell, A. E. (2006). Identification of glutathione-related quercetin metabolites in humans. *Chemical Research in Toxicology*, *19*, 1525-1532.

[150] Russell, W. R.; Labat, A.; Scobbie, L.; and Duncan, S. H. (2007). Availability of blueberry phenolics for microbial metabolism in the colon and the potential inflammatory implications. *Molecular Nutrition and Food Research*, *51*, 726-731.

[151] Gonthier, M. P.; Remesy, C.; Scalbert, A.; Cheynier, V.; Souquet, J. M.; Poutanen, K.; and Aura, A. M. (2006). Microbial metabolism of caffeic acid and its esters chlorogenic and caftaric acids by human faecal microbiota in vitro. *Biomedicine and Pharmacotherapy*, *60*, 536-540.

[152] Gonthier, M.-P.; Verny, M.-A.; Besson, C.; Remesy, C.; and Scalbert, A. (2003). Chlorogenic acid bioavailability largely depends on its metabolism by the gut microflora in rats. *Journal of Nutrition*, *133*, 1853-1859.

[153] Andreasen, M. F.; Kroon, P. A.; Williamson, G.; and Garcia-Conesa, M. T. (2001). Intestinal release and uptake of phenolic antioxidant diferulic acids. *Free Radical Biology and Medicine*, *31*, 304-314.

[154] Vitaglione, P.; Donnarumma, G.; Napolitano, A.; Galvano, F.; Gallo, A.; Scalfi, L.; and Fogliano, V. (2007). Protocatechuic acid is the major human metabolite of cyanidin-glucosides. *Journal of Nutrition*, *137*, 2043-2048.

[155] Kelebek, H.; Canbas, A.; and Selli, S. (2008). Determination of phenolic composition and antioxidant capacity of blood orange juices obtained from cvs. Moro and Sanguinello (Citrus sinensis (L.) Osbeck) grown in Turkey. *Food Chemistry*, *107*, 1710-1716.

[156] Nardini, M.; Natella, F.; Scaccini, C.; and Ghiselli, A. (2006). Phenolic acids from beer are absorbed and extensively metabolized in humans. *Journal of Nutritional Biochemistry*, *17*, 14-22.

[157] Konishi, Y.; Hitomi, Y.; and Yoshioka, E. (2004). Intestinal absorption of p-coumaric and gallic acids in rats after oral administration. *Journal of Agricultural and Food Chemistry*, *52*, 2527-2532.

[158] DuPont, M. S.; Bennett, R. N.; Mellon, F. A.; and Williamson, G. (2002). Polyphenols from alcoholic apple cider are absorbed, metabolized and excreted by humans. *Journal of Nutrition*, *132*, 172-175.

[159] Crespy, V.; Aprikian, O.; Morand, C.; Besson, C.; Manach, C.; Demigne, C.; and Remesy, C. (2001). Bioavailability of phloretin and phloridzin in rats. *Journal of Nutrition*, *131*, 3227-3230.

[160] He, J.; Magnuson, B. A.; and Giusti, M. M. (2005). Analysis of Anthocyanins in Rat Intestinal Contents-Impact of Anthocyanin Chemical Structure on Fecal Excretion. *Journal of Agricultural and Food Chemistry*, *53*, 2859-2866.

[161] Joannou, G. E.; Kelly, G. E.; Reeder, A. Y.; Waring, M.; and Nelson, C. (1995). A urinary profile study of dietary phytoestrogens. The identification and mode of metabolism of new isoflavonoids. *The Journal of Steroid Biochemistry and Molecular Biology*, *54*, 167-184.

[162] Yuan, J. P.; Wang, J. H.; and Liu, X. (2007). Metabolism of dietary soy isoflavones to equol by human intestinal microflora - implications for health. *Molecular Nutrition and Food Research*, *51*, 765-781.

[163] Hoey, L.; Rowland, I. R.; Lloyd, A. S.; Clarke, D. B.; and Wiseman, H. (2004). Influence of soya-based infant formula consumption on isoflavone and gut microflora metabolite concentrations in urine and on faecal microflora composition and metabolic activity in infants and children. *British Journal of Nutrition*, *91*, 607-616.

[164] Lee, H. C.; Jenner, A. M.; Low, C. S.; and Lee, Y. K. (2006). Effect of tea phenolics and their aromatic fecal bacterial metabolites on intestinal microbiota. *Research in Microbiology*, *157*, 876-884.

[165] Fleschhut, J.; Kratzer, F.; Rechkemmer, G.; and Kulling, S. E. (2006). Stability and biotransformation of various dietary anthocyanins in vitro. *European Journal of Nutrition*, *45*, 7-18.

[166] Hor-Gil Hur, F. R. (2000). Biotransformation of the isoflavonoids biochanin A, formononetin, and glycitein by Eubacterium limosum. *FEMS Microbiology Letters*, *192*, 21-25.

[167] Aura, A.-M.; Mattila, I.; Seppänen-Laakso, T.; Miettinen, J.; Oksman-Caldentey, K.-M.; and Oresic, M. (2008). Microbial metabolism of catechin stereoisomers by human faecal microbiota: Comparison of targeted analysis and a non-targeted metabolomics method. *Phytochemistry Letters*, *1*, 18-22.

[168] Meselhy, M. R.; Nakamura, N.; and Hattori, M. (1997). Biotransformation of (-)-epicatechin 3-O-gallate by human intestinal bacteria. *Chemical and Pharmaceutical Bulletin*, *45*, 888-893.

[169] Wang, L.-Q.; Meselhy, M. R.; Li, Y.; Nakamura, N.; Min, B.-S.; Qin, G.-W.; and Hattori, M. (2001). The Heterocyclic Ring Fission and Dehydroxylation of Catechins and Related Compounds by Eubacterium sp. Strain SDG-2, a Human Intestinal Bacterium. *Chemical and Pharmaceutical Bulletin*, *49*, 1640-1643.

[170] Rafii, F.; Jackson, L. D.; Ross, I.; Heinze, T. M.; Lewis, S. M.; Aidoo, A.; Lyn-Cook, L.; and Manjanathas, M. (2007). Metabolism of daidzein by fecal bacteria in rats. *Comparative Medicine*, *57*, 282-286.

[171] Labib, S.; Erb, A.; Kraus, M.; Wickert, T.; and Richling, E. (2004). The pig caecum model: A suitable tool to study the intestinal metabolism of flavonoids. *Molecular Nutrition and Food Research*, *48*, 326-332.

[172] Gao, K.; Xu, A. L.; Krul, C.; Venema, K.; Liu, Y.; Niu, Y. T.; Lu, J. X.; Bensoussan, L.; Seeram, N. P.; Heber, D.; and Henning, S. M. (2006). Of the major phenolic acids formed during human microbial fermentation of tea, citrus, and soy flavonoid supplements, only 3,4-dihydroxyphenylacetic acid has antiproliferative activity. *Journal of Nutrition*, *136*, 52-57.

[173] Matthies, A.; Clavel, T.; Gutschow, M.; Engst, W.; Haller, D.; Blaut, M.; and Braune, A. (2008). Conversion of daidzein and genistein by an anaerobic bacterium newly isolated from the mouse intestine. *Applied and Environmental Microbiology*, *74*, 4847-4852.

[174] Schoefer, L.; Mohan, R.; Braune, A.; Birringer, M.; and Blaut, M. (2002). Anaerobic C-ring cleavage of genistein and daidzein by Eubacterium ramulus. *FEMS Microbiology Letters*, *208*, 197-202.

[175] Deprez, S.; Brezillon, C.; Rabot, S.; Philippe, C.; Mila, I.; Lapierre, C.; and Scalbert, A. (2000). Polymeric Proanthocyanidins Are Catabolized by Human Colonic Microflora into Low-Molecular-Weight Phenolic Acids. *Journal of Nutrition*, *130*, 2733-2738.

[176] Schneider, H.; Schwiertz, A.; Collins, M. D.; and Blaut, M. (1999). Anaerobic transformation of quercetin-3-glucoside by bacteria from the human intestinal tract. *Archives of Microbiology*, *171*, 81-91.

[177] Aura, A. M.; O'Leary, K. A.; Williamson, G.; Ojala, M.; Bailey, M.; Puupponen-Pimia, R.; Nuutila, A. M.; Oksman-Caldentey, K. M.; and Poutanen, K. (2002). Quercetin derivatives are deconjugated and converted to hydroxyphenylacetic acids but not methylated by human fecal flora in vitro. *Journal of Agricultural and Food Chemistry*, *50*, 1725-1730.

[178] Justesen, U.; Arrigoni, E.; Larsen, B. R.; and Amado, R. (2000). Degradation of flavonoid glycosides and aglycones during in vitro fermentation with human faecal flora. *Lebensmittel-Wissenschaft und-Technologie*, *33*, 424-430.

[179] Braune, A.; Gutschow, M.; Engst, W.; and Blaut, M. (2001). Degradation of quercetin and luteolin by Eubacterium ramulus. *Applied and Environmental Microbiology*, *67*, 5558-5567.

[180] Schoefer, L.; Mohan, R.; Schwiertz, A.; Braune, A.; and Blaut, M. (2003). Anaerobic degradation of flavonoids by Clostridium orbiscindens. *Applied and Environmental Microbiology*, *69*, 5849-5854.

[181] Schneider, H.; Simmering, R.; Hartmann, L.; Pforte, H.; and Blaut, M. (2000). Degradation of quercetin-3-glucoside in gnotobiotic rats associated with human intestinal bacteria. *Journal of Applied Microbiology*, *89*, 1027-1037.

[182] Schneider, H.; and Blaut, M. (2000). Anaerobic degradation of flavonoids by Eubacterium ramulus. *Archives of Microbiology*, *173*, 71-75.

[183] Hein, E. M.; Rose, K.; Van't Slot, G.; Friedrich, A. W.; and Humpf, H. U. (2008). Deconjugation and degradation of flavonol glycosides by pig cecal microbiota characterized by fluorescence in situ hybridization (FISH). *Journal of Agricultural and Food Chemistry*, *56*, 2281-2290.

[184] McGhie, T. K.; Ainge, G. D.; Barnett, L. E.; Cooney, J. M.; and Jensen, D. J. (2003). Anthocyanin Glycosides from Berry Fruit Are Absorbed and Excreted Unmetabolized by Both Humans and Rats. *Journal of Agricultural and Food Chemistry*, *51*, 4539 - 4548.

[185] Moon, Y. J.; and Morris, M. E. (2007). Pharmacokinetics and bioavailability of the bioflavonoid biochanin A: Effects of quercetin and EGCG on biochanin A disposition in rats. *Molecular Pharmaceutics*, *4*, 865-872.

[186] Rechner, A. R.; Kuhnle, G.; Hu, H. L.; Roedig-Penman, A.; van den Braak, M. H.; Moore, K. P.; and Rice-Evans, C. A. (2002). The metabolism of dietary polyphenols and the relevance to circulating levels of conjugated metabolites. *Free Radical Research*, *36*, 1229-1241.

[187] Cooney, J. M.; Jensen, D. J.; and McGhie, T. K. (2004). LC-MS identification of anthocyanins in boysenberry extract and anthocyanin metabolites in human urine following dosing. *Journal of the Science of Food and Agriculture*, *84*, 237-245.

[188] Wu, X.; Pittman, H. E., III; McKay, S.; and Prior, R. L. (2005). Aglycones and sugar moieties alter anthocyanin absorption and metabolism after berry consumption in weanling pigs. *Journal of Nutrition*, *135*, 2417-2424.

[189] Wu, X.; Pittman, H. E., III; and Prior, R. L. (2004). Pelargonidin is absorbed and metabolized differently than cyanidin after marionberry consumption in pigs. *Journal of Nutrition*, *134*, 2603-2610.

[190] Baba, S.; Osakabe, N.; Natsume, M.; Muto, Y.; Takizawa, T.; and Terao, J. (2001). Absorption and urinary excretion of (-)-epicatechin after administration of different levels of cocoa powder or (-)-epicatechin in rats. *Journal of Agricultural and Food Chemistry*, *49*, 6050-6056.

[191] Roura, E.; Almajano, M. P.; Bilbao, M. L. M.; Andres-Lacueva, C.; Estruch, R.; and Lamuela-Raventos, R. M. (2007). Human urine: Epicatechin metabolites and antioxidant activity after cocoa beverage intake. *Free Radical Research*, *41*, 943-949.

[192] Roura, E.; Andres-Lacueva, C.; Estruch, R.; Mata-Bilbao, M. L.; Izquierdo-Pulido, M.; Waterhouse, A. L.; and Lamuela-Raventos, R. M. (2007). Milk does not affect the bioavailability of cocoa powder flavonoid in healthy human. *Annals of Nutrition and Metabolism*, *51*, 493-498.

[193] Valentova, K.; Stejskal, D.; Bednar, P.; Vostalova, J.; Cihalik, C.; Vecerova, R.; Koukalova, D.; Kolar, M.; Reichenbach, R.; Sknouril, L.; Ulrichova, J.; and Simanek, V. (2007). Biosafety, antioxidant status, and metabolites in urine after consumption of

dried cranberry juice in healthy women: A pilot double-blind placebo-controlled trial. *Journal of Agricultural and Food Chemistry*, *55*, 3217-3224.

[194] Meng, X.; Sang, S.; Zhu, N.; Lu, H.; Sheng, S.; Lee, M. J.; Ho, C. T.; and Yang, C. S. (2002). Identification and Characterization of Methylated and Ring-Fission Metabolites of Tea Catechins Formed in Humans, Mice, and Rats. *Chemical Research in Toxicology*, *15*, 1042-1050.

[195] Netzel, M.; Strass, G.; Bitsch, R.; Dietrich, H.; Herbst, M.; Bitsch, I.; and Frank, T. (2005). The excretion and biological antioxidant activity of elderberry antioxidants in healthy humans. *Food Research International*, *38*, 905-910.

[196] Natsume, M.; Osakabe, N.; Oyama, M.; Sasaki, M.; Baba, S.; Nakamura, Y.; Osawa, T.; and Terao, J. (2003). Structures of (-)-epicatechin glucuronide identified from plasma and urine after oral ingestion of (-)-epicatechin: differences between human and rat. *Free Radical Biology and Medicine*, *34*, 840-849.

[197] Coldham, N. G.; Howells, L. C.; Santi, A.; Montesissa, C.; Langlais, C.; King, L. J.; Macpherson, D. D.; and Sauer, M. J. (1999). Biotransformation of genistein in the rat: elucidation of metabolite structure by product ion mass fragmentologyn. *The Journal of Steroid Biochemistry and Molecular Biology*, *70*, 169-184.

[198] Li, C.; Lee, M. J.; Sheng, S.; Meng, X.; Prabhu, S.; Winnik, B.; Huang, B.; Chung, J. Y.; Yan, S.; Ho, C. T.; and Yang, C. S. (2000). Structural identification of two metabolites of catechins and their kinetics in human urine and blood after tea ingestion. *Chemical Research in Toxicology*, *13*, 177-184.

[199] Abd El Mohsen, M.; Marks, J.; Kuhnle, G.; Rice-Evans, C.; Moore, K.; Gibson, G.; Debnam, E.; and Srai, S. K. (2004). The differential tissue distribution of the citrus flavanone naringenin following gastric instillation. *Free Radical Research*, *38*, 1329-1340.

[200] Mennen, L. I.; Sapinho, D.; Ito, H.; Bertrais, S.; Galan, P.; Hercberg, S.; and Scalbert, A. (2007). Urinary flavonoids and phenolic acids as biomarkers of intake for polyphenol-rich foods. *British Journal of Nutrition*, *96*, 191-198.

[201] Felgines, C.; Texier, O.; Besson, C.; Fraisse, D.; Lamaison, J.-L.; and Remesy, C. (2002). Blackberry anthocyanins are slightly bioavailable in rats. *Journal of Nutrition*, *132*, 1249-1253.

[202] Milbury, P. E.; Cao, G.; Prior, R. L.; and Blumberg, J. (2002). Bioavailablility of elderberry anthocyanins. *Mechanisms of Ageing and Development*, *123*, 997-1006.

[203] Wu, X.; Cao, G.; and Prior, R. L. (2002). Absorption and metabolism of anthocyanins in elderly women after consumption of elderberry or blueberry. *Journal of Nutrition*, *132*, 1865-1871.

[204] Shoji, T.; Masumoto, S.; Moriichi, N.; Akiyama, H.; Kanda, T.; Ohtake, Y.; and Goda, Y. (2006). Apple procyanidin oligomers absorption in rats after oral administration: Analysis of procyanidins in plasma using the porter method and high-performance liquid chromatography/tandem mass spectrometry. *Journal of Agricultural and Food Chemistry*, *54*, 884-892.

[205] Gross, M.; Pfeiffer, M.; Martini, M.; Campbell, D.; Slavin, J.; and Potter, J. (1996). The quantitation of metabolites of quercetin flavonols in human urine. *Cancer Epidemiology Biomarkers and Prevention*, *5*, 711-720.

[206] Catterall, F.; King, L. J.; Clifford, M. N.; and Ioannides, C. (2003). Bioavailability of dietary doses of H-3-labelled tea antioxidants (+)-catechin and (-)-epicatechin in rat. *Xenobiotica, 33*, 743-753.

[207] Toshiyuki, K.; Natsuki, M.; Mana, Y.; Masayuki, S.; Fumio, N.; Yukihiko, H.; and Naoto, O. (2001). Metabolic fate of (-)-[4-3H]epigallocatechin gallate in rats after oral administration. *Journal of Agricultural and Food Chemistry, 49*, 4102 -4112.

[208] Heinonen, S. M.; Wahala, K.; and Adlercreutz, H. (2004). Identification of urinary metabolites of the red clover isoflavones formononetin and biochanin A in human subjects. *Journal of Agricultural and Food Chemistry, 52*, 6802-6809.

[209] Heinonen, S. M.; Wahala, K.; Liukkonen, K. H.; Aura, A. M.; Poutanen, K.; and Adlercreutz, H. (2004). Studies of the in vitro intestinal metabolism of isoflavones aid in the identification of their urinary metabolites. *Journal of Agricultural and Food Chemistry, 52*, 2640-2646.

[210] Bitsch, R.; Netzel, M.; Strass, G.; Frank, T.; and Bitsch, I. (2004). Bioavailability and biokinetics of anthocyanins from red grape juice and red wine. *Journal of Biomedicine and Biotechnology, 2004*, 293-298.

[211] Felgines, C.; Talavera, S.; Gonthier, M.-P.; Texier, O.; Scalbert, A.; Lamaison, J.-L.; and Remesy, C. (2003). Strawberry anthocyanins are recovered in urine as glucuro- and sulfoconjugates in humans. *Journal of Nutr*ition *133*, 1296-1301.

[212] Mullen, W.; Edwards, C. A.; Serafini, M.; and Crozier, A. (2008). Bioavailability of pelargonidin-3-O-glucoside and its metabolites in humans following the ingestion of strawberries with and without cream. *Journal of Agricultural and Food Chemistry, 56*, 713-719.

[213] Olthof, M. R.; Hollman, P. C. H.; Buijsman, M. N. C. P.; Amelsvoort, J. M. M. v.; and Katan, M. B. (2003). Chlorogenic acid, quercetin-3-rutinoside and black tea phenols are extensively metabolized in humans. *The Journal of Nutrition, 133*, 1806-1814.

[214] Baker, M. E. (2002). Albumin, steroid hormones and the origin of vertebrates. *Journal of Endocrinology, 175*, 121-127.

[215] Ames, B. N.; and Gold, L. S. (1997). Environmental pollution, pesticides, and the prevention of cancer: Misconceptions. *Faseb Journal, 11*, 1041-1052.

[216] Baker, M. E. (1995). Endocrine activity of plant-derived compounds - an evolutionary perspective. *Proceedings of the Society for Experimental Biology and Medicine, 208*, 131-138.

[217] Janisch, K. M.; Williamson, G.; Needs, P.; and Plumb, G. W. (2004). Properties of quercetin conjugates: Modulation of LDL oxidation and binding to human serum albumin. *Free Radical Research, 38*, 877-884.

[218] Kitson, T. M. (2004). Spectrophotometric and kinetic studies on the binding of the bioflavonoid quercetin to bovine serum albumin. *Bioscience Biotechnology and Biochemistry, 68*, 2165-2170.

[219] Papadopoulou, A.; Green, R. J.; and Frazier, R. A. (2005). Interaction of flavonoids with bovine serum albumin: A fluorescence quenching study. *Journal of Agricultural and Food Chemistry, 53*, 158-163.

[220] Dufour, C.; and Dangles, O. (2005). Flavonoid-serum albumin complexation: determination of binding constants and binding sites by fluorescence spectroscopy. *Biochimica et Biophysica Acta-General Subjects, 1721*, 164-173.

[221] Lancon, A.; Delmas, D.; Osman, H.; Thenot, J. P.; Jannin, B.; and Latruffe, N. (2004). Human hepatic cell uptake of resveratrol: involvement of both passive diffusion and carrier-mediated process. *Biochemical and Biophysical Research Communications*, *316*, 1132-1137.
[222] Fasano, M.; Curry, S.; Terreno, E.; Galliano, M.; Fanali, G.; Narciso, P.; Notari, S.; and Ascenzi, P. (2005). The extraordinary ligand binding properties of human serum albumin. *Iubmb Life*, *57*, 787-796.
[223] Hong, J.; Lambert, J. D.; Lee, S. H.; Sinko, P. J.; and Yang, C. S. (2003). Involvement of multidrug resistance-associated proteins in regulating cellular levels of (-)-epigallocatechin-3-gallate and its methyl metabolites. *Biochemical and Biophysical Research Communications*, *310*, 222-227.
[224] Hurst, R. D.; and Fritz, I. B. (1996). Properties of an immortalised vascular endothelial glioma cell co-culture model of the blood-brain barrier. *Journal of Cellular Physiology*, *167*, 81-88.
[225] Youdim, K. A.; Dobbie, M. S.; Kuhnle, G.; Proteggente, A. R.; Abbott, N. J.; and Rice-Evans, C. (2003). Interaction between flavonoids and the blood-brain barrier: in vitro studies. *Journal of Neurochemistry*, *85*, 180-192.
[226] Abd El Mohsen, M. M.; Kuhnle, G.; Rechner, A. R.; Schroeter, H.; Rose, S.; Jenner, P.; and Rice-Evans, C. A. (2002). Uptake and metabolism of epicatechin and its access to the brain after oral ingestion. *Free Radical Biology and Medicine*, *33*, 1693-1702.
[227] Youdim, K. A.; Qaiser, M. Z.; Begley, D. J.; Rice-Evans, C. A.; and Abbott, N. J. (2004). Flavonoid permeability across an in situ model of the blood-brain barrier. *Free Radical Biology and Medicine*, *36*, 592-604.
[228] Koga, T.; and Meydani, M. (2001). Effect of plasma metabolites of (+)-catechin and quercetin on monocyte adhesion to human aortic endothelial cells. *American Journal of Clinical Nutrition*, *73*, 941-948.
[229] Gläßer, G.; Graefe, E. U.; Struck, F.; Veit, M.; and Gebhardt, R. (2002). Comparison of antioxidative capacities and inhibitory effects on cholesterol biosynthesis of quercetin and potential metabolites. *Phytomedicine*, *9*, 33-40.
[230] Shirai, M.; Moon, J. H.; Tsushida, T.; and Terao, J. (2001). Inhibitory effect of a quercetin metabolite, quercetin 3-O-beta-D-Glucuronide, on lipid peroxidation in liposomal membranes. *Journal of Agricultural and Food Chemistry*, *49*, 5602-5608.
[231] Shirai, M.; Yamanishi, R.; Moon, J. H.; Murota, K.; and Terao, J. (2002). Effect of quercetin and its conjugated metabolite on the hydrogen peroxide-induced intracellular production of reactive oxygen species in mouse fibroblasts. *Bioscience Biotechnology and Biochemistry*, *66*, 1015-1021.
[232] Yoshizumi, M.; Tsuchiya, K.; Suzaki, Y.; Kirima, K.; Kyaw, M.; Moon, J.-H.; Terao, J.; and Tamaki, T. (2002). Quercetin glucuronide prevents VSMC hypertrophy by angiotensin II via the inhibition of JNK and AP-1 signaling pathway. *Biochemical and Biophysical Research Communications*, *293*, 1458-1465.
[233] O'Leary, K. A.; Pascual-Tereasa, S. d.; Needs, P. W.; Bao, Y.-P.; O'Brien, N. M.; and Williamson, G. (2004). Effect of flavonoids and Vitamin E on cyclooxygenase-2 (COX-2) transcription. *Mutation Research/Fundamental and Molecular Mechanisms of Mutagenesis*, *551*, 245-254.

[234] Lodi, F.; Jimenez, R.; Menendez, C.; Needs, P. W.; Duarte, J.; and Perez-Vizcaino, F. (2008). Glucuronidated metabolites of the flavonoid quercetin do not auto-oxidise, do not generate free radicals and do not decrease nitric oxide bioavailability. *Planta Medica*, *74*, 741-746.

[235] Loke, W. M.; Proudfoot, J. M.; McKinley, A. J.; Needs, P. W.; Kroon, P. A.; Hodgson, J. M.; and Croft, K. D. (2008). Quercetin and its in vivo metabolites inhibit neutrophil-mediated low-density lipoprotein oxidation. *Journal of Agricultural and Food Chemistry*, *56*, 3609-3615.

[236] Spencer, J. P. E.; Rice-Evans, C.; and Williams, R. J. (2003). Modulation of pro-survival Akt/Protein Kinase B and ERK1/2 signaling cascades by quercetin and Its in vivo metabolites underlie their action on neuronal viability. *Journal of Biological Chemistry*, *278*, 34783-34793.

[237] Day, A. J.; Bao, Y.; Morgan, M. R. A.; and Williamson, G. (2000). Conjugation position of quercetin glucuronides and effect on biological activity. *Free Radical Biology and Medicine*, *29*, 1234-1243.

[238] Kuo, H. M.; Ho, H. J.; Chao, P. D. L.; and Chung, J. G. (2002). Quercetin glucuronides inhibited 2-aminofluorene acetylation in human acute myeloid HL-60 leukemia cells. *Phytomedicine*, *9*, 625-631.

[239] Saito, A.; Sugisawa, A.; Umegaki, K.; and Sunagawa, H. (2004). Protective Effects of Quercetin and Its Metabolites on H2O2-Induced Chromosomal Damage to WIL2-NS Cells. *Bioscience, Biotechnology, and Biochemistry*, *68*, 271-276.

[240] Liu, W.; and Liang, N. (2000). Inhibitory effect of disodium qurecetin-7, 4'-disulfate on aggregation of pig platelets induced by thrombin and its mechanism. *Acta Pharmacologica Sinica*, *21*, 737-741.

[241] Fang, S.-H.; Hou, Y.-C.; Chang, W.-C.; Hsiu, S.-L.; Lee Chao, P.-D.; and Chiang, B.-L. (2003). Morin sulfates/glucuronides exert anti-inflammatory activity on activated macrophages and decreased the incidence of septic shock. *Life Sciences*, *74*, 743-756.

[242] Hsieh, C.-L.; Chao, P. D. L.; and Fang, S. H. (2005). Morin sulphates/glucuronides enhance macrophage function in microgravity culture system. *European Journal of Clinical Investigation*, *35*, 591-596.

[243] van Zanden, J. J.; van der Woude, H.; Vaessen, J.; Usta, M.; Wortelboer, H. M.; Cnubben, N. H. P.; and Rietjens, I. (2007). The effect of quercetin phase II metabolism on its MRP1 and MRP2 inhibiting potential. *Biochemical Pharmacology*, *74*, 345-351.

[244] Tseng, T.-H.; Wang, C.-J.; Kao, E.-S.; and Chu, h.-Y. (1996). Hibiscus protocatechuic acid protects against oxidative damage induced by tert-butylhydroperoxide in rat primary hepatocytes. *Chemico-Biological Interactions*, *101*, 137-148.

[245] Tseng, T.-H.; Kao, T.-W.; Chu, C.-Y.; Chou, F.-P.; Lin, W.-L.; and Wang, C.-J. (2000). Induction of apoptosis by Hibiscus protocatechuic acid in human leukemia cells via reduction of retinoblastoma (RB) phosphorylation and Bcl-2 expression. *Biochemical Pharmacology*, *60*, 307-315.

[246] Liu, C.-L.; Wang, J.-M.; Chu, C.-Y.; Cheng, M.-T.; and Tseng, T.-H. (2002). In vivo protective effect of protocatechuic acid on tert-butyl hydroperoxide-induced rat hepatotoxicity. *Food and Chemical Toxicology*, *40*, 635-641.

[247] Tarozzi, A.; Morroni, F.; Hrelia, S.; Angeloni, C.; Marchesi, A.; Cantelli-Forti, G.; and Hrelia, P. (2007). Neuroprotective effects of anthocyanins and their in vivo metabolites in SH-SY5Y cells. *Neuroscience Letters*, *424*, 36-40.

[248] Lu, H.; Meng, X.; Li, C.; Sang, S.; Patten, C.; Sheng, S.; Hong, J.; Bai, N.; Winnik, B.; Ho, C.-T.; and Yang, C. S. (2003). Glucuronides of Tea Catechins: Enzymology of Biosynthesis and Biological Activities. *Drug Metabolism and Disposition, 31*, 452-461.

[249] Spencer, J. P. E.; Schroeter, H.; Crossthwaithe, A. J.; Kuhnle, G.; Williams, R. J.; and Rice-Evans, C. (2001). Contrasting influences of glucuronidation and O-methylation of epicatechin on hydrogen peroxide-induced cell death in neurons and fibroblasts. *Free Radical Biology and Medicine, 31*, 1139-1146.

[250] Spencer, J. P. E.; Schroeter, H.; Kuhnle, G.; Srai, S. K. S.; Tyrrell, R. M.; Hahn, U.; and Rice-Evans, C. (2001). Epicatechin and its in vivo metabolite, 3 '-O-methyl epicatechin, protect human fibroblasts from oxidative-stress-induced cell death involving caspase-3 activation. *Biochemical Journal, 354*, 493-500.

[251] Li, S. M.; Sang, S. M.; Pan, M. H.; Lai, C. S.; Lo, C. Y.; Yang, C. S.; and Ho, C. T. (2007). Anti-inflammatory property of the urinary metabolites of nobiletin in mouse. *Bioorganic and Medicinal Chemistry Letters, 17*, 5177-5181.

[252] Stevenson, D.; Cooney, J.; Jensen, D.; Wibisono, R.; Adaim, A.; Skinner, M.; and Zhang, J. (2008). Comparison of enzymically glucuronidated flavonoids with flavonoid aglycones in an in vitro cellular model of oxidative stress protection. *In Vitro Cellular and Developmental Biology - Animal, 44*, 73-80.

[253] Cano, A.; Arnao, M. B.; Williamson, G.; and Garcia-Conesa, M. T. (2002). Superoxide scavenging by polyphenols: effect of conjugation and dimerization. *Redox Report, 7*, 379-383.

[254] Proteggente, A. R.; Basu-Modak, S.; Kuhnle, G.; Gordon, M. J.; Youdim, K.; Tyrrell, R.; and Rice-Evans, C. A. (2003). Hesperetin glucuronide, a photoprotective agent arising from Ffavonoid metabolism in human skin fibroblasts and para. *Photochemistry and Photobiology, 78*, 256-261.

[255] Spencer, J. P. E.; Kuhnle, G. G. C.; Williams, R. J.; and Rice-Evans, C. (2003). Intracellular metabolism and bioactivity of quercetin and its in vivo metabolites. *Biochemical Journal, 372*, 173-181.

[256] de Pascual-Teresa, S.; Johnston, K. L.; DuPont, M. S.; O'Leary, K. A.; Needs, P. W.; Morgan, L. M.; Clifford, M. N.; Bao, Y. P.; and Williamson, G. (2004). Quercetin metabolites downregulate cyclooxygenase-2 transcription in human lymphocytes ex vivo but not in vivo. *Journal of Nutrition, 134*, 552-557.

[257] Paulke, A.; Noldner, M.; Schubert-Zslavecz, M.; and Wurglics, M. (2008). St. John's wort flavonolds and their metabolites show antidepressant activity and accumulate in brain after multiple oral doses. *Pharmazie, 63*, 296-302.

[258] Hubbard, G. P.; Wolffram, S.; de Vos, R.; Bovy, A.; Gibbins, J. M.; and Lovegrove, J. A. (2006). Ingestion of onion soup high in quercetin inhibits platelet aggregation and essential components of the collagen-stimulated platelet activation pathway in man: a pilot study. *British Journal of Nutrition, 96*, 482-488.

[259] Kawai, Y.; Nishikawa, T.; Shiba, Y.; Saito, S.; Murota, K.; Shibata, N.; Kobayashi, M.; Kanayama, M.; Uchida, K.; and Terao, J. (2008). Macrophage as a target of quercetin glucuronides in human atherosclerotic arteries - Implication in the anti-atherosclerotic mechanism of dietary flavonoids. *Journal of Biological Chemistry, 283*, 9424-9434.

[260] Jackman, K. A.; Woodman, O. L.; and Sobey, C. G. (2007). Isoflavones, equol and cardiovascular disease: Pharmacological and therapeutic insights. *Current Medicinal Chemistry, 14*, 2824-2830.

[261] Nam Joo, K.; Ki Won, L.; Rogozin, E. A.; Yong-Yeon, C.; Yong-Seok, H.; Bode, A. M.; Hyong Joo, L.; and Zigang, D. (2007). Equol, a metabolite of the soybean isoflavone daidzein, inhibits neoplastic cell transformation by targeting the MEK/ERK/p90RSK/activator protein-1 pathway. *Journal of Biological Chemistry, 282*, 32856-32866.

[262] Zhang, Y.; Song, T. T.; Cunnick, J. E.; Murphy, P. A.; and Hendrich, S. (1999). Daidzein and genistein glucuronides in vitro are weakly estrogenic and activate human natural killer cells at nutritionally relevant concentrations. *The Journal of Nutrition, 129*, 399-405.

[263] Niculescu, M. D.; Pop, E. A.; Fischer, L. M.; and Zeisel, S. H. (2007). Dietary isoflavones differentially induce gene expression changes in lymphocytes from postmenopausal women who form equol as compared with those who do not. *Journal of Nutritional Biochemistry, 18*, 380-390.

[264] Rachon, D.; Seidlova-Wuttke, D.; Vortherms, T.; and Wuttke, W. (2007). Effects of dietary equol administration on ovariectomy induced bone loss in Sprague-Dawley rats. *Maturitas, 58*, 308-315.

[265] Rachon, D.; Vortherms, T.; Seidlova-Wuttke, D.; and Wuttke, W. (2007). Effects of dietary equol on body weight gain, intra-abdominal fat accumulation, plasma lipids, and glucose tolerance in ovariectomized Sprague-Dawley rats. *Menopause-the Journal of the North American Menopause Society, 14*, 925-932.

[266] Ohtomo, T.; Uehara, M.; Penalvo, J. L.; Adlercreutz, H.; Katsumata, S.; Suzuki, K.; Takeda, K.; Masuyama, R.; and Ishimi, Y. (2008). Comparative activities of daidzein metabolites, equol and O-desmethylangolensin, on bone mineral density and lipid metabolism in ovariectomized mice and in osteoclast cell cultures. *European Journal of Nutrition, 47*, 273-279.

[267] Rachon, D.; Menche, A.; Vortherms, T.; Seidlova-Wuttke, D.; and Wuttke, W. (2008). Effects of dietary equol administration on the mammary gland in ovariectomized Sprague-Dawley rats. *Menopause-the Journal of the North American Menopause Society, 15*, 340-345.

[268] Rechner, A. R.; and Kroner, C. (2005). Anthocyanins and colonic metabolites of dietary polyphenols inhibit platelet function. *Thrombosis Research, 116*, 327-334.

[269] Hiermann, A.; Schramm, H. W.; and Laufer, S. (1998). Anti-inflammatory activity of myricetin-3-O-beta-D-glucuronide and related compounds. *Inflammation Research, 47*, 421-427.

[270] Guo, J. M.; Qian, F.; Li, J. X.; Xu, Q.; and Chen, T. (2007). Identification of a new metabolite of astilbin, 3 '-O-methylastilbin, and its immunosuppressive activity against contact dermatitis. *Clinical Chemistry, 53*, 465-471.

[271] Bellion, P.; Hofmann, T.; Pool-Zobel, B. L.; Will, F.; Dietrich, H.; Knaup, B.; Richling, E.; Baum, M.; Eisenbrand, G.; and Janzowski, C. (2008). Antioxidant effectiveness of phenolic apple juice extracts and their gut fermentation products in the human colon carcinoma cell line caco-2. *Journal of Agricultural and Food Chemistry, 56*, 6310-6317.

[272] Chan, F. L.; Choi, H. L.; Chen, Z. Y.; Chan, P. S. F.; and Huang, Y. (2000). Induction of apoptosis in prostate cancer cell lines by a flavonoid, baicalin. *Cancer Letters, 160*, 219-228.

[273] Ueda, S.; Nakamura, H.; Masutani, H.; Sasada, T.; Takabayashi, A.; Yamaoka, Y.; and Yodoi, J. (2002). Baicalin induces apoptosis via mitochondrial pathway as prooxidant. *Molecular Immunology*, *38*, 781-791.

[274] Canali, R.; Ambra, R.; Stelitano, C.; Mattivi, F.; Scaccini, C.; and Virgili, F. (2007). A novel model to study the biological effects of red wine at the molecular level. *British Journal of Nutrition*, *97*, 1053-1058.

[275] Shukla, M.; Gupta, K.; Rasheed, Z.; Khan, K.; and Haqqi, T. (2008). Bioavailable constituents/metabolites of pomegranate (Punica granatum L) preferentially inhibit COX2 activity ex vivo and IL-1beta-induced PGE2 production in human chondrocytes in vitro. *Journal of Inflammation*, *5*, 9.

In: Flavonoids: Biosynthesis, Biological Effects... ISBN: 978-1-60741-622-7
Editor: Raymond B. Keller

Chapter 2

CYTOPROTECTIVE ACTIVITY OF FLAVONOIDS IN RELATION TO THEIR CHEMICAL STRUCTURES AND PHYSICOCHEMICAL PROPERTIES

Jingli Zhang* and Margot A. Skinner
The New Zealand Institute for Plant and Food Research Ltd,
Auckland, New Zealand

ABSTRACT

Flavonoids are widely distributed in fruit and vegetables and form part of the human diet. These compounds are thought to be a contributing factor to the health benefits of fruit and vegetables in part because of their antioxidant activities. Despite the extensive use of chemical antioxidant assays to assess the activity of flavonoids and other natural products that are safe to consume, their ability to predict an *in vivo* health benefit is debateable. Some are carried out at non-physiological pH and temperature, most take no account of partitioning between hydrophilic and lipophilic environments, and none of them takes into account bioavailability, uptake and metabolism of antioxidant compounds and the biological component that is targeted for protection. However, biological systems are far more complex and dietary antioxidants may function via multiple mechanisms. It is critical to consider moving from using 'the test tube' to employing cell-based assays for screening foods, phytochemicals and other consumed natural products for their potential biological activity. The question then remains as to which cell models to use. Human immortalized cell lines derived from many different cell types from a wide range of anatomical sites are available and are established well-characterized models.

The cytoprotection assay was developed to be a more biologically relevant measurement than the chemically defined antioxidant activity assay because it uses human cells as a substrate and therefore accounts for some aspects of uptake, metabolism and location of flavonoids within cells. Knowledge of structure activity relationships in the cytoprotection assay may be helpful in assessing potential *in vivo* cellular protective effects of flavonoids. This chapter will discuss the cytoprotective properties of flavonoids and focuses on the relationship between their cytoprotective activity, physicochemical properties such as lipophilicity (log P) and bond dissociation enthalpies (BDE), and their chemical structures. The factors influencing the ability of flavonoids to protect human gut cells are discussed, and these support the contention that the partition coefficients of flavonoids as well as their rate of reaction with the relevant radicals help define the protective abilities in cellular environments. By comparing the geometries of several flavonoids, we were able to explain the structural dependency of the antioxidant action of these flavonoids.

INTRODUCTION

The flavonoids are among the most numerous and widespread natural products found in plants and have many diverse applications and properties. Over the years, a wide range of beneficial properties related to human health have been reported. These include effects related to cancer (Colic and Pavelic, 2000; Eastwood, 1999; Middleton *et al.*, 2000), cardiovascular diseases (Riemersma *et al.*, 2001), including coronary heart disease (Eastwood, 1999; Giugliano, 2000; Middleton *et al.*, 2000) and atherosclerosis (Wedworth and Lynch, 1995); anti-inflammatory effects (Manthey, 2000; Middleton *et al.*, 2000), and other diseases in which an increase in oxidative stress have been implicated (Diplock *et al.*, 1998; Harborne and Williams, 2000; Packer *et al.*, 1999). A number of studies have shown that consumption of fruits and vegetables can reduce the risk of cardiovascular diseases and cancer, potentially through the biological actions of the phenolic components such as flavonoids.

The precise mechanisms by which flavonoids may protect different cell populations from oxidative insults are currently unclear. However, potential mechanisms that involve their classical antioxidant properties, interactions with mitochondria, modulation of intracellular signalling cascades, and stimulation of adaptive responses have been proposed. The effects of a flavonoid in a cellular environment may well extend beyond conventional antioxidant actions. In the cellular environment, the coexistence of other factors such as the bioavailability of the compound, the effectiveness of the compound within the cell, and the effectiveness of the compound in the body must also be considered. Therefore, using a cell-based assay format, these compounds react with cells and provide information regarding the cellular response, taking into account some aspects of uptake, metabolism, location of antioxidant compounds within cells and intracellular effects on signalling pathways and enzyme activity. These effects are likely to be the result of differential modulation of cellular activities such as signalling pathways, enzyme activity, transport and bioavailability, rather than simply a result of free radical scavenging. Furthermore, as cells from different anatomical sites respond differently to both stressors and treatments, it is important to use the appropriate cell types to test a particular cellular response, rather than a chemically-defined system for the antioxidant activity. Here, we employed and established cell-based assays using gut-derived cultured human cell lines. The rationale to use cultured human cell lines over primary cells is that human primary cells are not readily available, but human immortalized cell lines derived from many different cell types from a wide range of anatomical sites are available and are established well-characterized models.

The multiple biological activities of flavonoids as well as their structural diversity make this class of compounds a rich source for modelling lead compounds with targeted biological properties. Different classes of flavonoids are not equally physiologically active, presumably because they are structurally different. Despite the enormous interest in flavonoids and other polyphenolic compounds as potential protective agents against the development of human diseases, the real contribution of such compounds to health maintenance and the mechanisms through which they act are still unclear. Structure activity relationships (SARs) represent an attempt to correlate physicochemical or structural descriptors of a set of structurally related compounds with their biological activities or physical properties. Molecular descriptors usually include parameters accounting for electronic properties, hydrophobicity, topology, and steric effects. Activities include chemical and biological measurements. Once developed, SARs provide predictive models of biological activity and allow the identification of those molecular parameters responsible for the biological and physicochemical properties. These may shed light on the mechanism of action.

SARs of flavonoids have been previously reported for scavenging of peroxynitrite, hydroxyl radical and superoxide, and protection against lipid peroxidation (Chen *et al.*, 2002; Choi *et al.*, 2002; Cos *et al.*, 1998), inhibition of LDL oxidation (van Acker *et al.*, 1996; Vaya *et al.*, 2003), and the influence of flavonoid structure on biological systems has also been investigated, e.g., induction of DNA degradation; growth and proliferation of certain malignant cells; acute toxicity in isolated rat hepatocytes, and inhibition of gastric H^+, K^+-ATPase (Agullo *et al.*, 1997; Moridani *et al.*, 2002; Murakami *et al.*, 1999; Sugihara *et al.*, 2003).

CHEMICAL STRUCTURE OF FLAVONOIDS

The flavonoids are a group of phenolic compounds that share common structural features and physicochemical properties, which are important in determining their biological effects. Phenylpropanoid metabolism, which encompasses natural product metabolic pathways unique to plants, transforms phenylalanine into a variety of plant secondary metabolites, including lignins, sinapate esters, stilbenoids and flavonoids. Amongst these phenylpropanoids, flavonoids (C_6-C_3-C_6) have received significant attention in the past few decades because they appear to have diverse functions in plant defence systems and effects on human health such as antiallergic, anti-inflammatory, antithrombotic, anticancer, and antioxidant effects. Flavonoids constitute a relatively diverse family of aromatic molecules that are derived from phenylalanine via a *p*-coumaric acid (C_6-C_3) intermediate step (Figure 1) (Havsteen, 2002; Ververidis *et al.*, 2007; Winkel-Shirley, 2001). They account for a variety of colours in flowers, berries and fruits, from yellow to red and dark purple. The term "flavonoids" is generally used to describe a broad collection of natural products that include a C_6-C_3-C_6 carbon framework, which possess phenylbenzopyran functionality. Chalcones and dihydrochalcones are considered to be the primary C_6-C_3-C_6 precursors and constitute important intermediates in the synthesis of flavonoids. The nomenclature of flavonoids is with respect to the aromatic ring A condensed to the heterocyclic ring C and the aromatic ring B most often attached at the 2-position of the C-ring. The various attached substituents are listed first for the C-ring and A-ring and, as primed numbers, for the B-ring (Figure 1).

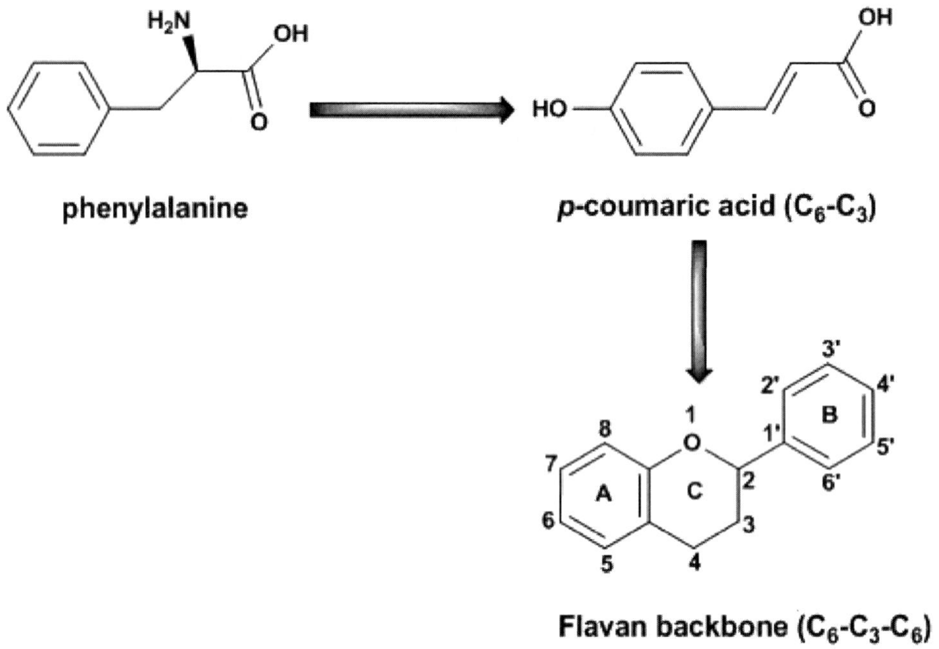

Figure 1. Diagram of biosynthetic formation of flavonoid backbone from phenylalanine. The basic flavonoid structure consists of the fused A and C-rings, with the phenyl B-ring attached through its 1′-position to the 2-position of the C-ring (numbered from the pyran oxygen).

Flavonoids differ in the arrangements of hydroxyl, methoxy, and glycosidic side groups, and in the configuration of the C-ring that joins the A- and B-rings. These give rise to a multitude of different compounds (Middleton *et al.*, 2000). In plants, the majority of the flavonoids are found as glycosides with different sugar groups linked to one or more of the hydroxyl groups. They are mainly found in the outer parts of the plants, such as leaves, flowers and fruits, whereas the content in stalks and roots is usually very limited. The flavonoids located in the upper surface of the leaf or in the epidermal cells have a role to play in the physiological survival of plants. They contribute to the disease resistance of the plant, either as constitutive antifungal agents or as induced phytoalexins (Harborne *et al.*, 2000). Multiple combinations of hydroxyl groups, sugars, oxygen atoms, and methyl groups attached to the basic ring structural skeleton create the various classes of flavonoids. According to the configuration of the C-ring, flavonoid can be classified as flavonol, flavonone, flavone, flavanol, anthocyanidin, chalcone, and isoflavone (Herrmann, 1976; Herrmann, 1989) as illustrated in Figure 2. It should be noted that chalcones contain an opened C-ring (Dziezak, 1986) and the numbering system for chalcones is reversed. Flavonoids comprise a large group of secondary plant metabolites. Presently more than 7000 individual compounds are known, which are based on very few core structures (Fossen and Andersen, 2006; Stack, 1997). Within each class, individual flavonoids may vary in the number and distribution of hydroxyl groups as well as in their degree of alkylation or glycosylation.

Flavones and flavonols occur as aglycones in foods. These compounds possess a double bond between C_2 and C_3. Flavones are a class of flavonoids based on the backbone of 2-phenylchromen-4-one, such as chrysin, apigenin, and luteolin. Flavones are lacking the 3-OH group on the backbone. Flavones are commonly found in fruit skins, celery, and parsley.

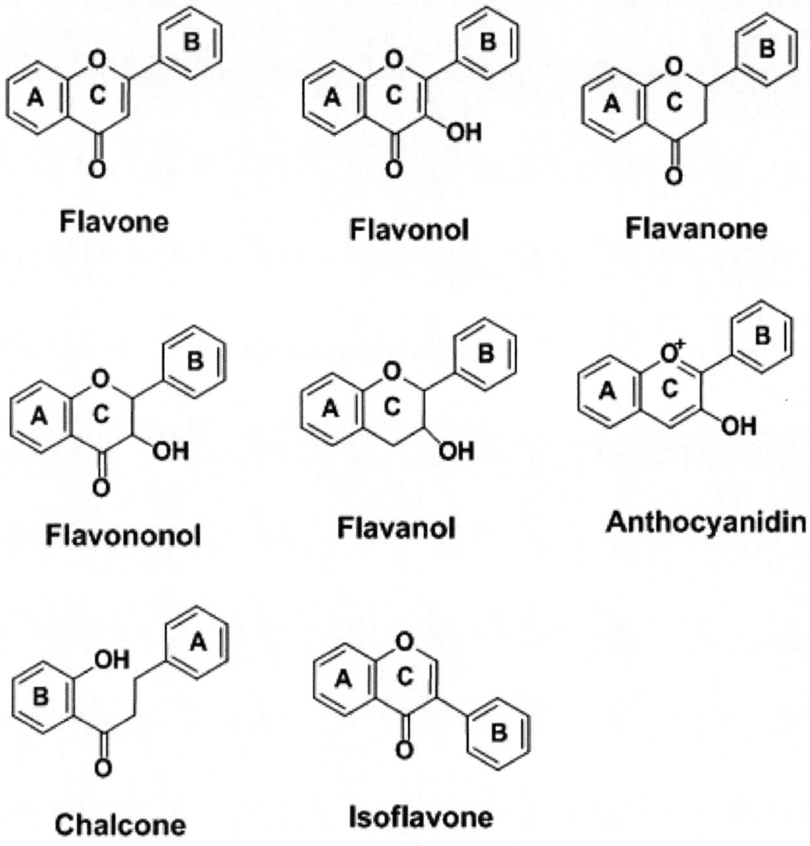

Figure 2. The basic ring structure of the subclasses of flavonoids.

Flavonols are a class of flavonoids that use the 3-hydroxyflavone backbone (3-hydroxy-2-phenylchromen-4-one (Figure 2). Flavonols are different from flavones in that they possess a hydroxyl group in the 3-position and can be regarded as 3-hydroxyflavones. The formation of flavonol and flavone glycosides depends on the action of light; therefore, they are found mainly in leaves and fruit skins with only trace amounts in parts of plants below the soil surface (Herrmann, 1976). In general, flavonols occur in the diet as glycosides (Hollman and Arts, 2000). Flavonols, such as galangin, kaempferol, quercetin, morin, rutin, myricetin, and isoquercetin, are found in plant-based foods, with onions, apples, berries, kale, and broccoli having the highest concentrations. Flavonols are present mainly as mono-, di- and triglycosides. The monoglycosides occur mainly as 3-O-glycosides. In the case of diglycosides, the two sugar moieties may be linked to the same or two different carbons.

Flavonones and flavononols are characterized by the presence of a saturated C_2–C_3 bond and an oxygen atom (carbonyl group) in the 4-position. Thus, flavonones may be referred to as dihydroflavones. Flavanones, such as hesperidin and naringin, have a more restricted distribution than other flavonoid compounds and are specific to citrus fruits. Naringin is the predominant flavanone in grapefruit (*Citrus paradisi*) (up to 10% of the dry weight) and is responsible for the bitterness of grapefruit juices. The flavonones in plants are often glycosylated in the 7-position with disaccharides rutinose and neohesperoside. Both of these disaccharides are made of rhamnose and glucose and differ only in their linkage type: 1→6 for rutinose and 1→2 for neohesperoside. It is worth noting that flavononol glycosides are good fungistatic and fungitoxic substances (Kefford and Chandler, 1970). Flavononols differ from flavanones by having a hydroxyl group in the 3-position and are often referred to as 3-hydroxyflavonones or dihydroflavonols, such as taxifolin. Flavonones have one centre of asymmetry in the 2-position, while flavononols possess a second centre of asymmetry in the 3-position.

Among flavonoids, anthocyanins and flavanols are known collectively as flavans because of lack of the carbonyl group in the 4-position. Flavanols are a class of flavonoids that use the 2-phenyl-3,4-dihydro-2H-chromen-3-ol skeleton. These compounds include catechin, epicatechin and its derivates. Flavanols are building blocks for proanthocyanidins. Proanthocyanidins consist of monomeric units of flavans linked through C-C and ether linkages. Fifteen subclasses of proanthocyanidins have been identified (Porter, 1993), however, only three appear to be prominent in human foods of plant origin, procyanidins (epicatechin or catechin polymers), prodelephinidins (epigallocatechin or gallocatechin polymers) and propelargonidins (epiafselechin or afselechin polymers) or their mixtures (Gu *et al.*, 2003). These proanthocyanidins are soluble up to a molecular weight of approximately 7000, corresponding to ca. 20 flavan units. The name proanthocyanidins, previously called leucoanthocyanidins, implies that these are colorless precursors of anthocyanidins. On heating in acidic solutions, the C-C bond made during formation is cleaved and terminal flavan units are released from the oligomers as carbocations, which are then oxidized to colored anthocyanidins by atmospheric oxygen. Anthocyanidins are naturally colored compounds occurring in the form of glycosides (anthocyanins), the largest group of water-soluble pigments in the plant kingdom. They are responsible for most of the red, blue, and purple colors of fruits, vegetables, flowers, and other plant tissues (Harborne *et al.*, 2000). Anthocyanidins are characterized by having the basic flavylium cation structure and different substituents on ring B. The electron deficiency of their structure makes anthocyanidins highly reactive, and their stability is both pH and temperature dependent. Their glycosides are usually much more stable than the aglycons (Delgado-Vargas *et al.*, 2000). The anthocyanins are all based chemically on the structure of cyanidin, and all are derived from this base structure by the addition or subtraction of hydroxyl groups, by the degree of methylation of these hydroxyl groups, and by the nature and number of sugars and their position on the aglycon (Harborne, 1962; Harborne and Williams, 2001). In aqueous media, most of the natural anthocyanins behave as pH indicators, being red at low pH, bluish at intermediate pH, and colorless at high pH. The nature of the chemical structures that these anthocyanins can adopt upon changes in pH has been described (Briviba *et al.*, 1993; Brouillard, 1983).

Chalcones are flavonoids lacking a heterocyclic C-ring. The chalcone structure contains an aromatic ketone that forms the central core for a variety of important biological compounds. The most common chalcones found in apples and other fruit of the Rosaceae family are phloretin and phloretin-7-glycoside (phloridzin).

PHYSICOCHEMICAL PROPERTIES OF FLAVONOIDS

The UV Absorption of Flavonoids

Studies on flavonoids by UV spectrophotometry have revealed flavonols exhibit two major absorption peaks in the region 240–400 nm, in which 300–380 nm (Band I) is considered to be associated with the absorption due to the B-ring cinnamoyl system, and 240–280 nm (Band II) with absorption involving the A-ring benzoyl system (Alonso-Salces *et al.*, 2004; Cook and Samman, 1996; Rice-Evans *et al.*, 1995). Functional groups attached to the flavonoid skeleton may cause a shift in absorption, such as from 367 nm in (3,5,7,4′-hydroxyl groups), to 371 nm in quercetin (3,5,7,3′,4′-hydroxyl groups), and to 374 nm in myricetin (3,5,7,3′,4′,5′-hydroxyl groups) (Cook *et al.*, 1996). The absence of a 3-hydroxyl group in flavones distinguishes them from flavonols. Thus, Band I occurs at a wavelength shorter by 20–30 nm, such as the 337 nm exhibited for apigenin (Rice-Evans *et al.*, 1995; Rice-Evans *et al.*, 1996). Flavanones have a saturated heterocyclic C ring, with no conjugation between the A and B rings, as determined by their UV spectral characteristics (Rice-Evans *et al.*, 1995). Flavanones and flavanonols exhibit a very strong Band II absorption maximum between 270 and 295 nm, namely 288 nm (naringenin) and 285 nm (taxifolin) and only a shoulder for Band I at 326 and 327 nm. As anthocyanins show distinctive Band I peaks in the 450–560-nm region due to the hydroxyl cinnamoyl system of the B-ring and Band II peaks in the 240–280-nm region due to the benzoyl system of the A-ring, the colour of the anthocyanins varies with the number and position of the hydroxyl groups (Wollenweber and Dietz, 1981).

Physical Properties of Flavonoids

Theoretical parameters employed to characterize radical scavenging activity of a flavonoid can be roughly grouped into the following classes: (1) indices reflecting O–H bond dissociation enthalpy (BDE), where a relatively low BDE value facilitates the H-abstraction reaction between antioxidant and radical (Dewar *et al.*, 1985; van Acker *et al.*, 1993; Zhang *et al.*, 2003b); (2) parameters representing electron-donating ability, such as ionization potential (IP) or relative adiabatic ionization potential (van Acker *et al.*, 1993), and enthalpy of single electron transfer (also defined as activation energy of the intermediate cation) (Vedernikova *et al.*, 1999); (3) factors stabilizing the corresponding radical after hydrogen-abstraction (Vedernikova *et al.*, 1999); (4) electrochemical properties, such as redox potentials (van Acker *et al.*, 1996; Vedernikova *et al.*, 1999); and (5) solubility, which controls the mobility of the antioxidant between lipid membranes (Gotoh *et al.*, 1996; Noguchi *et al.*, 1997), e.g. lipophilicity (logarithm of octanol/water partition coefficient).

Bond Dissociation Energy (BDE)

BDE is the measure of the energy change on bond making or bond breaking and is defined as the amount of energy required to break a given bond to produce two radical fragments when the molecule is in the gas phase at 25°C (298.15 °K) (McMurry, 1992).

$$A:B \xrightarrow{BDE} A^{\bullet} + B^{\bullet} \quad [1]$$

Bond dissociation energies have long been considered to provide the best quantitative measure of the stabilities of the radicals formed (Bordwell and Zhang, 1993). Since the rate constants of this reaction depend largely on the strength of the ArO-H bond (ArOH represents flavonoid molecule), the BDE of flavonoids is defined by the following equation:

$$A_rOH \xrightarrow{BDE} A_rO^{\bullet} + H^{\bullet} \quad [2]$$

BDE (ArO-H) can be obtained as:

$$BDE = H_{fr} + H_{fh} - H_{fp} \quad [3]$$

where H_{fr} is the enthalpy for radicals generated after H abstraction, H_{fh} is the enthalpy for the hydrogen atom, -0.49792 hartrees, and H_{fp} is the enthalpy of the parent molecule (Zhang *et al.*, 2003a).

The properties of the A_rO-H bond appear to be essential to understanding the chemical and biochemical behaviour of flavonoids. The A_rO-H bond must be broken to generate the truly active species, i.e. the phenoxy radical, in order to exhibit its antioxidant activity. There are a number of studies, using a diversity of modern experimental and computational tools, on the determinations of the BDEs of phenolic derivatives (Bordwell *et al.*, 1993; Lucarini and Pedulli, 1994; van Acker *et al.*, 1996). Their aim was to understand how the strength of the phenolic bond is affected by nature, position, and number of substituents. BDE can be experimentally determined in the gas phase using approaches such as radical kinetics, gas-phase acidity cycles and photoionization mass spectrometry (Berkowitz *et al.*, 1994) and in solutions using techniques such as photoacoustic calorimetry (PAC) (Mulder *et al.*, 1988), electrochemical (EC) (Wayner and Parker, 1993), and other measurements (Mahoney and DaRooge, 1975). It should be noted that neither the EC technique nor the PAC method for measuring BDEs is a stand-alone method. Both techniques are dependent upon at least one gas-phase measurement (Wayner *et al.*, 1995). However, all the above-mentioned methods are limited especially for the larger organic compounds since most of them are not stable in the gas phase. Moreover, these measurements require very sophisticated instruments. For these reasons, the number of experimentally known BDEs for flavonoids is very small (Denisov and Khydyakov, 1987).

Besides these experimental studies, a number of theoretical investigations of varying degrees of sophistication have also been reported in order to understand the structural factors determining the stability of the O-H phenolic bond. Both experimental and theoretical results indicate that the change of the O-H bond strength due to a given substituent is approximately constant in the variously substituted phenols and that, for each substituent in the *ortho, meta*, and *para* positions, an additive contribution may be derived that can be used to estimate the bond BDE of polysubstituted phenols for which experimental data are lacking (Wright *et al.*, 1997; Wright *et al.*, 2001).

As a fundamental chemical parameter (Borges dos Santos and Simoes, 1998), there have been several types of theoretical methods to estimate O-H BDE (Chipman *et al.*, 1994). The first is through the additive rule (Wright *et al.*, 2001). Although this is convenient to estimate the O-H BDEs for monophenols (Brigati *et al.*, 2002; Lucarini *et al.*, 1996), it has not been demonstrated as generally effective for catechols (Zhang *et al.*, 2003a). The second is through semi-empirical quantum chemical calculations by means of intermediate neglect of differential overlap (INDO) (Pople *et al.*, 1968), modified neglect of diatomic overlap (MNDO) (Dewar and Thiel, 1977), the Austin Model 1 (AM1) (Dewar *et al.*, 1985), and the parameterization method 3 (PM3) (Stewart, 1989). The third is through density functional theory (DFT) (Qin and Wheeler, 1995; Ziegler, 1991) or *ab initio* molecular dynamics (Bakalbassis *et al.*, 2001; Car, 2002) calculations.

The parameterization method 3 (PM3) uses nearly the same equations as the AM1 method along with an improved set of parameters. PM3 predicts energies and bond lengths more accurately than AM1 (Yong, 2001). Several computer programs, such as Gaussian, Hyperchem, and MOPAC have been developed based on these theories. All these programs can be employed to perform the calculation of BDEs. In this chapter, in order to investigate the cytoprotective mechanism, the BDEs of selected flavonoids were calculated using the PM3 method using the MOPAC2002 program through Chem3D Ultra 2008 (http://www.camsoft.com/). In this chapter, the difference (ΔH_f) between the heat of formation of a parent molecule (H_{fp}) and that of its phenoxyl radical (H_{fr}) is used to represent the BDE. As stated above, the heat of formation of the H atom (H_{fh}) is treated as a constant in order to simplify the calculations (Zhang, 1998; Zhang *et al.*, 1999) and can be ignored. Thus, BDE can be expressed:

$$BDE \approx \Delta H_f = H_{fr} - H_{fp} \qquad [4]$$

Therefore, ΔH_f was used in this chapter to approximate BDE and these two terms are interchangeable.

Lipophilicity (Log P)

Lipophilicity of compounds of bioactive interest is an important parameter in the understanding of transport processes across biological barriers (Lipinski *et al.*, 1997). The lipophilic behaviour of an antioxidant is determined by its partition between phases differing in polarity. The forces of interaction between molecules that result from attraction of different functional groups can lead to different partition behaviour (Schwarz *et al.*, 1996). It is possible to quantify the degree to which an antioxidant's action is moderated by its ability to enter the locus of autoxidation (Castle and Perkins, 1986; Porter *et al.*, 1989). Uptake of most organic chemicals to the site of action is by passive diffusion and is best modelled by lipophilicity (MacFarland, 1970). Lipophilicity characterizes the tendency of molecules (or parts of molecules) to escape contact with water and to move into a lipophilic environment.

Since Hansch *et al.* (Hansch *et al.*, 1968) recognized that the partition coefficient of a molecule in the n-octanol/water solvent system mimics molecule transport across biological membranes, the basic quantity to measure lipophilicity has been the logarithm of the partition coefficient, log P. The partition coefficient (P) is defined according to the Nernst Partition Law as the ratio of the equilibrium concentrations (C) of a dissolved substance in a two-phase system consisting of two largely-immiscible solvents, e.g. *n*-octanol and water (Eadsforth and

Moser, 1983). The partition coefficient is therefore dimensionless, being the quotient of two concentrations, and it is customary to express them in logarithmic form to base ten, i.e., as log P because P values commonly range over many orders of magnitude (Fujita *et al.*, 1964). The logarithm of the partition coefficient, log P, has been successfully used as a hydrophobic parameter (Leo, 1991).

Pioneering work by Leo and Hansch (Leo *et al.*, 1971) has led to the use of log P in quantitative structure-activity relation methods (QSAR), as a general description of cell permeability. In the field of drug development, log P has become a standard property determined for potential drug molecules (Lipinski *et al.*, 1997). The lipophilicity of the flavonoids is an important parameter in chemical toxicology as it can indicate metabolic fate, biological transport properties and intrinsic biological activity (Hansch *et al.*, 2000). Lipophilicity is of central importance for biological potency as it plays a role in the interaction of flavonoids with many of the targets in a biological system. Log P probably can be considered the most informative and successful physicochemical property in biochemistry and medicinal chemistry (Leo, 1991). Since log P is an additive, constitutive molecular property, it is possible to estimate the log P value of a molecule from the sum of its component molecular fragment values (Masuda *et al.*, 1997). Many programs developed to do this are based on substructure approaches such as ClogP (Leo, 1991; Leo, 1993), KOWWIN (Meylan and Howard, 1995), AB/LogP (Japertas et al., 2002), ACD/LogP (Buchwald and Bodor, 1998; Osterberg and Norinder, 2001), and KLOGP (Klopman and Zhu, 2001). The substructure methods usually require a long calculation time because a large number of structural parameters need to be taken into account (Mannhold and Petrauskas, 2003). An alternative approach for the computation of log P is based on additive atomic contributions. The Ghose-Crippen approach is the most widely used atom-based method (Ghose and Crippen, 1987). The parameters used in the calculation of log P can be obtained by first classifying atoms into different types according to their topological environments, which contribute differently to the global log P value. Several computer programs are developed based on atomic contribution techniques such as XLOG P (Wang *et al.*, 1997) and SMILOGP (Convard *et al.*, 1994). Since the whole is more than the sum of its parts, any method of calculating log P of a molecule from its parts has limitations. Thus, other methods have been proposed based on calculated molecular properties. Fewer programs are based on a whole-molecule approach compared with a substructure approach. The most widely available one is SciLogP Ultra (Bodor *et al.*, 1989). From a theoretical perspective, it is difficult to judge the validity of any particular method since it depends on the methodology used in data analysis and algorithm derivation.

Health Effects of Flavonoids

One of the most widely publicized properties of flavonoids is their capability to scavenge reactive oxygen species (ROS). Although this has been known for some time, flavonoids are gaining more and more attention because of the impact of ROS on human (Guarnieri *et al.*, 2007) and plant metabolism and physiology (Reddy *et al.*, 2007). ROS such as singlet oxygen ($^1O_2$), super oxide ($O_2^{\bullet}$), hydrogen peroxide (H_2O_2) and hydroxyl radical ($HO^{\bullet}$) are implicated in membrane function and permeability, in oxidative degradation of proteins and DNA, in oxidation of pigments, in reduction of photosynthetic activity and respiration, and in senescence and cell death (Potapovich and Kostyuk, 2003; Williams *et al.*, 2004). It is well established that the ability that some the flavonoids and stilbenoids exert in inhibiting free-radical mediated events mainly depends on the arrangement of substituents in their structure. Such protective properties, particularly of flavonoids against oxidative stress, have been reported to be structure dependent (Barbouti *et al.*, 2002; Lien *et al.*, 1999; Rastija and Medic-Saric, 2008; Rice-Evans *et al.*, 1996; Zhang *et al.*, 2008; Zhang *et al.*, 2006a). The biochemical activities of flavonoids and their metabolites depend on their chemical structure and relative orientation of various moieties attached to the molecule. For a flavonoid to be defined as an antioxidant it should meet two basic criteria: first, when present in low concentrations, related to the substrate to be oxidized, it can delay, retard, or prevent the oxidation process (Halliwell, 1990); second, the resulting radical formed after scavenging should be stable (Shahidi and Wanasundara, 1992).

Usually inflammation is part of an immune response caused by bacterial infection, injury, trauma or UV light irradiation. As such, it is a necessary reaction of the body for protection from bacterial infection and to facilitate wound healing. Chronic inflammation on the other hand is associated with several degenerative diseases such as arthritis, atherosclerosis, heart disease, Alzheimer's disease and cancer (Brod, 2000; Kumazawa *et al.*, 2006; O'Byrne and Dalgleish, 2001). Formation of ROS and subsequent activation of the transcription factor nuclear factor-κB (NF-κB) plays a key role in triggering inflammation (Schreck *et al.*, 1991). Many of the naturally occurring anti-inflammatory substances are also antioxidants and/or inhibitors of the NF-κB signaling pathway. As mentioned previously, since most flavonoids are quickly metabolized to less potent antioxidants, their main mode of action may rather be their influence on cell signaling than their antioxidant properties (Williams *et al.*, 2004).

It is likely that the polyphenols that are the most common in the human diet are not necessarily the most active within the body, either because they have a lower intrinsic activity or because they are poorly absorbed from the intestine, highly metabolized, or rapidly eliminated. During metabolism, hydroxyl groups of flavonoids are added, methylated, sulphated or glucuronidated. In addition, the metabolites that are found in blood and target organs and that result from digestive or hepatic activity may differ from the native substances in terms of biological activity. Extensive knowledge of the bioavailability of polyphenols is thus essential if their health effects are to be understood. Metabolism of polyphenols occurs via a common pathway (Scalbert and Williamson, 2000). The aglycones can be absorbed from the small intestine. However, most polyphenols are present in food in the form of esters, glycosides, or polymers that cannot be absorbed in their native form. These compounds must be hydrolyzed by intestinal enzymes or by the colonic microflora before they can be absorbed. When the flora are involved, the efficiency of absorption is often reduced because the flora also degrade the aglycones that they release and produce various simple aromatic acids in the process.

During the course of absorption, polyphenols are conjugated in the small intestine and later in the liver. This process mainly includes methylation, sulphation, and glucuronidation (Spencer *et al.*, 2004; Spencer *et al.*, 2003). This is a metabolic detoxication process common to many xenobiotics that restricts their potential toxic effects and facilitates their biliary and urinary elimination by increasing their lipophilicity. The conjugation mechanisms are highly efficient, and aglycones are generally either absent in blood or present in low concentrations after consumption of nutritional doses. Circulating flavonoids are conjugated derivatives that are extensively bound to albumin. Flavonoids are able to penetrate tissues, particularly those in which they are metabolized, but their ability to accumulate within specific target tissues needs to be further investigated. Flavonoids and their derivatives are eliminated chiefly in urine and/or bile, and are secreted via the biliary route into the duodenum, where they are subjected to the action of bacterial enzymes, especially ß-glucuronidase, in the distal segments of the intestine, after which they may be reabsorbed. This enterohepatic recycling may lead to a longer presence of polyphenols within the body.

Anthocyanins can be absorbed intact as glycosides. The mechanism of absorption is not clear. However, it has been found that anthocyanins can serve as ligands for bilitranslocase, an organic anion membrane carrier found in the epithelial cells of gastric mucosa (Passamonti *et al.*, 2002). This finding suggested that bilitranslocase could play a role in the bioavailability of anthocyanins. Considering the physiological implications, the interaction of anthocyanins with bilitranslocase suggests that, at the gastric level, it could promote the transport of these compounds from the lumen into the epithelial layers of the gastric mucosa, thus favoring their transfer to the portal blood, and then, at the hepatic level, from the portal blood into the liver cell. At this level, anthocyanins could also be transported by other organic anion carriers.

It has been reported that procyanidin dimmer (B2), epicatechin, and catechin were detected in the plasma of human subjects as early as 30 min (16, 2.61, 0.13 μM, respectively) after acute cococa consumption and reached maximal concentrations by 2 h (41, 5.92, and 0.16 μM, respectively) (Holt *et al.* 2002).

CYTOPROTECTION ASSAY

Oxidative stress refers to the cytopathological consequences of an imbalance between the production of free radicals and the ability of the cell to neutralize them. Reactive oxygen species (ROS) have been suggested to be a major cause of neurodegenerative disorders, such as Alzheimer's disease, Parkinson's disease and Huntington's disease (Simonian and Coyle, 1996). Hydrogen peroxide (H_2O_2) can traverse membranes and exerts cytotoxic effects on cells in the proximity of those responsible for its production (Halliwell, 1992). Although H_2O_2 is not a free radical and has a limited reactivity, it is thought to be the major precursor of the highly reactive hydroxyl radical ($HO^{\bullet}$). Recent studies have shown a close association between H_2O_2 and neurodegenerative disease, and it has been suggested that H_2O_2 levels are increased during pathological conditions such as ischemia (Behl *et al.*, 1994; Hyslop *et al.*, 1995).

ROS such as H_2O_2 and $HO^{\bullet}$ readily damage biological molecules that can eventually lead to apoptotic or necrotic cell death (Gardner *et al.*, 1997). Exposure of cells to oxidative stress induces a range of cellular events that can result in apoptosis or necrosis (Davies, 1999). Apoptotic cells can be evaluated based on the measurement of the loss of plasma membrane asymmetry (van Engeland *et al.*, 1998). Under normal physiological conditions, a cell maintains a strictly asymmetric distribution of phospholipids in the two leaflets of the cellular membranes with phosphatidylserine (PS) facing the cytosolic side (Devaux, 1991). However, during early apoptosis this membrane asymmetry is rapidly lost without concomitant loss of membrane integrity (van Engeland *et al.*, 1998). Cell surface exposure of PS, which precedes the loss of membrane integrity, can be detected by fluorescein isothiocyanate (FITC)-labelled annexin V, a reagent that has high affinity for PS residues in the presence of millimolar concentrations of calcium (Ca^{2+}) (Andree *et al.*, 1990). By simultaneous probing of membrane integrity by means of exclusion of the nuclear dye propidium iodide (PI), apoptotic cells can be discriminated from necrotic cells (Darzynkiewicz *et al.*, 1997). The importance of apoptosis in the regulation of cellular homeostasis has mandated the development of accurate assays capable of measuring this process. Apoptosis assays based on flow cytometry have proven particularly useful; they are rapid, quantitative, and provide an individual cell-based mode of analysis (rather than a bulk population).

In this chapter, the relationship between physicochemical properties, chemical structures and cytoprotective capacity of twenty-four different flavonoids was established using human colon adenocarcinoma (HT-29) cells.

Materials and Methods

Materials

4-[3-(4-iodophenyl)-2-(4-nitrophenyl)-2H-5-tetrazolio]-1, 3-benzene disulphonate (WST-1 reagent) was obtained from Roche (Basel, Switzerland). Hydrogen peroxide was obtained from BDH Chemicals (Poole, England). Annexin V-FITC and binding buffer were obtained from BD Biosciences (San Diego, CA). All other chemicals were obtained from Sigma (St. Louis, MO). All solvents were of HPLC grade. Deionized water (MilliQ) was used in all experiments. All cell culture media were obtained from Invitrogen-Life Technologies (Carlsbad, CA). Cultured human colon adenocarcinoma HT-29) were obtained from the ATCC (American Type Culture Collection; Manassas, VA).

Assessment of Cell Viability

Cell viability was assessed using the WST-1 assay. The WST-1 assay is based on the cleavage of the tetrazolium salt WST-1 by mitochondrial dehydrogenases to form dark red formazan, which absorbs at 450 nm. Cultured human cells were seeded in 96-well plates (in 0.1 ml medium) at a density of 5×10^5 cells/ml with various concentrations (0.25-20 μM) of testing compounds. Tested compounds were either dissolved in DMSO or deionised water depending on their solubility (the amount of DMSO in cell culture was limited to 0.1%). Equivalent amounts of the DMSO vehicle had no effect compared with results in control cells. After 24 h of incubation in a humidified 5% CO_2, 95% air atmosphere at 37°C, 10 μl WST-1 tetrazolium salt was added to each well and the cells were incubated for 2 h to allow the reaction between the mitochondrial dehydrogenase released from viable cells and the tetrazolium salt of the WST-1 reagent.

The absorbance was measured at 450 nm with a reference at 690 nm using a microplate reader (Synergy HT, BioTEK Instruments, Winooski, VT). The level of absorbance directly correlates to viable cell numbers. Each assay was performed in triplicate and the cell viability was expressed as a percentage of the absorbance of cells exposed to test samples compared with that of controls (cells only).

Culture and Treatment of HT-29 Cells

HT-29 cells were grown in McCoy's 5A medium (modified) supplemented with 10% fetal bovine serum (FBS) in the presence of 100 U/ml penicillin and 0.1 g/l streptomycin at 37°C in humidified air with 5% CO2. Cultured HT-29 cells were plated in 24-well plates at a density of 5 × 10^5 cells/ml. A range of non-toxic concentrations (0-20 μM) of testing compounds were added together with 150 μM H_2O_2. Cells were incubated for 24 h at 37°C in humidified air with 5% CO2.

Annexin V Staining and Flow Cytometric Analysis

Annexin V coupled with fluorescein isothiocyanate (FITC) is typically used in conjunction with a vital dye such as propidium iodide (PI) to identify different stages of apoptotic and necrotic cells using flow cytometry. This assay was performed according to the method described by Vermes and co-workers (Vermes *et al.*, 2000) with slight modifications. After 24 h of incubation, cells were harvested and stained with both annexin V and propidium iodide to identify different stages of apoptotic and necrotic cell death using flow cytometry.

Briefly, the washed cells were resuspended in 100 μl of 1X binding buffer containing Annexin V-FITC (5 μl per test according to the manufacturer's instruction) and incubated in the dark for 20 min. Then, another 400 μl binding buffer containing PI (5 μl per test from 1 mg/ml stock solution) was added and incubated for a further 10 min. Flow cytometric analysis was performed within 1 h using a Cytomics FC500 MPL (Beckman Coulter, Miami, FL). The total cell count was set to 35,000 cells per sample.

Calculation of Results

Cell Death Index (CDI)

The percentages of viable, early, late apoptotic and necrotic cells were determined as illustrated in the cytogram (Figure 3).

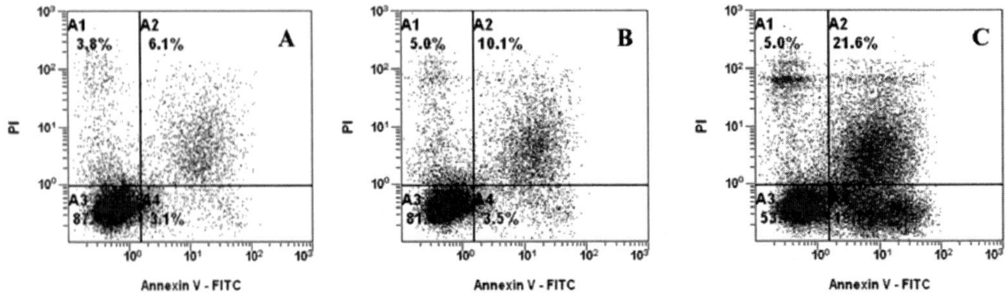

Figure 3. Cytograms of control (prior to incubation) (A), incubated control (B) and 150 μM H_2O_2 treated (C) human colon adenocarcinoma (HT-29) cells.

The viable cells are located in the lower left corner (negative in both annexin V-FITC and propidium iodide) (A3). Early apoptotic cells are in the lower right corner (annexin V-FITC positive only) (A4). Late apoptotic cells that show progressive cellular membrane and nuclear damage are in the upper right corner (both annexin V-FITC and PI positive) (A2). Necrotic cells are located in the upper left corner (PI positive only) (A1). The total percentage of damaged cells (both apoptotic and necrotic) was considered as (A1+A2+A4). The cell death index (CDI) was calculated based on the cytogram by the following equation (equation 1):

$$\mathrm{CDI} = \frac{(\mathrm{A1+A2+A4})}{\mathrm{A3}} \times 100 \qquad (5)$$

The CDI is the ratio of total damaged cells to viable cells and is used to remove inter-experimental variations in cell density. The net cell damage ($\Delta\mathrm{CDI}$) is derived by subtracting the CDI of incubated control cells (Figure 3B) from that of treated cells (Figure 3C) (equation 4-2).

$$\Delta\mathrm{CDI} = (\mathrm{CDI}_{\mathrm{Treated\ cells}} - \mathrm{CDI}_{\mathrm{Incubated\ control\ cells}}) \qquad (6)$$

Calculation of 50% Reduction in Cell Death (EC_{50})

The cytoprotective effects of test compounds were measured by the inhibition of the cytotoxic effects of H_2O_2 using both apoptosis and necrosis endpoints (approximately causing 50% total cell death). The percentage of inhibition of cell death was calculated by equation 7:

$$\%\ \text{Inhibition of cell death} = \frac{\Delta\mathrm{CDI}_{\mathrm{HP}} - \Delta\mathrm{CDI}_{\mathrm{Sample}}}{\Delta\mathrm{CDI}_{\mathrm{HP}}} \times 100 \qquad (7)$$

where $\Delta\mathrm{CDI}_{\mathrm{HP}}$ and $\Delta\mathrm{CDI}_{\mathrm{Sample}}$ are the net cell damage caused by H_2O_2 and test sample, respectively. The EC_{50} values were calculated from the dose-response relationship between the concentrations of antioxidant and % inhibition of cell death.

Quantum Chemical Calculations

Calculation of Heat of Formation

All geometry calculations of flavonoid were performed by using PM3 of the MOPAC2002 molecular package through Chem3D Ultra 2008 interface. The procedures were as follows. The molecular geometries were optimized by MM2 and then by the semiempirical quantum chemical method (PM3), and energies were minimized by using the EF algorithm. After the calculation of the heat of formation of the parent molecules (H_{fp}), the phenolic H was removed to get its free radical and a restricted Hartree-Fock optimization was performed on the phenoxyl radical. The differences in heat of formation was calculated by calculated by $\Delta H_f = H_{fr} - H_{fp}$.

Calculation of Log P

The log P of flavonoids was obtained by using ClogP in the Chem3D Ultra 2008 molecular package.

Results And Discussion

Cytotoxic Effects of H_2O_2

Hydrogen peroxide is known to be able to induce both apoptosis and necrosis in cells (Antunes and Cadenas, 2001; Barbouti *et al.*, 2002; Kim *et al.*, 2000), with the required concentrations and exposure time dependent on the cell type being investigated. The response of cultured human cells to H_2O_2 in terms of both concentration and exposure time was determined to calculate the dosage required to kill approximately half the cells. The CDI increased with increasing concentrations of H_2O_2 on HT-29 cells (Figure 4).

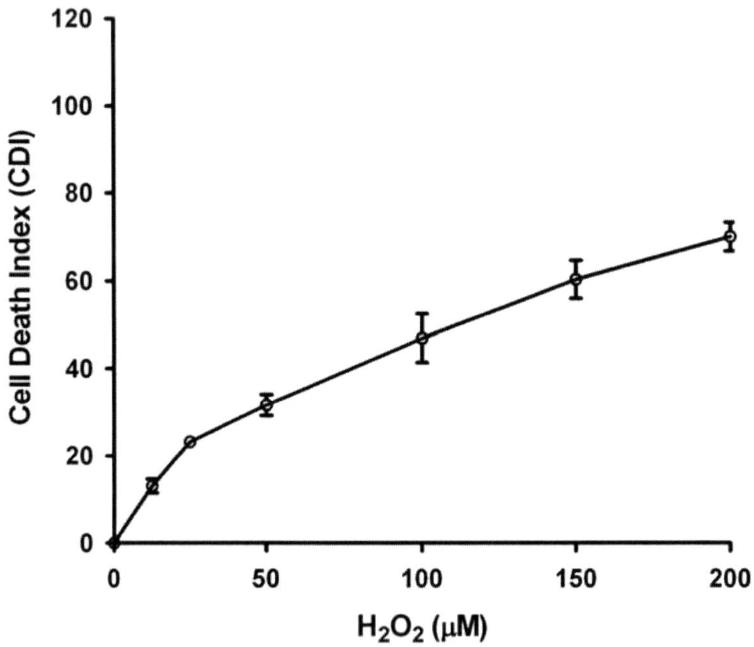

Figure 4. Cell death responses of cultured human HT-29 cells exposed to increasing concentrations of hydrogen peroxide (H_2O_2). HT-29 cells (5 x 10^5 cells per ml) were exposed to different concentrations of H_2O_2 and incubated at 37°C in humidified air with 5% CO_2 for 24 h. Bars indicate standard deviation from the mean of two separate determinations.

A concentration of 150 μM H_2O_2 was selected for the cytoprotection assay using HT-29 cells (CDI of 63.5 ± 2.7) with a 24-hour exposure to H_2O_2. These conditions were used in this assay to investigate the protective effects of antioxidants against H_2O_2-induced total cell death. Although H_2O_2 itself is a relatively unreactive species and easily scavenged by cellular catalase (Gille and Joenje, 1992), it can cause membrane damage by increasing the release of arachidonic acid from the cell membrane, which may account for the prolonged damage caused by H_2O_2 even after being scavenged (Cantoni *et al.*, 1989). Thus, even at low concentrations, H_2O_2 can cause damage to cultured cells. These facts demonstrate that the cytoprotection assay can be used to screen for and compare the protective effects of flavonoids in a biologically relevant cellular environment.

Cytotoxicity of Flavonoids

The cytotoxicities of Trolox, catechol, pyrogallol and selected flavonoids were tested on cultured human HT-29 cells at different concentrations for 24 h using the WST-1 assay (data not shown). None of the compounds tested affected the viability of HT-29 cells within the concentration range used (0–20.0 μM) in this study.

The Influence of Trolox on Cytotoxic Effects of H_2O_2

As described above, Trolox is a common compound used as a standard for most antioxidant assays. Trolox was co-incubated with cultured HT-29 cells at doses of 0, 0.25, 0.5, 1.0, 5.0, 10.0, 20.0 μM immediately prior to the addition of the H_2O_2. Trolox protected HT-29 cells against H_2O_2-induced cell death in a dose dependent manner (Figure 5).

The EC_{50} value (7.91 ± 0.22 μM) of Trolox was calculated from its dose-response curve. Trolox could thus be used as a standard antioxidant in this cytoprotection assay for comparison with other antioxidant compounds.

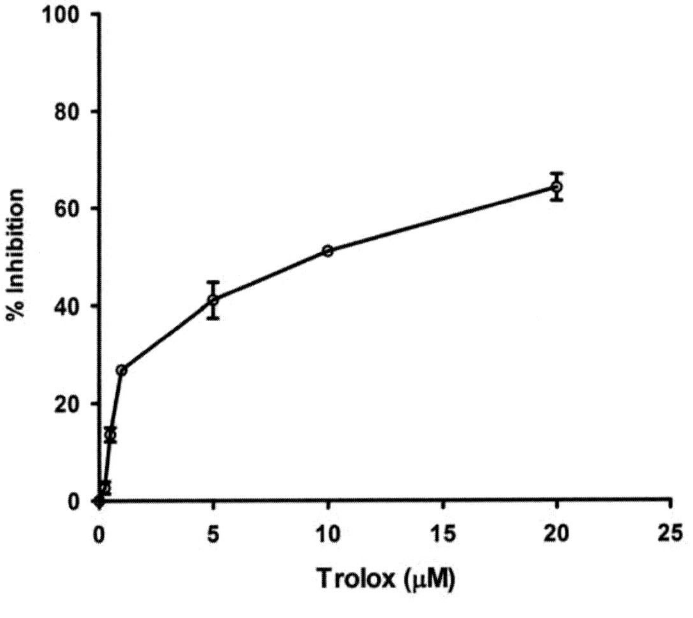

Figure 5. The concentration-response curve of Trolox for protection of HT-29 cells from 150 μM hydrogen peroxide. HT-29 cells (5 x 10^5 cells per well) were incubated at 37°C in humidified air with 5% CO_2 for 24 h. After incubation, cells were stained with both Annexin V-FITC and PI and analyzed by flow cytometry. Bars indicate standard deviation from the mean of two separate determinations.

Structural Related Cytoprotective Activity of Flavonoids

In the present Chapter, the cytoprotective activities (EC_{50}) of a range of structurally diverse flavonoids were measured (Table 1). Structural variations within the rings subdivide the flavonoids into several families (Figure 2). Measurement of the potential health effects of dietary-derived phenolic compounds needs to be undertaken at concentration ranges that are relevant to levels that might be achieved *in vivo*. Maximum plasma concentrations attained after a polyphenol-rich meal are thought to be in the range of 0.1–10 μM (Kroon *et al.*, 2004). In this work gut-derived cells were used but general bioavailability was taken into account. Hence, the 24 flavonoids, catechol and pyrogallol were added to HT-29 cells at doses of 0, 0.25, 0.5, 1.0, 5.0, 10.0, 20.0 μM immediately prior to the addition of the H_2O_2.

Table 1. Calculated differences of heat of formation (ΔH_f) between the parent flavonoid, catechol, and pyrogallol and each possible corresponding relative radical, the lipophilities (log P) and their cytoprotective activities

Compounds	EC_{50}	Least OH	3-OH	3'-OH	4'-OH	5'-OH	Log P
	(μM)	ΔH_f (KJ/mol)	ΔH_f (KJ/mol)	ΔH_f (KJ/mol)	ΔH_f (KJ/mol)	ΔH_f (KJ/mol)	
Chrysin	15.42 ± 1.99	162.83					3.56
Apigenin	12.87 ± 0.94	149.84			149.84		2.91
Luteolin	4.05 ± 0.48	127.03		127.03	137.14		2.31
Galangin	16.64 ± 2.30	167.08	105.67				2.76
Kaempferol	10.98 ± 1.17	154.25	104.87		154.25		2.10
Quercetin	2.11 ± 0.40	125.80	103.06	125.80	138.53		1.50
Isoquercetin	2.72 ± 0.50	110.17		124.61	110.17		-0.34
Rutin	4.14 ± 0.40	109.91		109.91	137.32		-2.68
Morin	9.98 ± 1.07	154.18	104.29	154.18		158.51	1.43
Myricetin	4.47 ± 0.53	123.43	104.06	133.34	123.43	140.68	0.84
Naringenin	12.27 ± 0.87	149.91			149.91		2.44
Naringin	16.50 ± 2.25	158.11			158.11		-0.09
Hesperitin	6.86 ± 0.69	135.31		135.31			2.29
Hesperidin	7.73 ± 1.29	124.38		124.38			-0.29
Taxifolin	4.79 ± 0.22	124.86	210.59	139.16	124.86		0.77
Catechin	5.01 ± 0.47	123.12	211.65	124.65	123.12		0.53
Phloretin	7.26 ± 0.71	141.91	163.29		141.91		2.22
Phloridzin	9.57 ± 1.00	137.90	159.37		137.90		0.79
Cyanidin	5.48 ± 0.53	144.49		144.49	159.40		1.76
Idaein	6.36 ± 0.87	143.06		143.06	159.64		0.19
Keracyanin	9.63 ± 1.81	144.67	157.04	144.67	165.47		-0.84
Delphinidin	8.33 ± 0.98	140.03		146.39	140.03	158.62	1.10
Callistephin	18.69 ± 1.52	184.06	151.50		184.06		0.78
Pelargonidin	17.95 ± 2.11	182.16			182.16		2.36
Catechol	6.61 ± 0.78	126.93		126.93	126.93		0.88
Pyrogallol	3.22 ± 0.25	119.87		137.26	119.87	125.70	0.21

Notes: Structural optimization of each flavonoid and its radical was determined by calculating the minimum energy conformation by the MM2 method. MOPAC2002 in Chem3D Ultra was used to determine the final minimum energy conformation of the flavonoids and was calculated by applying the semi-empirical Hamiltonian PM3 calculation to obtain the final heat of formation of each compound. The lowest ΔH_f of chrysin and galangin were obtained from their hydroxyl groups in the A ring. All other flavonoids were calculated from their B ring hydroxyl groups.

Effects of Hydroxyl Groups in the B Ring

The manipulation of the hydroxyl substitutions in the B-ring in flavones (with the 2,3-double bond and 4-keto function in the C-ring, but no 3-OH group) allows the observation of the contribution of these hydroxyl groups to their cytoprotective activities. With the 3′,4′-dihydroxyl group, the EC_{50} value of luteolin is 4.05 μM. Dehydroxylation at the 3′-position as in apigenin increases the value to 12.87 μM, making the cytoprotective activity of apigenin only one-third of luteolin (Figure 6). The EC_{50} value of chrysin is further increased because of the lack of any hydroxyl group in its B-ring. The cytoprotective activity of chrysin can be reasonably attributed to the 5,7-*meta*-dihydroxyl groups of its A-ring.

As a group of flavonols, galangin, quercetin, morin and myricetin have the same structures on the A and C-rings but the number of hydroxyl groups in the B-ring increases from zero to three (Figure 7).

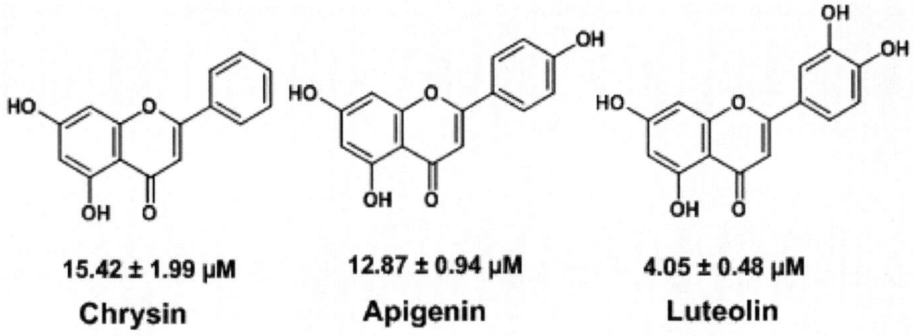

Figure 6. The influences of hydroxylation in the B ring on the cytoprotective activity of the flavones.

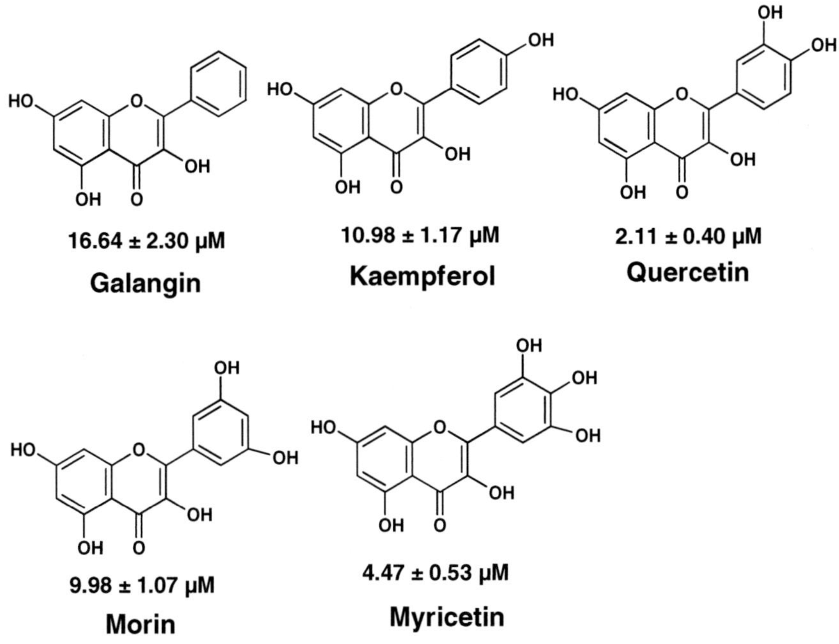

Figure 7. The influences of hydroxylation in the B ring on the cytoprotective activity of the flavanols.

As the number of hydroxyl groups increases the EC_{50} value decreases except for quercetin, which is more active than myricetin. With morin, the dihydroxyl groups in the B-ring are arranged *meta* to each other. This significantly reduces its cytoprotective activity compared with quercetin (the EC_{50} value of morin was four times than that of quercetin). This result confirms that the presence of two adjacent hydroxyl groups in the B-ring plays a significant role in the high cytoprotective activity of flavonoids. Possibly, the two adjacent hydroxyl groups at position 3′ and 4′ in quercetin are more vulnerable to loss of a proton than the two hydroxyl groups at position 3′ and 5′ in morin. Myricetin, which possesses *ortho*-trihydroxyl (pyrogallol) groups in the B-ring, is much less active than quercetin. This suggests that the additional 5′-hydroxyl group has a negative impact on its cytoprotective activity. However, the cytoprotective activity of pyrogallol is much more active than that of catechol as illustrated in Figure 8. This may be the result of the rest of the quercetin structure (C- and A-rings) stabilizing the oxidation product (*o*-quninoe) as shown in Figure 9.

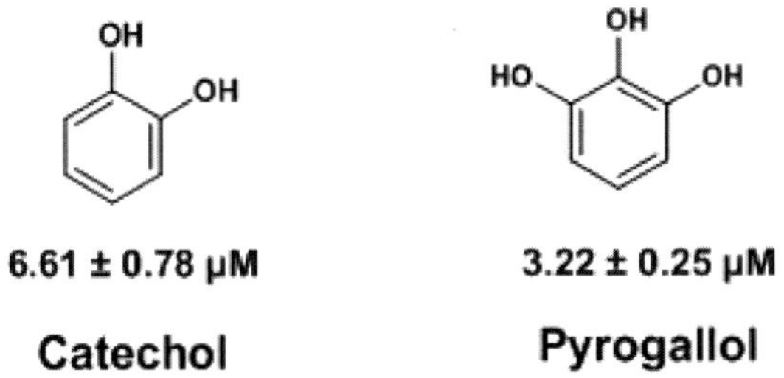

Figure 8. The cytoprotective activity of catechol and pyrogallol.

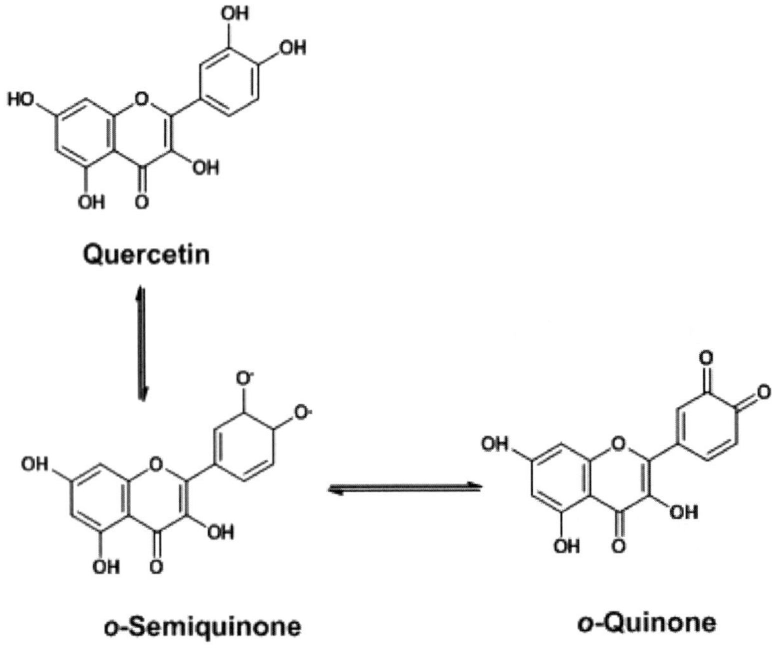

Figure 9. Quercetin oxidation and its possible consequences.

A fairly stable *ortho*-semiquinone radical can be formed by oxidation of a flavonoid on the B ring, when the 3′4′-catechol structure is present facilitating electron delocalization (Arora *et al.*, 1998; Mora *et al.*, 1990). The formation of flavonoid aroxyl radicals is an essential step after initial scavenging of an oxidizing radical (Bors *et al.*, 1990). The stability of aroxyl radicals strongly depends on their bimolecular disproportionation reaction and electron delocalization. For instance the oxidation of quercetin can form an *o*-semiquinone radical and then an *o*-quinone radical (Awad *et al.*, 2001; Awad *et al.*, 2003; Boersma *et al.*, 2000; Metodiewa *et al.*, 1999) as illustrated in Figure 9. However, with only one hydroxyl group in the B-ring the EC_{50} value of kaempferol was significantly increased. Without any hydroxyl substitutions in its B-ring, the cytoprotective activity of galangin was almost negligible like that of chrysin. The flavanone, naringenin, with only a single 4′-OH group in the B-ring has a EC_{50} value twice than that of hesperitin, which has an identical structure to naringenin except for the 3′-OH, 4′-methoxy substitution in the B-ring (Figure 10).

This finding suggested that methoxylation does not destroy cytoprotective activity. Repeated studies have shown that flavonoids having greater numbers of hydroxyl groups, or hydroxyl groups localized *ortho* to one another, are more effective antioxidants. The B-ring of most flavonoids is usually the initial target of oxidants, as it is more electron-rich than the A- and C-rings, whose electron densities are somewhat drained away by the carbonyl group.

These properties are consistent with the expected mechanisms of oxidation of phenols; electron-donating substitutes, such as hydroxyl groups, should lower the oxidation potential for a compound, and *ortho* hydroxylation should stabilize phenoxyl radicals.

The cytoprotective activity pattern of pelargonidin, cyanidin and delphinidin (Figure 11) shows a similar trend to that revealed by kaempferol, quercetin and myricetin (Figure 7). The EC_{50} value of cyanidin is much lower than that of delphinidin, and the cytoprotective activity of pelargonidin, which has a lone 4′-OH, is almost negligible. With the anthocyanin C-ring, the cytoprotective activity of cyanidin is only half of that of quercetin. The same trend also applies to delphinidin and myricetin.

The presence of a third OH group in the B-ring does not enhance the effectiveness against H_2O_2-induced cell death. This is also supported by the findings that myricetin was less active in protecting liposome oxidation (Zhang *et al.*, 2006b).

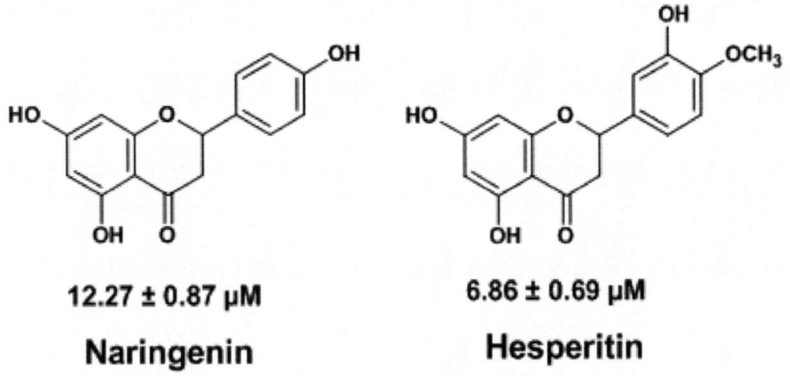

Figure 10. The influences of hydroxylation and methoxylation in the B-ring on the cytoprotective activity of the flavanones.

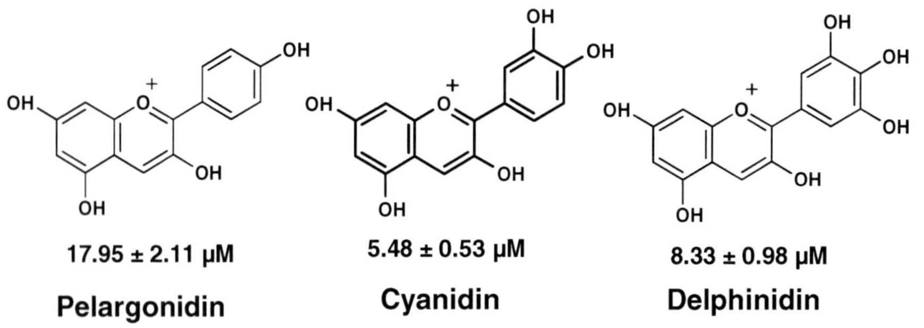

Figure 11. The influences of hydroxylation in the B-ring on the cytoprotective activity of the anthocyanins.

In acidic or neutral media, four anthocyanin structures exist in equilibrium (Figure 12): the flavylium cation, the quinonoidal base, the carbinal pseudobase, and the chalcone (Borkowski *et al.*, 2005; Brouillard, 1983).

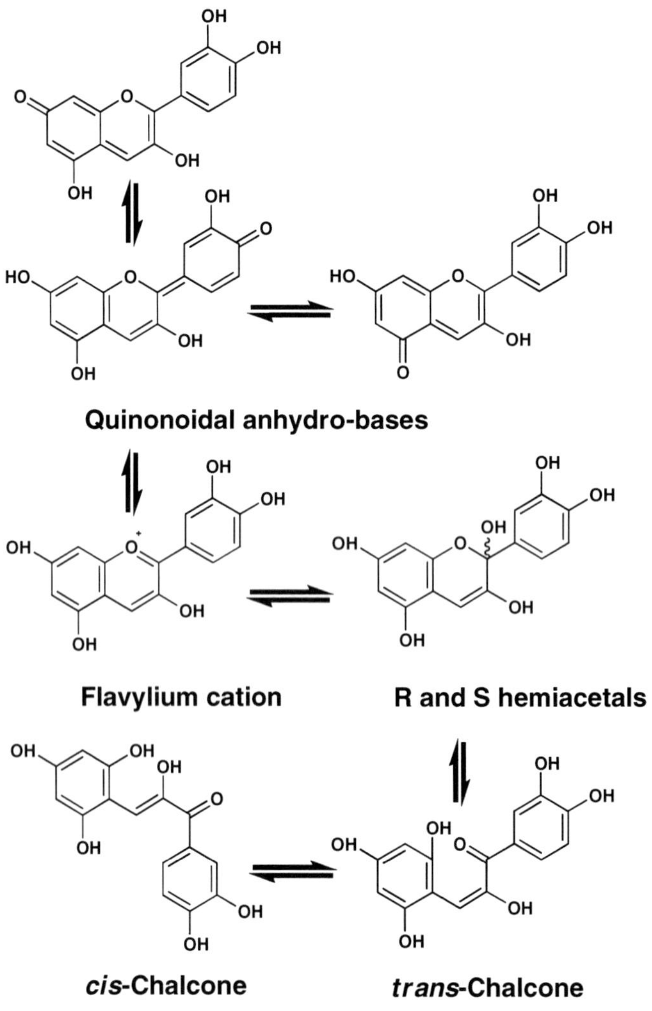

Figure 12. Structural transformations of cyanidin in acidic to alkaline aqueous media.

The equilibrium among the four different structural conformations of anthocyanin is illustrated in Figure 12 (using cyanidin as an example).

At pH less than 2, the anthocyanin exists primarily in the form of the red (with a 3-O-sugar substitute) or yellow (with a 3-OH) flavylium cation. As the pH is raised, there is a rapid proton loss to yield the red or blue quinonoidal forms. At higher pH, hydration of the flavylium cation occurs to give the colorless carbinol or pseudobase. The relative amounts of flavylium cation, quinonoidal forms, pseudobases and chalcones at equilibrium vary with both pH and the structure of the anthocyanin. At pH 3.5-4.5, a mixture of the flavylium ion and the neutral quinonoidal anhydro-base is found. At pH 4.5-6.0, the concentration of the flavylium ion becomes vanishingly small, the quinonoidal anhydro-base increasingly predominates and there is a mixture of both the neutral and the ionized (blue anionic) quinonoidal anhydro-base forms present at pH 7.0 (around neutrality) (Brouillard and Dubois, 1977b). As their quinonoidal anhydro-base or as their flavylium cations, anthocyanins could be strongly stabilized by neutral salts such as magnesium chloride and sodium chloride in concentrated aqueous solutions. The anthocyanidin structural transformation path is very sensitive to the substitution pattern of the pyrilium ring, especially the C_3 position. The 3-OH substituted anthocyanidins are significantly shifted towards colorless pseudobase forms causing color instability (Timberlake and Bridle, 1967). In addition, an increase in the number of hydroxyl groups tends to deepen the color to a more bluish shade. The hydroxyl groups at C_5, C_7 on the A-ring and $C_{4'}$ on the B-ring of the flavylium cation can lose a proton at pH values close to equilibrium.

It must be emphasized that the interpretation of the cytoprotective properties of anthocyanins is complicated by the relatively complex pathway of reversible structural transformations of anthocyanins in aqueous solution (Brouillard and Delaporte, 1977a; Brouillard *et al.*, 1977b), which not only includes proton transfer between coloured forms but also water addition to the pyrylium ring leading to colourless hemiacetal and chalcone forms. Hence, the EC_{50} values of anthocyanins measured here are actually a reflection of the cytoprotective properties of the transformed products, i.e. the quinonoidal anhydro-base (Hoshino, 1991; Hoshino and Goto, 1990; Hoshino *et al.*, 1981).

Effect of the 3-OH Group, 2,3-Double Bond and 4-Keto Group

Without the 3-OH group in the C-ring, the EC_{50} values of apigenin and luteolin are increased compared with those of kaempferol and quercetin, respectively (Figure 13). However, the EC_{50} value is reduced for chrysin compared with that of galangin. The results presented in Figure 13 demonstrate that when the 3-hydroxyl group is absent, its contribution to electron dislocation is substantially reduced and so consequently is the flavonoid cytoprotective activity, although this reduction is smaller when the catechol structure is absent in the B ring. This fact indicated that 3-OH is required to stabilize the catechol structure in the B ring. A distinguishing feature among the flavonoid structural classes is the presence or absence of an unsaturated 2,3-double bond in conjugation with a 4-keto group.

Comparison of naringenin with apigenin shows that the 2,3-double bond in the C-ring has a slightly negative influence on the cytoprotective activity (Figure 13). On the other hand, the introduction of a 2,3-double bound and 4-keto group to catechin with the existing 3-hydroxyl group decreases the EC_{50} value as in quercetin. This fact indicates that the presence of the 3-hydroxyl group is an important factor in neutralizing the negative impact of the 2,3-double bond on the cytoprotective activity. This may also indicate that the combined effect of the

2,3-double bond in the C-ring and the *ortho*-hydroxyl groups in the B-ring have positive effect on cytoprotective activity as demonstrated by the comparison of apigenin and luteolin.

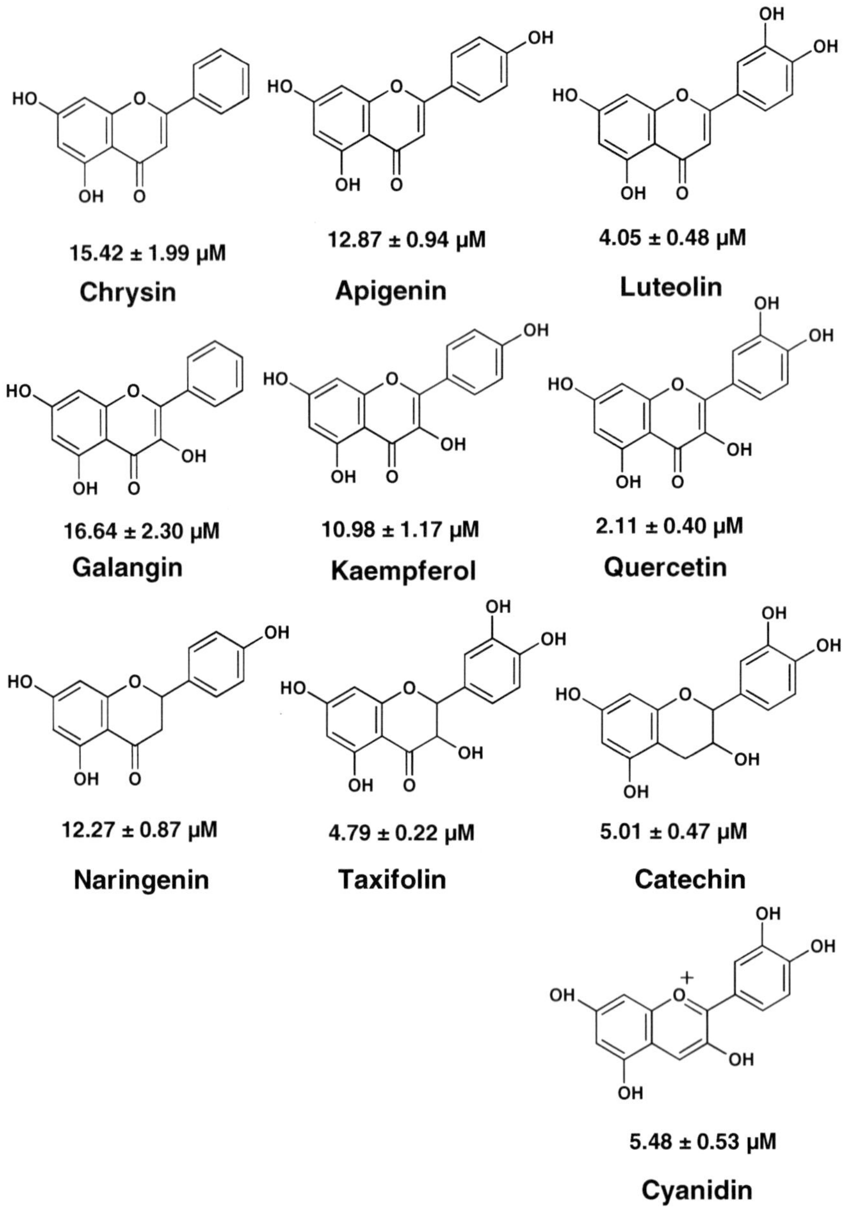

Figure 13. Structure-cytoprotective activity comparisons of the 3-OH, 2,3-double bond and 4-keto group of flavonoids.

However, the presence of a 2,3-double bond when the 3-hydroxyl group is absent (apigenin and luteolin) does not significantly change the cytoprotective activity of flavonoids relative to those that do not contain this double bond (naringenin and taxifolin). When the 3-hydroxyl group is present (quercetin), it significantly enhances cytoprotective activity compared with those that do not contain this double bond (taxifolin). The loss of the 4-keto group at the C-ring and introduction of a positive charge decreases cytoprotective activities as seen in cyanidin and quercetin. As shown in Figure 13, quercetin, catechin and cyanidin have identical A- and B-rings, but quercetin is more than twice as cytoprotective as catechin and cyanidin. This observation indicates the important contribution of the 2,3-double bond and 4-keto group to the cytoprotective activity.

Effect of the Carbohydrate Moieties

Blocking the 3-hydroxyl group in the C-ring of quercetin as a glycoside (while retaining the 3′,4′-dihydroxy structure in the B-ring) as in isoquercetin (quercetin-3-glucoside) decreases the cytoprotective activities. Replacement of the hydroxyl group at the C_3 position of quercetin by the disaccharide rutinose in rutin further decreases cytoprotective activity (Figure 14).

The presence of the 3-OH group on the C-ring double bond undoubtedly contributes to attack by free radicals. If the 3-OH is replaced by an O-sugar group (as in the glycoside rutin or isoquercetin, for example), reactivity is decreased by about a factor of 2-3 (Briviba *et al.*, 1993; Tournaire *et al.*, 1993). The results shown in Figure 14 also indicate that when the 3-hydroxyl group is substituted, the reduction in cytoprotective activity of the flavonoids depends on the nature of the substituted sugar group. This reduction can be smaller when this hydroxyl group is substituted (isoquercetin) than when it is just absent (luteolin).

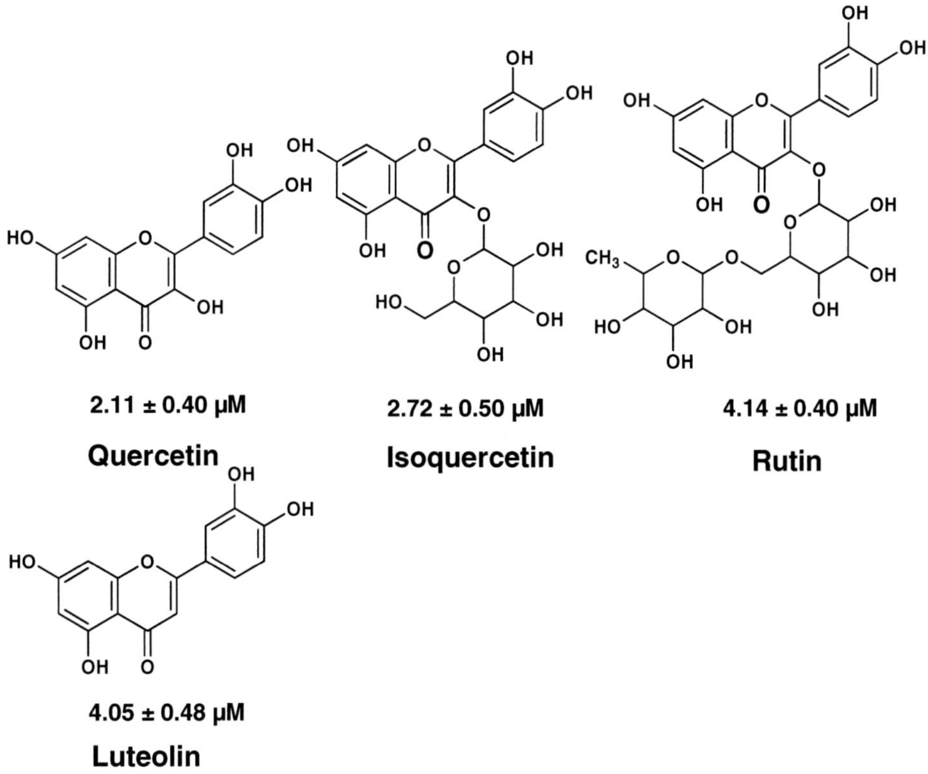

Figure 14. Influences of glycosylation of flavanols on their cytoprotective activity.

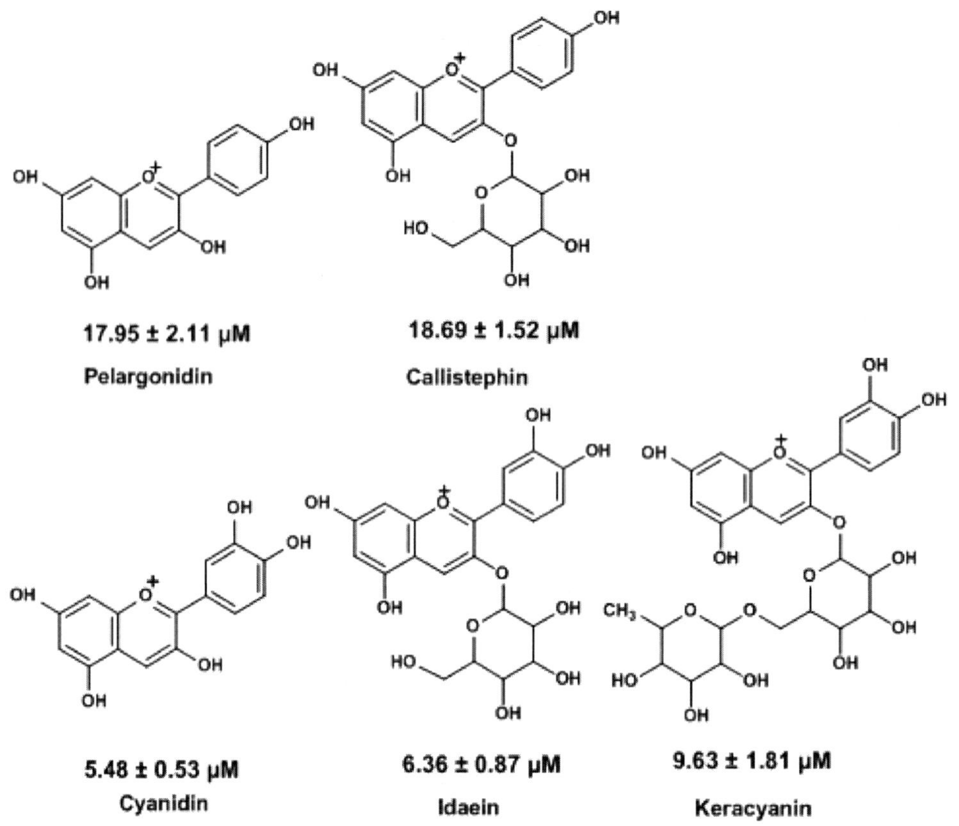

Figure 15. Influences of glycosylation of anthocyandins on their cytoprotective activity.

Similar effects are observed when cyanidin is compared with its 3-glucoside, idaein and its 3-rutinoside, keracyanin, and when pelargonidin is compared with its 3-glucoside, callistephin (Figure 15).

Comparison of naringenin with naringin shows that glycosylation of the 7-hydroxyl group in a structure with a saturated heterocyclic C-ring and with a single hydroxyl group on the B-ring has a significant negative impact on the EC_{50} values. Similar trends are observed with hesperitin when a 4′-hydroxyl group in the B-ring is replaced by a methoxy and 3′-hydroxyl group, in contrast to naringenin, compared with its rhamnoside, hesperidin, which has a glycosylated 7-hydroxyl group. However, hesperidin is much more cytoprotective than that of naringin because of its B-ring configuration (Figure 16).

The results presented in Figure 16 and 17 demonstrate that the presence of both 3- and 5-hydroxyl groups is also necessary to maximize cytoprotective activity of flavonoids.

The sugar moiety is reported to have a negative effect on the oxidizability of flavonoid glycosides (Hedrickson *et al.*, 1994). The oxidation rate of compounds decreased as the substituent at the 3-position became a poorer leaving group. Disaccharides are a poorer leaving group than monosaccharides, thus rutin is less oxidizable than isoquercetin (Hopia and Heinonen, 1999). This observation may explain why rutin displays a lower cytoprotective activity than quercetin and isoquercetin.

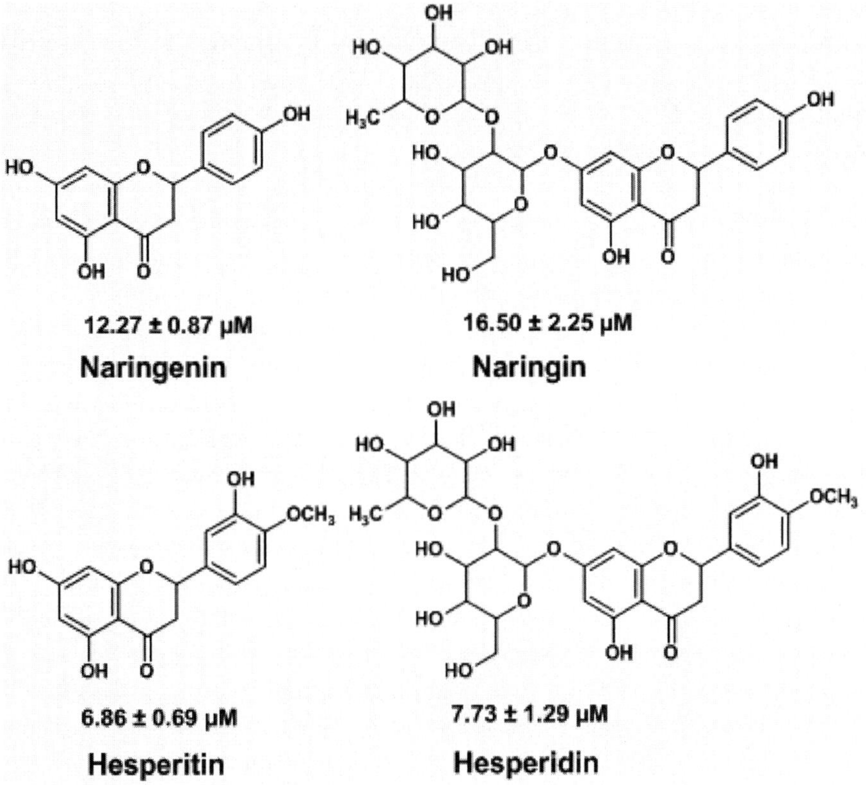

Figure 16. Influences of glycosylation of flavanones on their cytoprotective activity.

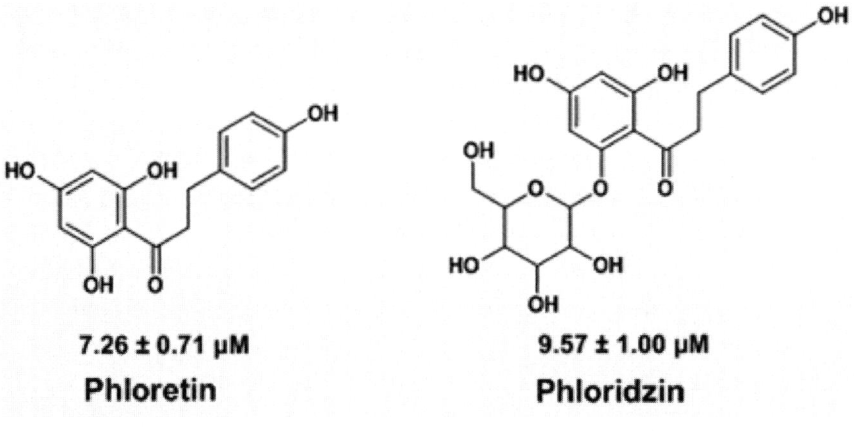

Figure 17. Influences of glycosylation of chalcones on their cytoprotective activity.

The structural criteria for the very high cytoprotective activity by flavonoids can be summarized as: 1) the *o*-dihydroxy (catechol) structure in the B-ring; 2) the 2,3-double bond in conjugation with the 4-keto group in the C-ring; and 3) the 3-hydroxyl group in the C-ring. Thus, quercetin, for example, satisfies all the above-mentioned determinants and has the highest cytoprotective activities among 24 flavonoids tested.

Cytoprotective Activities and Physicochemical Properties of Flavonoids

Correlation between O-H Bond Dissociation Enthalpy (BDE) and Cytoprotective Activity (EC_{50}) of Flavonoids

Possible explanations of the cytoprotective capacity of flavonoids obtained from cell-based assay could be derived by calculating the heat of formation differences (ΔH_f) between radicals and their parent molecules (bond dissociation energy approximation) of flavonoids. Quantum chemical calculations of the geometry of the flavonoids and their corresponding radicals give their heat of formation. The ΔH_f calculated between each flavonoid and its corresponding radicals provides an estimation of the ease with which radicals may be formed (Lien *et al.*, 1999). The ΔH_f of a given compound represents the difference between the parent compound and the appropriate radical, which was constructed by an abstraction of a hydrogen atom from assigned hydroxyl moiety (Zhang, 1998). This value may represent the relative stability of a radical with respect to its parent compound, and it enables a comparison to be made between the stabilization achieved by hydrogen abstraction (toward radical formation) (Sun *et al.*, 2002; Zhang, 1998; Zhang *et al.*, 2002a; Zhang and Wang, 2002b). Generally speaking , the smaller the ΔH_f, the more stable the phenoxyl radical and the weaker the O-H bond in the molecule, so the more active is the flavonoid (van Acker *et al.*, 1993).

A summary of calculated ΔH_f for the H-abstraction from hydroxyl groups (in the B ring and 3-OH) in all the flavonoids tested is shown in Table 1. All heat of formations were calculated or selected by the PM3 semi-empirical method, for energy-optimized species as described in the method section.

The ΔH_f of chrysin and galangin were calculated from the hydroxyl groups in their A-ring because there are no hydroxyl groups in their B-ring. The calculated ΔH_f shows that the least energy required for abstracting a hydrogen atom is from the 3-OH, when the C-ring contains the 2,3-double bond and the 4-keto group (flavonols). In the absence of flavonol structure, the most favored position for donating a hydrogen atom is from the two adjacent hydroxyls in the B-ring, with 3′-OH preferred over 4′-OH. In myricetin and delphinidin, in which 4′-OH is adjacent to two hydroxyl groups (3′-OH and 5′-OH), the donation of a hydrogen atom from 4′-OH is favored over 3′-OH or 5′-OH. The calculated ΔH_f of 5′-OH is larger than that of 3′-OH (Table 1). However, the 3-hydroxyl group is not the determining factor for the cytoprotective activity of flavonoids and this is better demonstrated by galangin, which showed a very weak cytoprotective activity. The ΔH_f of flavonols (galangin, kaempferol, quercetin, morin and myricetin) is almost identical regardless of their cytoprotective activities. Therefore, the least ΔH_f of flavonoids was obtained from their hydroxyl groups in the B ring, and then the A ring.

As shown in previous work, flavonoids with a catechol group in the B ring are the most active free radical scavengers (Zhang *et al.*, 2006b). It appears that the rest of the hydroxyl groups of the flavonoid are of little importance to the antioxidant activity, except for quercetin and its derivatives, in which the combination of the catechol moiety with a 2,3-double bond at the C-ring and a 3-hydroxyl group results in an extremely active scavenger. Therefore, the ΔH_f values were calculated from the O-H bond in the B-ring, and only the most stable phenoxyl radical is considered (lowest ΔH_f) to derive the correlation with the cytoprotective activity of flavonoids (Figure 18).

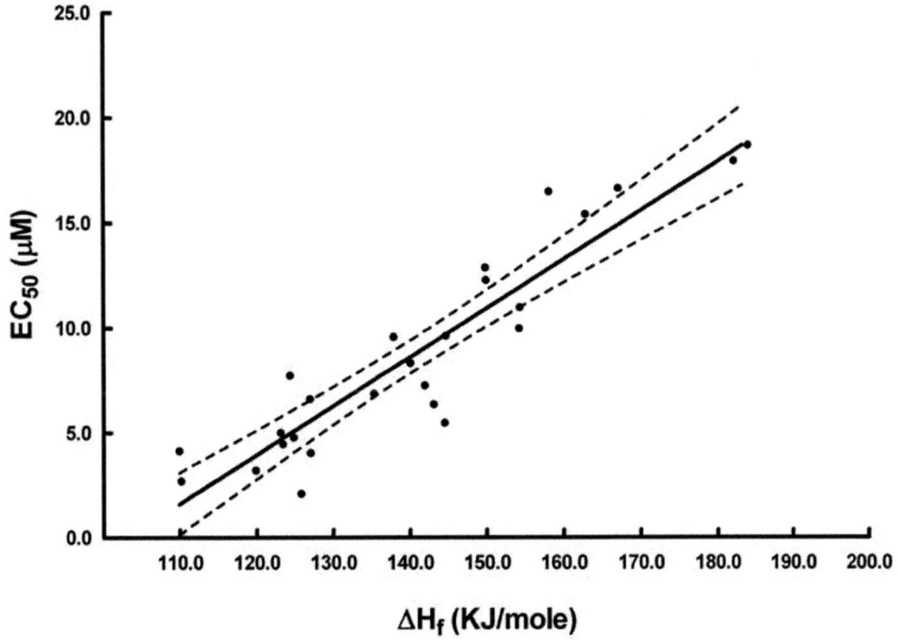

Figure 18. Correlation between EC_{50} (cytoprotective activity of flavonoids) and ΔH_f (the lowest heat of formation of the ArO-H bond of flavonoids from the A- or B-ring hydroxyl group) ($r^2 = 0.85$, n = 26).

As illustrated in Figure 18, a correlation was demonstrated between the calculated ΔH_f (the lowest differences in the enthalpy between each flavonoid's parent compound and its radical) values and the experimentally determined cytoprotective activity of flavonoids. There is a strong linear correlation between the lowest ΔH_f and the EC_{50} values and from the regression analysis a correlation with $r^2 = 0.85$ (n = 26) was obtained for the following equation 8:

$$EC_{50} = 0.23\ (\pm\ 0.02)\ \Delta H_f - 23.97\ (\pm\ 2.81)\ (n = 26) \qquad [8]$$

These findings suggest that a relatively low O-H bond dissociation enthalpy (BDE, approximation by the lowest ΔH_f), which facilitates the H-abstraction reaction between flavonoids and reactive oxygen species (ROS) and other hydroxyl groups may well have contributed to this reaction in the consequent steps. However, substitution of the hydroxyl group at the C_3 position of quercetin by the monosaccharide glucose in isoquercetin and disaccharide rutinose in rutin decreases the lowest ΔH_f values, but this does not result in an increase in the cytoprotective activity. This is probably due to the fact that glycosylation decreases the lipophilicity, and to the loss of the free hydroxyl group at the 3-position of the C-ring. An appropriate solubility, which improves the mobility of the antioxidant across cell membranes, is another important factor in explaining the cytoprotective effects of flavonoids.

Correlation between Partition Coefficient (Log P) and Cytoprotective Activity (EC_{50}) of Flavonoids

As shown in Table 1, flavonoids with log P values that were high (log P > 3.0) or low (log P <1.0) had low cytoprotective activity, indicating that the cytoprotective activity of flavonoids is associated with their affinity and distribution in lipid membranes. This is presumably because a) at high values of log P, the flavonoid is dispersed in a lipid phase and not located at the lipid-water interface and, b) at low values of log P, the flavonoid is located in an aqueous phase and has insufficient solubility in the lipid phase. This can be important in terms of paracellular transport of flavonoids and the ability to enter the cell to participate in intracellular protection from oxidative damage. It has long been recognized that for a chemical to be biologically active, it must first be transported from its site of administration to its site of action and then it must bind to or react with its receptor or target, i.e. biological activity is a function of partitioning and reactivity (Barratt, 1998). It should be noted that the effect of membrane partitioning is not necessarily a direct relationship with lipophilicity. Beyeler and coworkers (Beyeler *et al.*, 1988), for example, reported that the effects of cianidanols on rat hepatic monooxygenase increased with lipophilicity, reached a plateau, decreased and then leveled off for the most lipophilic compounds.

As illustrated in Figure 19, for the 26 compounds tested, no correlation could be found between EC_{50} and log P (equation 9).

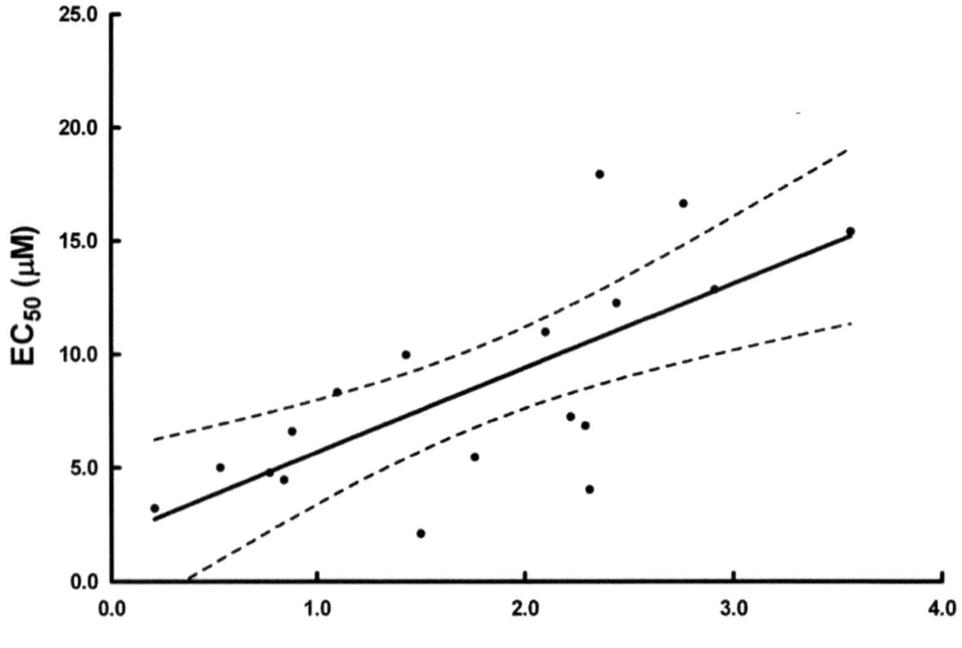

Figure 19. Correlation between EC_{50} (cytoprotective activity of flavonoids) and log P (calculated by CLogP program) of flavonoids ($r^2 = 0.15$, n = 26).

$$EC_{50} = 1.42\ (\pm\ 0.68)\ \log P + 7.23\ (\pm\ 1.20) \qquad [9]$$

$n = 26$, $r^2 = 0.15$, $p = 0.048$

As mentioned above, glycosylation decreased the lipophilicity of flavonoid aglycones significantly and also decreased their cytoprotective activity depending on the nature of the sugar involved. Therefore, the balance of lipophilicity and lipophobicity allowing concentration at the interface is an important factor in the estimation of the antioxidant activity of flavonoids.

As demonstrated in Figure 20, there is a moderate linear correlation between the cytoprotective activities (EC_{50} values) and the partition coefficient (log P) values of flavonoid aglycones and from the regression analysis a correlation with $r^2 = 0.51$ ($n = 18$) was obtained for the following equation 10:

$$EC_{50} = 3.72\ (\pm\ 0.92)\ \log P + 1.97\ (\pm\ 1.82)\ (n = 18) \qquad [10]$$

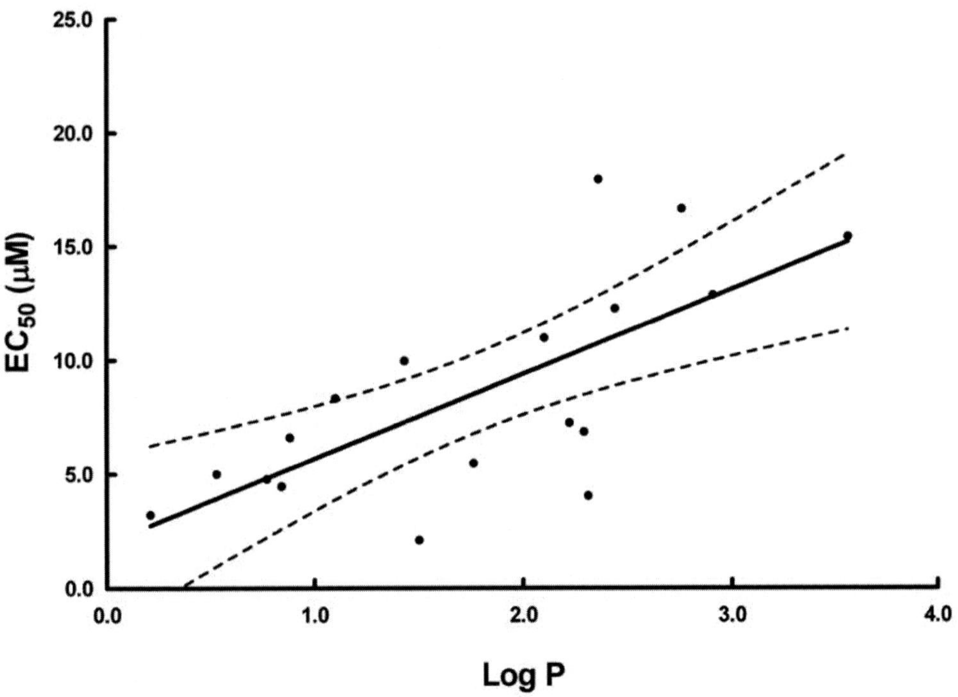

Figure 20. Correlation between EC_{50} (cytoprotective activity of flavonoids) and log P (calculated by CLogP program) of flavonoid aglycones (without sugar substitution) ($r^2 = 0.51$, $n = 18$).

Generally speaking, the cytoprotective activity of flavonoid aglycones decreases with increasing log P. However, this result also demonstrated that the cytoprotective activity of flavonoid aglycones is not solely dependant on their partition coefficient.

Quantitative Structure-Activity Relationship (QSAR) Model

The QSAR paradigm has been useful in elucidating the mechanisms of chemical-biological interactions in various biomolecules, particularly enzymes, membranes, organelles and cells (Hansch and Gao, 1997; Zhang *et al.*, 2002a; Zhang *et al.*, 2002b). The description of QSARs has been undertaken in order to find predictive models and/or mechanistic explanations for chemical as well as biological activities (Soffers *et al.*, 2001). The underlying premise of SARs and QSARs is that the properties of a chemical are implicit in its molecular structure and the behavior of chemical compounds is dominated by their physicochemical properties (Hansch *et al.*, 2000). If a QSAR model is deficient in modeling either partition or reactivity, only a partial correlation with the *in vivo* response is likely to be observed. The ΔH_f represents the stability of the free radical formed after H-abstraction and log P is an important parameter in chemical toxicology as it can indicate metabolic fate and biological transport properties.

The cytoprotection assay is a more biological measurement that accounts for some aspects of uptake, metabolism and location of flavonoids within cells. Here, a QSAR is modeled by starting from log P values and then incorporating ΔH_f.

With the introduction of ΔH_f (ease of H-abstraction) into equation 9, a two-parameter predictive model in the cytoprotection system could be derived based on the 26 compounds tested by step-wise regression as shown in equation 11.

$$EC_{50} = -0.45\ (\pm 0.33)\ \log P + 0.25\ (\pm 0.02)\ \Delta H_f - 25.75\ (\pm 3.04) \qquad [11]$$

$$n = 26,\ r^2 = 0.86,\ p = 0.0000000001$$

The use of the new parameter (ΔH_f) increased the correlation coefficient r^2-value from 0.15 to 0.86. The significant increase in correlation coefficient upon the introduction of ΔH_f confirmed the importance of O-H bond strength (bond dissociation energy approximated by ΔH_f), which contributed most to the model. However, log P gave a negative contribution to the EC_{50} values in this model.

A QSAR model could also be derived by the introduction of ΔH_f to equation 9 for flavonoid aglycones through step-wise regression as shown in equation 12.

$$EC_{50} = 0.38\ (\pm 0.65)\ \log P + 0.24\ (\pm 0.03)\ \Delta H_f - 26.25\ (\pm 4.04) \qquad [12]$$

$$n = 18,\ r^2 = 0.88,\ p = 0.000000072$$

Equation 12 indicated that log P gave a positive contribution to the EC_{50} values of flavonoid aglycones.

In conclusion, a QSAR model was derived from the cytoprotective activity and calculated theoretical parameters (enthalpy of hemolytic O-H bond cleavage ΔH_f and the partition coefficient). It demonstrated that the H-abstraction was not the sole mechanism responsible for the cytoprotective activity of flavonoids. It seems that the relative contribution of lipophilicity (log P) is much smaller than that of ΔH_f. These results demonstrated that it is feasible to estimate the cytoprotective activities of a flavonoid from the lipophilicity and the difference of heat of formations by using equation 11. The lipophilicity and heat of formation can be calculated purely by computer programs. Therefore, the QSAR model derived here could be useful in the selection of natural flavonoids with potential cytoprotective effects.

Conclusion

In summary, the cytoprotection assay provides information regarding cellular activity of antioxidants, which is important to our understanding of this area of antioxidant research. Traditionally, the antioxidant activity of phytochemicals has been measured using a range of chemically-defined laboratory-based assays. A cytoprotection assay that is a more biologically relevant method than the chemical antioxidant assays has been developed and can be adapted for use in other cell lines appropriate to tissues of interest. Using the cytoprotection assay, the effects of compounds on cells is determined, providing information regarding the cellular response to antioxidants, taking into account some aspects of uptake, metabolism, location of antioxidant compounds within cells and intracellular effects on signalling pathways and enzyme activity.

In the present study we showed that with a cell-based bioassay it is possible to identify natural-occurring flavonoids that are gastroprotective in a model of oxidant injury. By directly evaluating the effects of different classes of flavonoids using a lower dose of H_2O_2 and more chronic exposure, we showed that removal of excess ROS or suppression of their generation by flavonoids may be effective in preventing oxidative cell death.

In this study, we carried out a theoretical investigation into the possible mechanisms governing the cytoprotective activity of 24 different subclasses of flavonoids by computational chemistry, and explored the correlation between experimentally determined cytoprotective activities and physicochemical properties. It is reasonable to conclude that multiple mechanisms regulate the protective actions of flavonoid compounds although they contribute to the cytoprotective activity to different degrees. The cytoprotective activities of flavonoids were strongly correlated to their calculated enthalpy of hemolytic O-H bond cleavage (ΔH_f) but weakly correlated to their lipophilicity. It is concluded that the relative contribution of lipophilicity is much smaller than that of ΔH_f to their cytoprotective capacity. However, the balance of lipophilicity and lipophobicity is still critical in determining their abilities to protect human cells from oxidative damage.

Judging from the improvement in the correlation coefficient in the stepwise multiple-linear regression, we can conclude that the more precise the mechanistic information included in the QSAR model, the better the coefficient of relation that is obtained. It is reasonable to conclude that multiple mechanisms regulate the cytoprotection actions of flavonoids although they contribute to cytoprotective activity to different degrees. These results suggest the possibility of predicting the degree of contribution of different physicochemical factors among flavonoids by their *in vitro* actions against oxidative stress-induced cellular damage.

Acknowledgments

This work was funded by the Foundation for Research Science and Technology Wellness Food Programme Contract C06X0405. We thank Dr. Tony McGhie and Dr. Jeffery Greenwood for critically reviewing the manuscript.

References

Agullo G., Gamet-Payrastre L., Manenti S., Viala C., Rémésy C., Chap H., and Payrastre B. (1997). Relationship between flavonoid structure and inhibition of phosphatidylinositol 3-kinase: A comparison with tyrosine kinase and protein kinase C inhibition. *Biochemical Pharmacology* 53, 1649-1657.

Alonso-Salces R. M., Ndjoko K., Queiroz E. F., Ioset J. R., Hostettmann K., Berrueta L. A., Gallo B., and Vicente F. (2004). On-line characterisation of apple polyphenols by liquid chromatography coupled with mass spectrometry and ultraviolet absorbance detection. *Journal of Chromatography A* 1046, 89-100.

Andree H. A., Reutelingsperger C. P., Hauptmann R., Hemker H. C., Hermens W. T., and Willems G. M. (1990). Binding of vascular anticoagulant alpha (VAC alpha) to planar phospholipid bilayers. *Journal of Biological Chemistry* 265, 4923-4928.

Antunes F., and Cadenas E. (2001). Cellular titration of apoptosis with steady state concentrations of H_2O_2: submicromolar levels of H_2O_2 induce apoptosis through fenton chemistry independent of the cellular thiol state. *Free Radical Biology and Medicine* 30, 1008-1018.

Arora A., Nair M. G., and Strasburg G. M. (1998). Structure-activity relationships for antioxidant activities of a series of flavonoids in a liposomal system. *Free Radical Biology and Medicine* 24, 1355-1363.

Awad H. M., Boersma M. G., Boeren S., van Bladeren P. J., Vervoort J., and Rietjens I. M. (2001). Structure-activity study on the quinone/quinone methide chemistry of flavonoids. *Chemical Research in Toxicology* 14, 398-408.

Awad H. M., Boersma M. G., Boeren S., Van Bladeren P. J., Vervoort J., and Rietjens I. M. (2003). Quenching of quercetin quinone/quinone methides by different thiolate scavengers: Stability and reversibility of conjugate formation. *Chemical Research in Toxicology* 16, 822-831.

Bakalbassis E. G., Chatzopoulou A., Melissas V. S., Tsimidou M., Tsolaki M., and Vafiadis A. (2001). Ab initio and density functional theory studies for the explanation of the antioxidant activity of certain phenolic acids. *Lipids* 36, 181-190.

Barbouti A., Doulias P. T., Nousis L., Tenopoulou M., and Galaris D. (2002). DNA damage and apoptosis in hydrogen peroxide-exposed Jurkat cells: bolus addition versus continuous generation of H_2O_2. *Free Radical Biology and Medicine* 33, 691-702.

Barratt M. D. (1998). Integrating computer prediction systems with *in vitro* methods towards a better understanding of toxicology. *Toxicology Letters* 102-103, 617-621.

Behl C., Davis J. B., Lesley R., and Schubert D. (1994). Hydrogen peroxide mediates amyloid β–protein toxicity. *Cell* 77, 817-827.

Berkowitz J., Ellison G. B., and Gutman D. (1994). Three methods to measure RH bond energies. *Journal of Physical Chemistry* 98, 2744-2765.

Beyeler S., Testa B., and Perrissoud D. (1988). Flavonoids as inhibitors of rat liver monooxygenase activities. *Biochemical Pharmacology* 37, 1971-1979.

Bodor N., Gabanyi Z., and Wong C. K. (1989). A new method for the estimation of partition coefficient. *Journal of the American Chemical Society* 111, 3783-3786.

Boersma M. G., Vervoort J., Szymusiak H., Lemanska K., Tyrakowska B., Cenas N., Segura-Aguilar J., and Rietjens I. M. (2000). Regioselectivity and reversibility of the glutathione conjugation of quercetin quinone methide. *Chemical Research in Toxicology* 13, 185-191.

Bordwell F. G., and Zhang X.-M. (1993). From equilibrium acidities to radical stabilization energies. *Account in Chemical Research* 26, 510-517.

Borges dos Santos R. M., and Simoes J. A. M. (1998). Energetics of the O-H bond in phenol and substituted phenols: A critical evaluation of literature data. *Journal of Physical Chemistry Reference Data* 27, 707-739.

Borkowski T., Szymusiak H., Gliszczynska-Swiglo A., and Tyrakowska B. (2005). The effect of 3-O-[beta]-glucosylation on structural transformations of anthocyanidins. *Food Research International* 38, 1031-1037.

Bors W., Heller W., Michel C., and Saran M. (1990). Radical chemistry of flavonoid antioxidants. *Advances in Experimental Medicine and Biology* 264, 165-170.

Brigati G., Lucarini M., Mugnaini V., and Pedulli G. F. (2002). Determination of the substituent effect on the O-H bond dissociation enthalpies of phenolic antioxidants by the EPR radical equilibration technique. *Journal of Organic Chemistry* 67, 4828-4832.

Briviba K., Devasagayam T. P., Sies H., and Steenken S. (1993). Selective para hydroxylation of phenol and aniline by singlet molecular oxygen. *Chemical Research in Toxicology* 6, 548-553.

Brod S. A. (2000). Unregulated inflammation shortens human functional longevity. *Inflammation Research* 49, 561-570.

Brouillard R. (1983). The in vivo expression of anthocyanin colour in plants. *Phytochemistry* 22, 1311-1323.

Brouillard R., and Delaporte B. (1977a). Chemistry of anthocyanin pigments. 2. Kinetic and thermodynamic study of proton transfer, hydration, and tautomeric reactions of malvidin 3-glucoside. *Journal of the American Chemical Society* 99, 8461-8468.

Brouillard R., and Dubois J.-E. (1977b). Mechanism of the structural transformations of anthocyanins in acidic media. *Journal of the American Chemical Society* 99, 1359-1364.

Buchwald P., and Bodor N. (1998). Octanol-water partition of nonzwitterionic peptides: predictive power of a molecular size-based model. *Proteins* 30, 86-99.

Cantoni O., Cattabeni F., Stocchi V., Meyn R. E., Cerutti P., and Murray D. (1989). Hydrogen peroxide insult in cultured mammalian cells: Relationships between DNA single-strand breakage, poly(ADP-ribose) metabolism and cell killing. *Biochimica et Biophysica Acta* 1014, 1-7.

Car R. (2002). Introduction to density-functional theory and *ab-Initio* molecular mynamics. *Quantitative Structure-Activity Relationships* 21, 97-104.

Castle L., and Perkins M. J. (1986). Inhibition kinetics of chain-breaking phenolic antioxidants in SDS micelles. Evidence that intermicellar diffusion rates may be rate-limiting for hydrophobic inhibitors such as α-tocopherol. *Journal of the American Chemical Society* 108, 6382-6384.

Chen J. W., Zhu Z. Q., Hu T. X., and Zhu D. Y. (2002). Structure-activity relationship of natural flavonoids in hydroxyl radical-scavenging effects. *Acta Pharmacologica Sinica* 23, 667-672.

Chipman D. M., Liu R., Zhou X., and Pulay P. (1994). Structure and fundamental vibrations of phenoxyl radical. *Journal of Chemical Physics* 100, 5023-5035.

Choi J. S., Young C. H., Sik K. S., Jung J. M., Won K. J., Kyung N. J., and Ah J. H. (2002). The structure-activity relationship of flavonoids as scavengers of peroxynitrite. *Phytotherapy Research* 16, 232-235.

Colic M., and Pavelic K. (2000). Molecular mechanisms of anticancer activity of natural dietetic products. *Journal of Molecular Medicine* 78, 333-336.

Convard T., Dubost J. P., Le Solleu H., and Kummer E. (1994). SmilogP: A program for a fast evaluation of theoretical log P from smiles code of a molecule. *Quantitative Structure-Activity Relationships* 13, 34-37.

Cook N. C., and Samman S. (1996). Flavonoids--Chemistry, metabolism, cardioprotective effects, and dietary sources. *The Journal of Nutritional Biochemistry* 7, 66-76.

Cos P., Ying L., Calomme M., Hu J. P., Cimanga K., Van Poel B., Pieters L., Vlietinck A. J., and Berghe D. V. (1998). Structure-activity relationship and classification of flavonoids as inhibitors of xanthine oxidase and superoxide scavengers. *Journal of Natural Products* 61, 71-76.

Darzynkiewicz Z., Juan G., Li X., Gorczyca W., Murakami T., and Traganos F. (1997). Cytometry in cell necrobiology: analysis of apoptosis and accidental cell death (necrosis). *Cytometry* 27, 1-20.

Davies K. J. (1999). The broad spectrum of responses to oxidants in proliferating cells: a new paradigm for oxidative stress. *IUBMB Life* 48, 41-47.

Delgado-Vargas F., Jimenez A. R., Paredes-Lopez O., and Francis F. J. (2000). Natural pigments: Carotenoids, anthocyanins, and betalains - Characteristics, biosynthesis, processing, and stability. *Critical Reviews in Food Science and Nutrition* 40, 173-289.

Denisov E. T., and Khydyakov I. V. (1987). Mechanisms of action and reactivities of the free radicals of inhibitors. *Chemical Review* 87, 1313-1357.

Devaux P. F. (1991). Static and dynamic lipid asymmetry in cell membranes. *Biochemistry* 30, 1163-1173.

Dewar M. J. S., and Thiel W. (1977). Ground states of molecules. 38. The MNDO-method approximations and parameters. *Journal of the American Chemical Society* 99, 4899-4907.

Dewar M. J. S., Zoebisch E. G., Healy E. F., and Stewart J. J. P. (1985). AM1: A new general purpose quantum mechanical molecular model. *Journal of the American Chemical Society* 107, 3902-3909.

Diplock A. T., Charleux J. L., Crozier-Willi G., Kok F. J., Rice-Evans C., Roberfroid M., Stahl W., and Vina-Ribes J. (1998). Functional food science and defence against reactive oxidative species. *British Journal of Nutrition* 80 Suppl 1, S77-112.

Dziezak J. D. (1986). Preservatives: Antioxidants, the ultimate answer to oxidation. *Food Technology* 40 (9), 94-106.

Eadsforth C. V., and Moser P. (1983). Assessment of reverse-phase chromatographic methods for determining partition coefficients. *Chemosphere* 12, 1459-1475.

Eastwood M. A. (1999). Interaction of dietary antioxidants in vivo: how fruit and vegetables prevent disease? *Quarterly Journal of Medicine* 92, 527-530.

Fossen T., and Andersen Ø. M. (2006) Spectroscopic techniques applied to flavonoids, in *Flavonoids : Chemistry, biochemistry, and applications* (Andersen VM and Markham KR eds) pp 37-142, Taylor and Francis Group, Boca Raton, FL.

Fujita T., Iwasa J., and Hansch C. (1964). A new substituent constant, T, derived from partition coefficients. *Journal of the American Chemical Society* 86, 5175-5180.

Gardner A. M., Xu F. H., Fady C., Jacoby F. J., Duffey D. C., Tu Y., and Lichtenstein A. (1997). Apoptotic vs. nonapoptotic cytotoxicity induced by hydrogen peroxide. *Free Radical Biology and Medicine* 22, 73-83.

Ghose A. K., and Crippen G. M. (1987). Atomic physicochemical parameters for three-dimensional-structure-directed quantitative structure-activity relationships. 2. Modeling dispersive and hydrophobic interactions. *Journal of Chemical Information and Computer Sciences* 27, 21-35.

Gille J. J. P., and Joenje H. (1992). Cell culture models for oxidative stress: Superoxide and hydrogen peroxide versus normobaric hyperoxia. *Mutation Research/DNAging* 275, 405-414.

Giugliano D. (2000). Dietary antioxidants for cardiovascular prevention. *Nutrition, Metabolism and Cardiovascular Diseases* 10, 38-44.

Gotoh N., Noguchi N., Tsuchiya J., Morita K., Sakai H., Shimasaki H., and Niki E. (1996). Inhibition of oxidation of low density lipoprotein by vitamin E and related compounds. *Free Radical Research* 24, 123-134.

Gu L., kelm M. A., Hammerstone J. F., Beecher G., Holden J., Haytowitz D., and Prior R. L. (2003). Screening foods containing proanthocyanidins and their structural characterization using LC-MS/MS and thiolytic degradation. *Journal of Agriculture and Food Chemistry* 51, 7513-7521.

Guarnieri S., Riso P., and Porrini M. (2007). Orange juice vs vitamin C: effect on hydrogen peroxide-induced DNA damage in mononuclear blood cells. *British Journal of Nutrition* 97, 639-643.

Halliwell B. (1990). How to characterize a biological antioxidant. *Free Radical Research Communication* 9, 1-32.

Halliwell B. (1992). Reactive oxygen species and the central nervous system. *Journal of Neurochemistry* 59, 1609-1623.

Hansch C., and Gao H. (1997). Comparative QSAR: Radical reactions of benzene derivatives in chemistry and biology. *Chemical Review* 97, 2995-3060.

Hansch C., McKarns S. C., Smith C. J., and Doolittle D. J. (2000). Comparative QSAR evidence for a free-radical mechanism of phenol-induced toxicity. *Chemico-Biological Interactions* 127, 61-72.

Hansch C., Quinlan J. E., and Lawrence G. L. (1968). The linear free energy relationship between partition coefficients and the aqueous solubility of organic liquids. *Journal of Organic Chemistry* 33, 347-350.

Harborne J. B. (1962). Anthocyanins and their sugar components. *Fortschritte der Chemie Organischer Naturstoffe (Vienna)* 20, 165-199.

Harborne J. B., and Williams C. A. (2000). Advances in flavonoid research since 1992. *Phytochemistry* 55, 481-504.

Harborne J. B., and Williams C. A. (2001). Anthocyanins and other flavonoids. *Natural Product Reports* 18, 310-333.

Havsteen B. H. (2002). The biochemistry and medical significance of the flavonoids. *Pharmacology and Therapeutics* 96, 67-202.

Hedrickson H. P., Kaufman A. D., and Lunte C. E. (1994). Electrochemistry of catechol-containing flavonoids. *Journal of Pharmaceutical and Biomedical Analysis* 12, 325-334.

Herrmann K. M. (1976). Flavonoids and flavones in food plants: A review. *Journal of Food Technology* 11, 443-448.

Herrmann K. M. (1989). Occurrence and content of hydrocinnamic and hydrobenzoic acid compounds in foods. *Critical Review of Food Science and Nutrition* 28, 315-347.

Hollman P. C. H., and Arts I. C. W. (2000). Flavonols, flavones and flavanols - nature, occurrence and dietary burden. *Journal of the Science of Food and Agriculture* 80, 1081-1093.

Holt R. R., Lazarus S. A., Sullards M. C., Zhu Q. Y., Schramm D. D., Hammerstone J. F., Fraga C. G., Schmitz H. H., and Keen C. L. (2002). Procyanidin dimmer B2 [epicatechin-(4β-8)-epicatechin] in human plasma after the consumption of a flavanol-rich cococa. *Amercian Journal of Clinical Nutrition* 76, 798-804.

Hopia A., and Heinonen M. (1999). Antioxidant activity of flavonol aglycones and their glycosides in methyl linoleate. *Journal of the American Chemical Society* 76, 139-144.

Hoshino T. (1991). An approximate estimate of self-association constants and the self-stacking conformation of Malvin quinonoidal bases studied by 1H NMR. *Phytochemistry* 30, 2049-2055.

Hoshino T., and Goto T. (1990). Effects of pH and concentration on the self-association of malvin quinonoidal base -- electronic and circular dichroic studies. *Tetrahedron Letters* 31, 1593-1596.

Hoshino T., Matsumoto U., and Goto T. (1981). Self-association of some anthocyanins in neutral aqueous solution. *Phytochemistry* 20, 1971-1976.

Hyslop P. A., Zhang Z., Pearson D. V., and Phebus L. A. (1995). Measurement of striatal H_2O_2 by microdialysis following global forebrain ischemia and reperfusion in the rat: Correlation with the cytotoxic potential of H_2O_2 *in vitro*. *Brain Research* 671, 181-186.

Japertas P., Didziapetris R., and Petrauskas A. (2002). Fragmental methods in the design of new compounds. Applications of the advanced algorithm builder. *Quantitative Structure-Activity Relationships* 21, 23-37.

Kefford J. F., and Chandler B. V. (1970) *The chemical constituents of citrus fruits.* Academic Press, New York, NY.

Kim D. K., Cho E. S., and Um H. D. (2000). Caspase-dependent and -independent events in apoptosis induced by hydrogen peroxide. *Experimental Cell Research* 257, 82-88.

Klopman G., and Zhu H. (2001). Estimation of the aqueous solubility of organic molecules by the group contribution approach. *Journal of Chemical Information and Computer Sciences* 41, 439-445.

Kroon P. A., Clifford M. N., Crozier A., Day A. J., Donovan J. L., Manach C., and Williamson G. (2004). How should we assess the effects of exposure to dietary polyphenols *in vitro*? *American Journal of Clinical Nutrition* 80, 15-21.

Kumazawa Y., Kawaguchi K., and Takimoto H. (2006). Immunomodulating effects of flavonoids on acute and chronic inflammatory responses caused by tumor necrosis factor alpha. *Current Pharmaceutical Design* 12, 4271-4279.

Leo A., Hansch C., and Elkins D. (1971). Partition coefficients and their uses. *Chemical Review* 71, 525-616.

Leo A. J. (1991). Hydrophobic parameter: Measurement and calculation. *Methods in Enzymology* 202, 544-591.

Leo A. J. (1993). Calculating log P_{oct} from structures. *Chemical Review* 93, 1281-1306.

Lien E. J., Ren S., Bui H.-H., and Wang R. (1999). Quantitative structure-activity relationship analysis of phenolic antioxidants. *Free Radical Biology and Medicine* 26, 285-294.

Lipinski C. A., Lombardo F., Dominy B. W., and Feeney P. J. (1997). Experimental and computational approaches to estimate solubility and permeability in drug discovery and development settings. *Advanced Drug Delivery Reviews* 23, 3-25.

Lucarini M., Pedrielli P., and Pedulli G. F. (1996). Bond dissociation energies of O-H bonds in substituted from equilibration studies. *Journal of Organic Chemistry* 61, 9259-9263.

Lucarini M., and Pedulli F. (1994). Bond dissociation enthalpy of α–tocopherol and other phenolic antioxidants. *Journal of Organic Chemistry* 59, 5063-5070.

MacFarland J. W. (1970). On the parabolic relationship between drug potency and hydrophobicity. *Journal of Medicinal Chemistry* 13, 1192-1196.

Mahoney L. R., and DaRooge M. A. (1975). Kinetic behavior and thermochemical properties of phenoxy radicals. *Journal of the American Chemical Society* 97, 4722-4731.

Mannhold R., and Petrauskas A. (2003). Substructure versus whole-molecule approaches for calculating log P. *QSAR and Combinatorial Science* 22, 466-475.

Manthey J. A. (2000). Biological properties of flavonoids pertaining to inflammation. *Microcirculation* 7, S29-34.

Masuda J., Nakamura K., Kimura A., Takagi T., and Fujiwara H. (1997). Introduction of solvent-accessible surface area in the calculation of the hydrophobicity parameter log P from an atomistic approach. *Journal of Pharmaceutical Sciences* 86, 57-63.

McMurry J. (1992) Describing a reaction: Bond dissociation energies., in *McMurry Organic Chemistry.* (McMurry J eds) pp 156-159, Brooks/Cole Publishing Company, Belmont, California.

Metodiewa D., Jaiswal A. K., Cenas N., Dickancaite E., and Segura-Aguilar J. (1999). Quercetin may act as a cytotoxic prooxidant after its metabolic activation to semiquinone and quinoidal product. *Free Radical Biology and Medicine* 26, 107-116.

Meylan W. M., and Howard P. H. (1995). Atom/fragment contribution method for estimating octanol-water partition coefficients. *Journal of Pharmaceutical Sciences* 84, 83-92.

Middleton E., Jr., Kandaswami C., and Theoharides T. C. (2000). The effects of plant flavonoids on mammalian cells: Implications for inflammation, heart disease, and cancer. *Pharmacological Reviews* 52, 673-751.

Mora A., Paya M., Rios J. L., and Alcaraz M. J. (1990). Structure-activity relationships of polymethoxyflavones and other flavonoids as inhibitors of non-enzymic lipid peroxidation. *Biochemical Pharmacology* 40, 793-797.

Moridani M. Y., Galati G., and O'Brien P. J. (2002). Comparative quantitative structure toxicity relationships for flavonoids evaluated in isolated rat hepatocytes and HeLa tumor cells. *Chemico-Biological Interactions* 139, 251-264.

Mulder P., Saastad O. W., and Griller D. (1988). O-H bond dissociation energies in *para*-substituted phenols. *Journal of the American Chemical Society* 110, 4090-4092.

Murakami S., Muramatsu M., and Tomisawa K. (1999). Inhibition of gastric H+,K+-ATPase by flavonoids: A structure-activity study. *Journal of Enzyme Inhibition* 14, 151-166.

Noguchi N., Okimoto Y., Tsuchiya J., Cynshi O., Kodama T., and Niki E. (1997). Inhibition of oxidation of low-density lipoprotein by a novel antioxidant, BO-653, prepared by theoretical design. *Archives of Biochemistry and Biophysics* 347, 141-147.

O'Byrne K. J., and Dalgleish A. G. (2001). Chronic immune activation and inflammation as the cause of malignancy. *British Journal of Cancer* 85, 473-483.

Osterberg T., and Norinder U. (2001). Prediction of drug transport processes using simple parameters and PLS statistics: The use of ACD/logP and ACD/ChemSketch descriptors. *European Journal of Pharmaceutical Sciences* 12, 327-337.

Packer L., Rimbach G., and Virgili F. (1999). Antioxidant activity and biologic properties of a procyanidin-rich extract from pine (Pinus maritima) bark, pycnogenol. *Free Radical Biology and Medicine* 27, 704-724.

Passamonti S., Vrhovsek U., and Mattivi F. (2002). The interaction of anthocyanins with bilitranslocase. *Biochemical and Biophysical Research Communications* 296, 631-636.

Pople J. A., Beveridge D. L., and Doboshlc P. A. (1968). Molecular orbital theory of the electronic structure of organic compounds. 11. Spin densities in paramagnetic species. *Journal of the American Chemical Society* 90, 4201-4209.

Porter L. J. (1993). Flavans and proanthocyanidins. In: *The Flavonoids. Advances in Research since 1986* (Harborne JB eds), pp 23-55. Chapman & Hall, London, UK.

Porter W. L., Black E. D., and Drolet A. M. (1989). Use of polyamide oxidative fluorescence test on lipid emulsions: Contrast in relative effectiveness of antioxidants in bulk versus dispersed systems. *Journal of Agricultural and Food Chemistry* 37, 615-624.

Potapovich A. I., and Kostyuk V. A. (2003). Comparative study of antioxidant properties and cytoprotective activity of flavonoids. *Biochemistry (Mosc)* 68, 514-519.

Qin Y., and Wheeler R. A. (1995). Density-functional methods give accurate vibrational frequencies and spin densities for phenoxyl radical. *Journal of Chemical Physics* 102, 1689-1698.

Rastija V., and Medic-Saric M. (2009). QSAR study of antioxidant activity of wine polyphenols. *European Journal of Medicinal Chemistry* 44, 400-408.

Reddy A. M., Reddy V. S., Scheffler B. E., Wienand U., and Reddy A. R. (2007). Novel transgenic rice overexpressing anthocyanidin synthase accumulates a mixture of flavonoids leading to an increased antioxidant potential. *Metabolic Engineering* 9, 95-111.

Rice-Evans C. A., Miller N. J., Bolwell P. G., Bramley P. M., and Pridham J. B. (1995). The relative antioxidant activities of plant-derived polyphenolic flavonoids. *Free Radical Research* 22, 375-383.

Rice-Evans C. A., Miller N. J., and Paganga G. (1996). Structure-antioxidant activity relationships of flavonoids and phenolic acids. *Free Radical Biology and Medicine* 20, 933-956.

Riemersma R. A., Rice-Evans C. A., Tyrrell R. M., Clifford M. N., and Lean M. E. J. (2001). Tea flavonoids and cardiovascular health. *Quarterly Journal of Medicine* 94, 277-282.

Scalbert A., and Williamson G. (2000). Dietary Intake and Bioavailability of Polyphenols. *Journal of Nutrition* 130, 2073S-2085.

Schreck R., Rieber P., and Baeuerle P. A. (1991). Reactive oxygen intermediates as apparently widely used messengers in the activation of the NF-kappa B transcription factor and HIV-1. *Embo Journal* 10, 2247-2258.

Schwarz K., Frankel E. N., and German J. B. (1996). Partition behaviour of antioxidative phenolic compounds in heterophasic systems. *Lipid -Fett.* 98, 115-121.

Shahidi F., and Wanasundara P. K. (1992). Phenolic antioxidants. *Critical Review of Food Science and Nutrition* 32, 67-103.

Simonian N. A., and Coyle J. T. (1996). Oxidative stress in neurodegenerative diseases. *Annual Review of Pharmacology and Toxicology* 36, 83-106.

Soffers A. E. M. F., Boersma M. G., Vaes W. H. J., Vervoort J., Tyrakowska B., Hermens J. L. M., and Rietjens I. M. C. M. (2001). Computer-modeling-based QSARs for analyzing experimental data on biotransformation and toxicity. *Toxicology In Vitro* 15, 539-551.

Spencer J. P. E., Abd El Mohsen M. M., and Rice-Evans C. (2004). Cellular uptake and metabolism of flavonoids and their metabolites: implications for their bioactivity. *Archives of Biochemistry and Biophysics* 423, 148-161.

Spencer J. P. E., Kuhnle G. G., Williams R. J., and Rice-Evans C. (2003). Intracellular metabolism and bioactivity of quercetin and its in vivo metabolites. *Biochemical Journal* 372, 173-181.

Stack D. (1997) Phenolic metabolism., in *Plant Biochemistry* (Dey PM and Harborne JB eds) pp 387-417, Academic Press, London, UK.

Stewart J. P. J. (1989). Optimization of parameters for semiempirical methods. II. Applications. *Journal of Computational Chemistry* 10, 221-264.

Sugihara N., Kaneko A., and Furuno K. (2003). Oxidation of flavonoids which promote DNA degradation induced by bleomycin-Fe complex. *Biological and Pharmaceutical Bulletin* 26, 1108-1114.

Sun Y. M., Zhang H. Y., Chen D. Z., and Liu C. B. (2002). Theoretical elucidation on the antioxidant mechanism of curcumin: A DFT study. *Organic Letters* 4, 2909-2911.

Timberlake C. F., and Bridle P. (1967). Flavylium salts, anthocyanidins and anthocyanins. I. - Structural transformations in acid solutions. *Journal of the Science of Food and Agriculture* 18, 473-478.

Tournaire C., Croux S., Maurette M. T., Beck I., Hocquaux M., Braun A. M., and Oliveros E. (1993). Antioxidant activity of flavonoids: efficiency of singlet oxygen (1 delta g) quenching. *Journal of Photochemistry and Photobiology B* 19, 205-215.

van Acker S. A., de Groot M. J., van den Berg D. J., Tromp M. N., Donne-Op den Kelder G., van der Vijgh W. J., and Bast A. (1996). A quantum chemical explanation of the antioxidant activity of flavonoids. *Chemical Research in Toxicology* 9, 1305-1312.

van Acker S. A., Koymans L. M., and Bast A. (1993). Molecular pharmacology of vitamin E: Structural aspects of antioxidant activity. *Free Radical Biology and Medicine* 15, 311-328.

van Engeland M., Nieland L. J., Ramaekers F. C., Schutte B., and Reutelingsperger C. P. (1998). Annexin V-affinity assay: a review on an apoptosis detection system based on phosphatidylserine exposure. *Cytometry* 31, 1-9.

Vaya J., Mahmood S., Goldblum A., Aviram M., Volkova N., Shaalan A., Musa R., and Tamir S. (2003). Inhibition of LDL oxidation by flavonoids in relation to their structure and calculated enthalpy. *Phytochemistry* 62, 89-99.

Vedernikova I., Tollenaere J. P., and Haemers A. (1999). Quantum mechanical evaluation of the anodic oxidation of phenolic compounds. *Journal of Physical Organic Chemistry* 12, 144-150.

Vermes I., Haanen C., and Reutelingsperger C. (2000). Flow cytometry of apoptotic cell death. *Journal of Immunological Methods* 243, 167-190.

Ververidis F., Trantas E., Carl D., Guenter V., Georg K., and Panopoulos N. (2007). Biotechnology of flavonoids and other phenylpropanoid-derived natural products. Part I: Chemical diversity, impacts on plant biology and human health. *Biotechnology Journal* 2, 1214-1234.

Wang R., Fu Y., and Lai L. (1997). A new atom-additive method for calculating partition coefficients. *Journal of Chemical Information and Computer Sciences* 37, 615-621.

Wayner D. D., Lusztyk J. E., Page D., Ingold K. U., Mulder P., Laarhoven L. J. J., and Aldrichs H. S. (1995). Effects of solvation on the enthalpies of reaction of *tert*-butoxyl radicals with phenol and on the calculated O-H bond strength in phenol. *Journal of the American Chemical Society* 117, 8738-8744.

Wayner D. D. M., and Parker V. D. (1993). Bond energies in solution from electrode potentials and thermochemical cycles. A simplified and general approach. *Account in Chemical Research* 26, 287-294.

Wedworth S. M., and Lynch S. (1995). Dietary flavonoids in atherosclerosis prevention. *The Annals of Pharmacotherapy* 29, 627-628.

Williams R. J., Spencer J. P. E., and Rice-Evans C. (2004). Flavonoids: Antioxidants or signalling molecules? *Free Radical Biology and Medicine* 36, 838-849.

Winkel-Shirley B. (2001). Flavonoid Biosynthesis. A Colorful Model for Genetics, Biochemistry, Cell Biology, and Biotechnology. *Plant Physiology* 126, 485-493.

Wollenweber E., and Dietz V. H. (1981). Occurrence and distribution of free flavonoid aglycones in plants. *Phytochemistry* 20, 869-932.

Wright J. S., Carpenter D. J., McKay D. J., and Ingold K. U. (1997). Theoretical calculation of substituent effects on the O-H bond strength of phenolic antioxidants related to vitamin E. *Journal of the American Chemical Society* 119, 4245-4252.

Wright J. S., Johnson E. R., and DiLabio G. A. (2001). Predicting the activity of phenolic antioxidants: Theoretical method, analysis of substituent effects, and application to major families of antioxidants. *Journal of the American Chemical Society* 123, 1173-1183.

Yong D. C. (2001) *Computational chemistry: A practical guide for applying techniques to real-world problems.* Wiley Interscience, New York.

Zhang H.-Y., You-Min S., and Xiu-Li W. (2003a). Substituent Effects on O-H Bond Dissociation Enthalpies and Ionization Potentials of Catechols: A DFT Study and Its Implications in the Rational Design of Phenolic Antioxidants and Elucidation of Structure-Activity Relationships for Flavonoid Antioxidants. *Chemistry - A European Journal* 9, 502-508.

Zhang H. Y. (1998). Selection of theoretical parameter characterizing scavenging activity of antioxidants on free radicals. *Journal of the American Oil Chemists' Society* 75, 1705-1709.

Zhang H. Y., Ge N., and Zhang Z. Y. (1999). Theoretical elucidation of activity differences of five phenolic antioxidants. *Zhongguo Yao Li Xue Bao* 20, 363-366.

Zhang H. Y., Sun Y. M., and Wang X. L. (2002a). Electronic effects on O-H proton dissociation energies of phenolic cation radicals: A DFT study. *Journal of Organic Chemistry* 67, 2709-2712.

Zhang H. Y., and Wang L. F. (2002b). Theoretical elucidation on structure-antioxidant activity relationships for indolinonic hydroxylamines. *Bioorganic and Medicinal Chemistry Letters* 12, 225-227.

Zhang H. Y., Wang L. F., and Sun Y. M. (2003b). Why B-ring is the active center for genistein to scavenge peroxyl radical: A DFT study. *Bioorganic and Medicinal Chemistry Letters* 13, 909-911.

Zhang J., Melton L., Adaim A., and Skinner M. (2008). Cytoprotective effects of polyphenolics on H2O2-induced cell death in SH-SY5Y cells in relation to their antioxidant activities. *European Food Research and Technology* 228, 123-131.

Zhang J., Stanley R. A., Adaim A., Melton L. D., and Skinner M. A. (2006a). Free radical scavenging and cytoprotective activities of phenolic antioxidants. *Molecular Nutrition and Food Research* 50, 996-1005.

Zhang J., Stanley R. A., and Melton L. D. (2006b). Lipid peroxidation inhibition capacity assay for antioxidants based on liposomal membranes. *Molecular Nutrition and Food Research* 50, 714-724.

Ziegler T. (1991). Approximate density functional theory as a practical tool in molecular energetics and dynamics. *Chemical Review* 91, 651-667.

In: Flavonoids: Biosynthesis, Biological Effects... ISBN: 978-1-60741-622-7
Editor: Raymond B. Keller

Chapter 3

OLIGOMERIC NATURE, COLLOIDAL STATE, RHEOLOGY, ANTIOXIDANT CAPACITY AND ANTIVIRAL ACTIVITY OF POLYFLAVONOIDS

A.Pizzi

ENSTIB-LERMAB, University Henry Poincare – Nancy 1,
Epinal, France

ABSTRACT

The determination by Matrix-Assisted Laser Desorption/Ionization time–of-flight (MALDI-TOF) mass spectroscopy of the oligomeric nature of the two major industrial polyflvonoid tannins which exist, namely mimosa and quebracho tannins, and some of their modified derivatives indicates that: (i) mimosa tannin is predominantly composed of prorobinetinidins while quebracho is predominantly composed of profisetinidins, that (ii) mimosa tannin is heavily branched due to the presence of considerable proportions of "angular" units in its structure while quebracho tannin is almost completely linear. These structural differences also contribute to the considerable differences in viscoity of water solutions of the two tannins. (iii) the interflavonoid link is more easily hydrolysable, and does appear to sometime hydrolyse in quebracho tannin and profisetinidins, partly due to the linear structure of this tannin, and confirming NMR findings that this tannin is subject to polymerisation/depolymerisation equilibria. This tannin hydrolysis does not appear to occur in mimosa tannin in which the interflavonoid link is completely stable to hydrolysis. (iv) Sulphitation has been shown to influence the detachment of catechol B-rings much more than pyrogallol-type B-rings. (vi) The distribution of tannin oligomers, and the tannins number average degree of polymerisation obtained by MALDI-TOF, up to nonamers and decamers, appear to compare well with the results obtained by other techniques. As regards procyanidin tannins, it has been possible to determine for mangrove polyflavonoid tannins that: (i) procyanidins oligomers formed by catechin/epicatechin, epigallocatechin and epicatechin gallate monomers are present in great proportions. (ii) oligomers, up to nonamers, in which the repeating unit at 528-529 Da is a catechin gallate dimer that has lost both the gallic acid residues and an hydroxy group are the predominant species. (iii) oligomers of the two types covalently linked to each other also occur.

Water solution of non-purified polyflavonoid extracts appear to be incolloidal state, this being due mainly to the hydrocolloid gums extracted with the tannin as well as to the tannin itself.

Commercial, industrially produced mimosa, quebracho, pine and pecan polyflavonoid tannin extracts water solutions of different concentrations behave mainly as viscous liquids at the concentrations which are generally used for their main industrial applications. Clear indications of viscoelastic response are also noticeable, among these the cross-over of the elastic and viscous moduli curves at the lower concentrations of the range investigated, with some differences being noticeable between each tannin and the others, pine and quebracho tannin extracts showing the more marked viscoelastic behaviour. Other than pH dependence (and related structural considerations), the parameters which were found to be of interest as regards the noticeable viscoelastic behaviour of the tannin extracts were the existence in the solutions of labile microstructures which can be broken by applied shear. This is supported by the well known thixotropic behaviour of concentrated, commercial polyflavonoid tannin extracts water solutions.

Such microstructures appear to be due or (i) to the known colloidal interactions of these materials, or (ii) to other types of secondary interactions between tannin oligomers and particularly between tannin and carbohydrate oligomers. The latter is supported by the dependence of this effect from both the average molecular masses of the tannin and of the carbohydrate oligomers.

The behaviour of polyflavonoid tannins as regards their antioxydant capacity and radical scavenging ability has been examined. Radical formation and radical decay reactions of some polyflavonoid and hydrolysable tannins has been followed, and comparative kinetics determined, for both light induced radicals and by radical transfer from a less stable chemical species to the tannin as part of an investigation of the role of tannin as antioxidants.

The five parameters which appear to have a bearing on the very complex pattern of the rates of tannin radical formation and radical decay were found to be (i) the extent of the colloidal state of the tannin in solution (ii) the stereochemical structure at the interflavonoid units linkage (iii) the ease of heterocyclic pyran ring opening, (iv) the relative numbers of A- and B-rings hydroxy groups and (v) solvation effects when the tannin is in solution. It is the combination of these five factors which appears to determine the behaviour as an antioxidant of a particular tannin under a set of application conditions.

The chapter ends with some recent results on the antiviral activity of polyflavonoid tannins for a great variety of viruses.

INTRODUCTION

Polyflavonoids also called condensed tannins are natural polyphenolic materials. Industrial polyflavonoid tannin extracts are mostly composed of flavan-3-ols repeating units, and smaller fractions of polysaccharides and simple sugars. Two types of phenolic rings having different reactivities are present on each flavan-3-ol repeating unit, namely A-rings and B-rings, with each repeating unit being linked 4,6 or 4,8 with the units which precede and follow it.

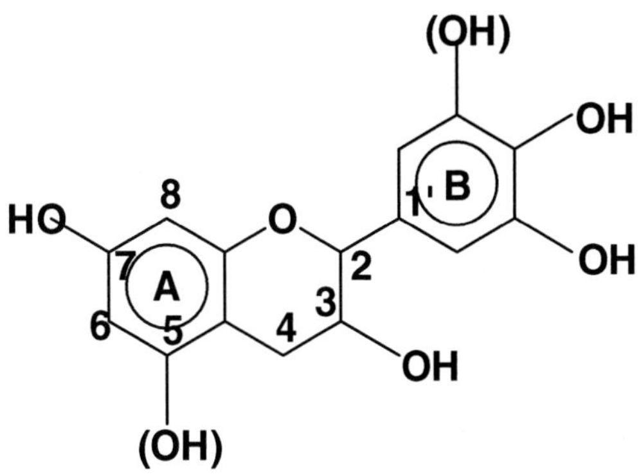

Recently, the radical and ionic mechanisms of the reaction of autocondensation and networking of polyflavonoid tannins induced by bases and by weak Lewis acids has been described [2-8]. Different polyflavonoid tannins however present different structures and different average molecular masses, and as a consequence often present peculiarly different behaviour in their application [10]. The most common method of examination of the relative structures of polyflavonoid tannins, and of their differences, is by ^{13}C NMR [10].

THE OLIGOMERIC NATURE OF POLYFLAVONOIDS

Since its introduction by Karas and Hillenkamp in 1987 [11], Matrix-Assisted Laser Desorption/Ionization (MALDI) mass spectrometry has greatly expanded the use of mass spectrometry towards large molecules and has revealed itself to be a powerful method for the characterization of both synthetic and natural polymers [12-17]. Fragmentation of analyte molecules upon laser irradiation can be substantially reduced by embedding them in a light absorbing matrix. As a result intact analyte molecules are desorbed and ionized along with the matrix and can be analysed in a mass spectrometer. This soft ionization technique is mostly combined with time-of-flight (TOF) mass analysers. This is so as TOF-MS present the advantage of being capable to provide a complete mass spectrum per event, for its virtually unlimited mass range, for the small amount of analyte necessary and the relatively low cost of the equipment.

Matrix-Assisted Laser Desorption/Ionization Time-of-Flight (MALDI-TOF) mass spectrometry (MS) is a technique that has revealed itself to be a very useful tool in defining the oligomeric structure of polyflavonoids, much more pointed than other techniques used before. As an example even oligomers up to and even of more than 10 flavonoid repeating units have been clearly detected in commercial polyflavonoid extracts by using such a technique. The technique was used to compare the structures of the most common industrial polyflavonoid condensed tannins.

Profisetinindin and Prorobinetinidin Type Polyflavonoids

The profisetinidin/prorobinetinidin type of polyflavonoid tannins are the most common extracted industrially [1]. The great majority of the flavonoid units are linked C4 to C6 to form the oligomers, but certain units, in the minority are also linked C4 to C8. Quebracho tannin and Mimosa tannin are the two main exponents of this class. Quebracho gave clear spectra showing the degree of polymerization of the building units and oligomer series with masses of the repeat units of 272 Da and 288 Da (Figure 1a; Table 1). For each oligomer, substructures with mass increments of 16 Da appear, indicating different combinations of various substructures. As quebracho is mainly based on combinations of resorcinol, catechol and pyrogallol building blocks the following monoflavonoids and their oligomers can be expected to be present:

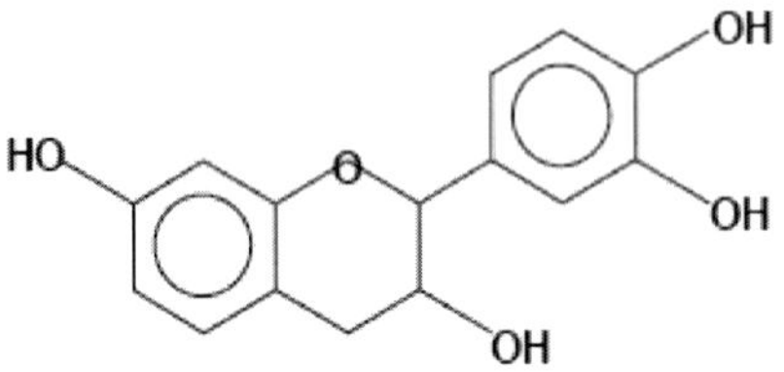

A

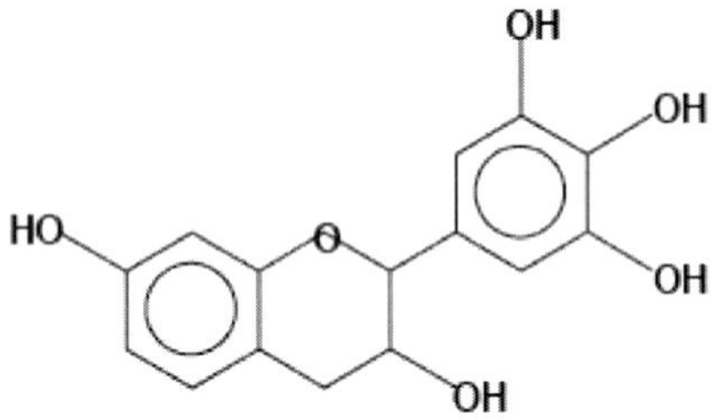

B

The masses of units A and B are 274 Da and 290 Da respectively. Combinations of these masses can be used to calculate the masses of the oligomer peaks in the spectra according to the expression $M+Na^{+} = 23(Na) + 2$ (endgroups, 2xH) + 272A +288B (Table 1). As can be seen in the spectra, there are more peak series which are due to different endgroups. They have the same repeat units, for example 683-956 Da and 1555-1827 Da in Figure 1. The peak at 683 is very near to a result of 688 Da which would be obtained by the loss of both a B-ring plus the three-carbons chain from the heterocycle of the lower terminal repeat unit, be this of type B or of type A, to yield two flavonoid units linked to a resorcinol phenoxy anion.

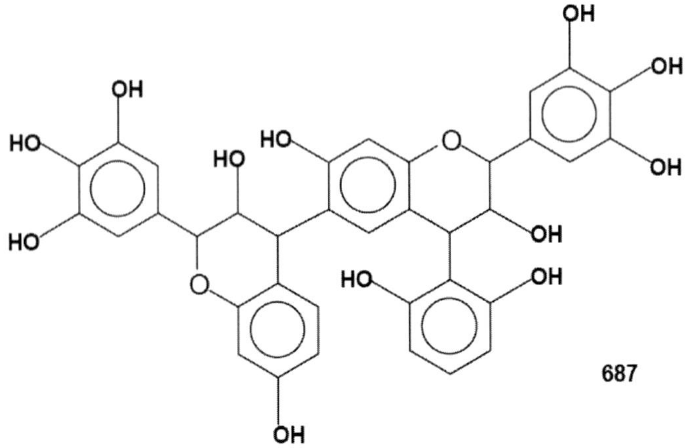

687

The peak at 585 Da is also explained by the presence of a dimer according to the same equation above composed of a A-unit plus a B-unit plus 2 H endgroups plus Na^{+}. The peak at 375 Da is obtained from the 585 Da dimer by elimination of a catecholic B-ring (585-110 = 375).

There is however an alternate, and more correct explanation for the 683 Da peak. Industrial quebracho tannin extract is sulphited/bisulphited, which introduces a sulphite or sodium sulphite group on the C1 of the flavonoid structure and causes the opening of the heterocycle ring. Thus, if one of the flavonoid units of a 857 Da trimer loses its catechol B-ring (-110) from a type A repeat unit as well as the $-SO_2^-$ group (-64), the 683 Da signal is obtained.

Table 1. MALDI fragmentation peaks for industrial quebracho tannin extract. Note that the predominant repeat units in this tannin is 272 Da, indicating that this tannin is predominantly a profisetinidin

M+Na+	M+Na+	Unit type	
(exp) (calc.) A			B
Dimers			
585	586	1	1
601	601	--	2
Trimers			
842	841	3	--
*857	857	2	1
874	873	1	2
Tetramers			
1114	1113	4	--
*1130	1129	3	1
1146	1145	2	2
Pentamers			
1387	1385	5	--
*1402	1401	4	1
1420	1417	3	2
1435	1433	2	3
Hexamers			
1658	1659	6	--
1675	1673	5	1
*1692	1689	4	2
1708	1705	3	3
Heptamers			
1948	1945	6	1
*1965	1961	5	2
1982	1977	4	3
Octamers			
*2237	2233	6	2
Nonamers			
*2510	2505	7	2
Decamers			
*2782	2777	8	2
2798	2793	7	3

*Dominant fragment.

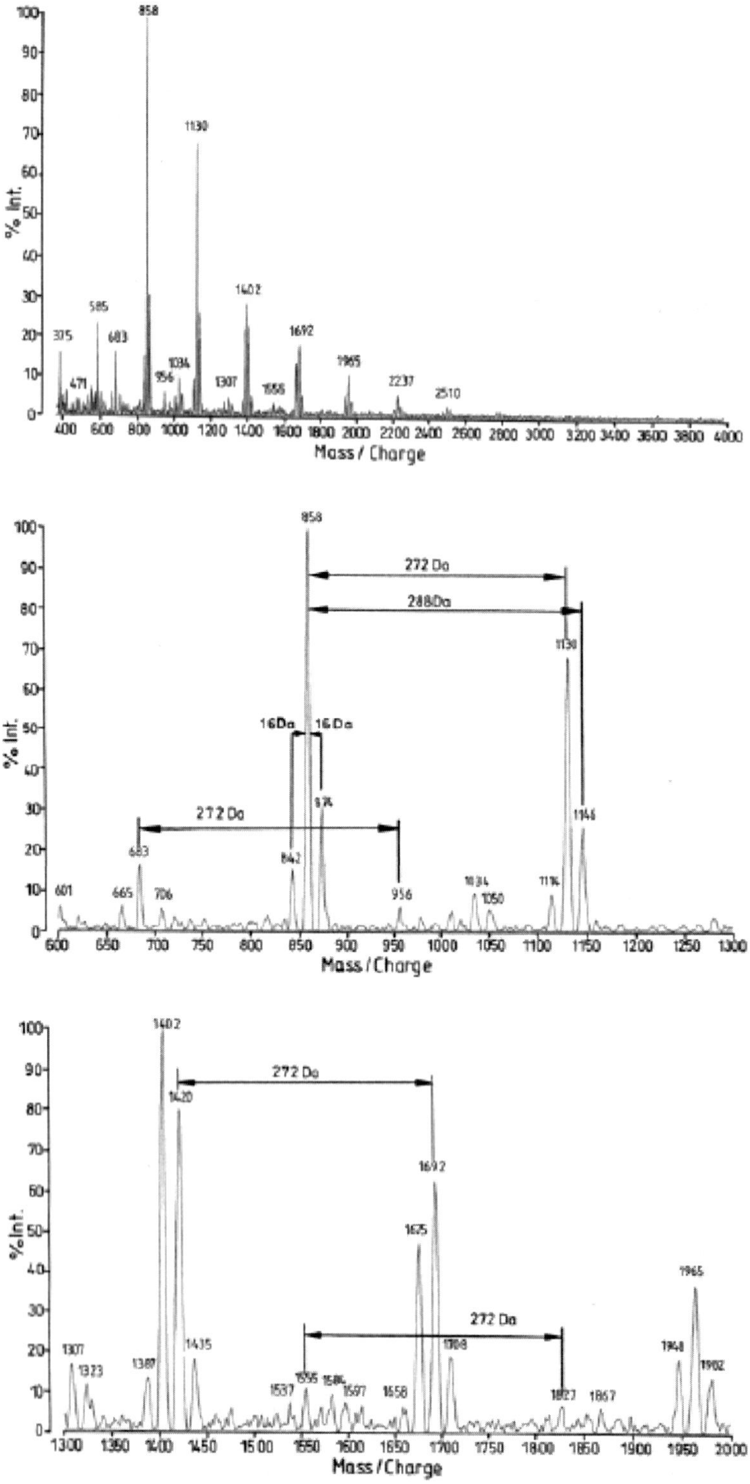

Figure 1. MALDI mass spectrum of (A) natural sulphited quebracho tannin extract. (B) details of the 600-1300 Da range with indication of the relevant 272 Da repeat unit. (C) details of the 1300-2000 Da range with indication of the relevant 272 Da repeat unit.

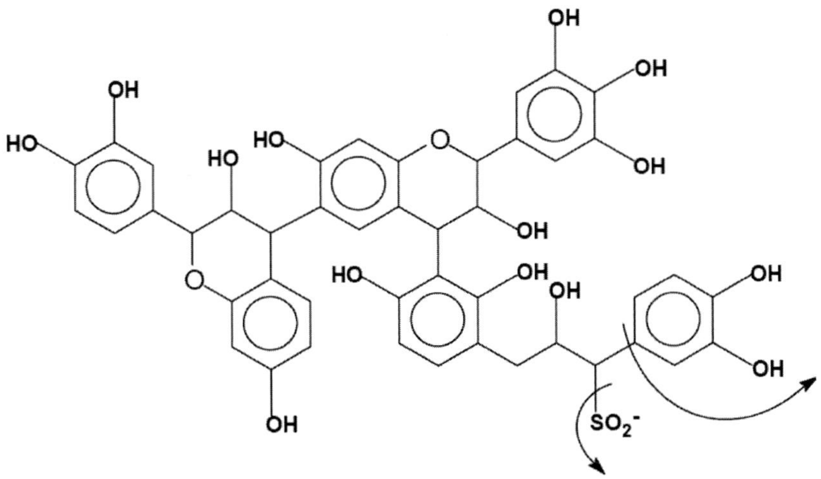

This is more likely as the introduction of the $-SO_2^-$ group should favour under certain conditions the elimination of the B-ring of the unit. The origin of the much smaller 665 Da peak is the same but by elimination of the $-SO_2H$ group (-65) and of a pyrogallol B-ring (-126) from a type B repeat unit. The fact that the intensity of the 665 Da peak is considerably lower than that of the 683 Da peak indicates the novel finding that as a consequence of sulphitation catechol rings appear to be much more easily detached than pyrogallol ones from a flavonoid unit. That the 683 peak is caused by the presence of the sulphonic group on C1 and the relative ease of decomposition indicated above is shown by the fact that in mimosa tannin which in general is not sulphited the 683 Da peak does not exist while presenting a very small peak at 687 Da which come from the first explanation (Figure 2a).

Also of interest are the existence of peaks at 1965, 2237, 2510 and 2800 Da for commercial quebracho tannin, these representing respectively heptamers, octamers, nonamers and decamers (Figure 1). Tannins are not easily water soluble at this higher molecular weight and thus it is of interest to find definite proof of the existence of such higher molecular weight oligomers in a commercial tannin extract. The sample in question had been found by ^{13}C NMR to have a number average degree of polymerization of 6.74 [19,20] which appears to confirm the existence of such higher molar mass oligomers in this commercial tannin extract. The same type of pattern is obtained for solvent purified commercial quebracho extract (MALDI spectrum not reported here), in which all the carbohydrates have been eliminated, confirming that the patterns observed are really due to the polyflavonoid components of the tannin extract. It is, however, of interest to note that the tannin extract which has undergone an acid/base treatment [18] to obtain an adhesive intermediate gives at best a pentamer at 1967 Da, see Figure 2. This is accompanied by a considerable increase in the proportion of the 858 Da trimers, of the 727 degraded trimers (2 flavonoid units + 1 A-ring + its C4), of degradation product composed of a single flavonoid unit linked to a single A-ring of another flavonoid unit (375 da) and also an increase in the 1130 Da tetramers confirming that the treatment to yield a tannin adhesive intermediate clearly induces some level of hydrolysis of the interflavonoid bond and hence some level of depolymerization in quebracho tannin.

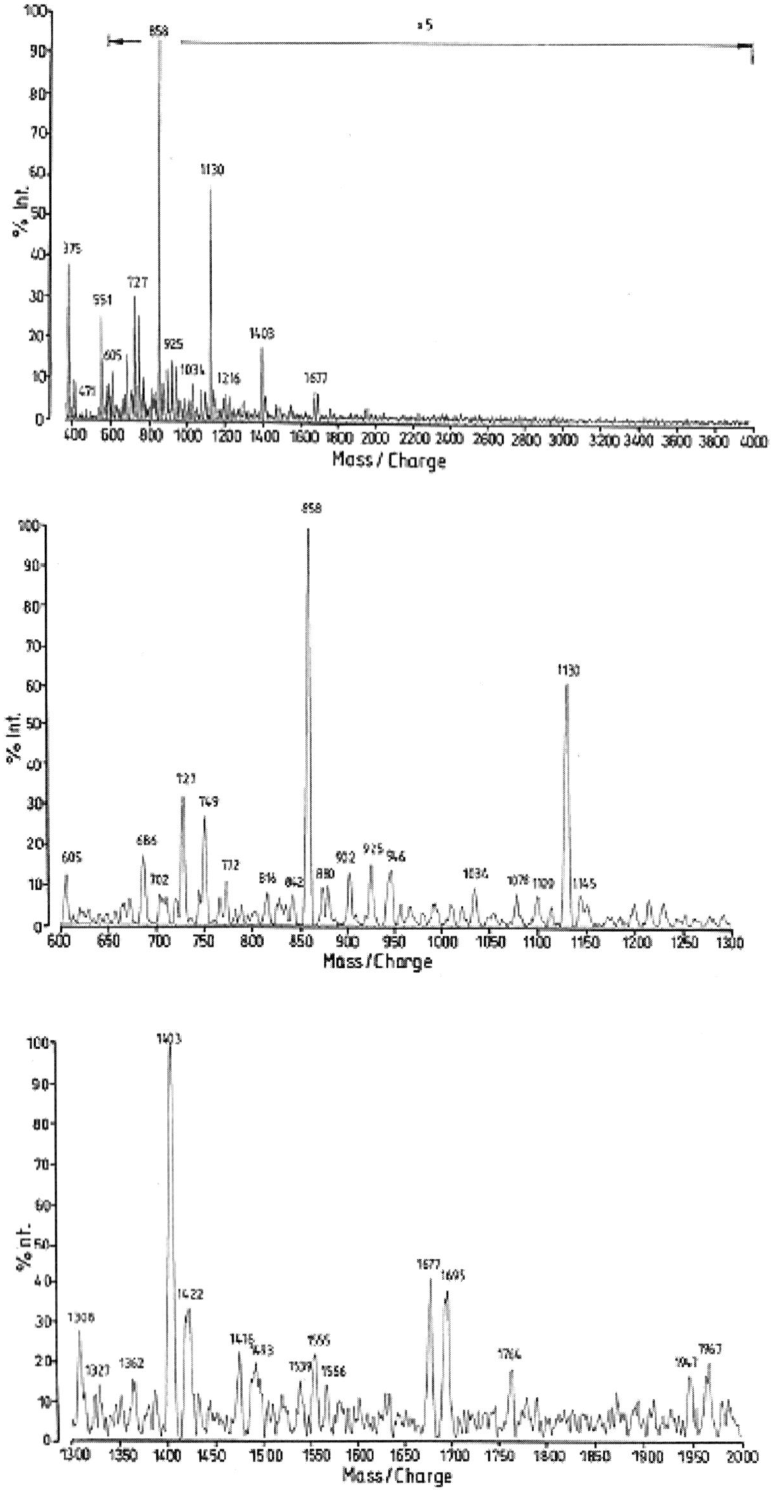

Figure 2. MALDI mass spectrum of (a) acid/base treated modified quebracho tannin extract. (b) details of the 600-1300 Da range, (c) details of the 1300-2000 Da range.

This confirms previous findings [6-8,18] obtained by ^{13}C NMR that contrary to what widely thought the interflavonoid bond in the profisetinidins/prorobinetinidins of quebracho tannin are fairly labile and that this particular type of tannin can be subject to some depolymerization. It also confirms what has been up to now only a suspicion, namely that the decrease in viscosity [18] of tannin solutions as a consequence of acid/base treatments is not only due to hydrolysis of the hydrocolloid polymeric carbohydrates present in the extract, but also to the decrease in degree of polymerization of the tannin itself, this at least in the case of quebracho tannin. It is also interesting to observe a definite, clear peak at 605 Da (see Figure 2) which can only belong to a pure robinetinidin dimer (289+289+25 = 605), MALDI-TOF analysis appearing to indicate here that it is the interflavonoid inter-fisetinidin link, or at least links in which fisetinidin units are involved which appear to be more sensitive to cleavage. The acid/base treatment to produce a tannin adhesive intermediate involves the use of acetic anhydride or maleic anhydride for the acid hydrolysis phase. As the treatment is done in water solution but being the tannin extract strongly colloidal in nature a question of interest is to know if some of the tannin –OH groups have been acetylated within the micelles present in the solution and before the induced hydrolysis has drastically decreased the level of colloidality of the system. Past investigations by ^{13}C NMR and by other techniques [18] indicate that a certain amount (small) of acetylation appears also to occur, this being of importance in accelerating subsequently, on application, the polycondensation of tannins with aldehydes. MALDI-TOF appears to confirm this by the presence of small but detected peaks at 772 Da (in theory 769) and 902 Da (see Figure 2), respectively a flavonoid dimer and a flavonoid trimer both monoacetylated.

The MALDI-TOF analysis of mimosa tannin extract (Figure 3) indicates the presence in the tannin of oligomers to the maximum of octamers (2333 Da) in line with the lower number average degree of polymerzation of 4.90 obtained by other means for this tannin [19,20], and the distribution obtained is shown in Table 2. The flavonoid repeating units present in this tannin extract are of type A and B as for quebracho but with a relatively important proportion of units of type C.

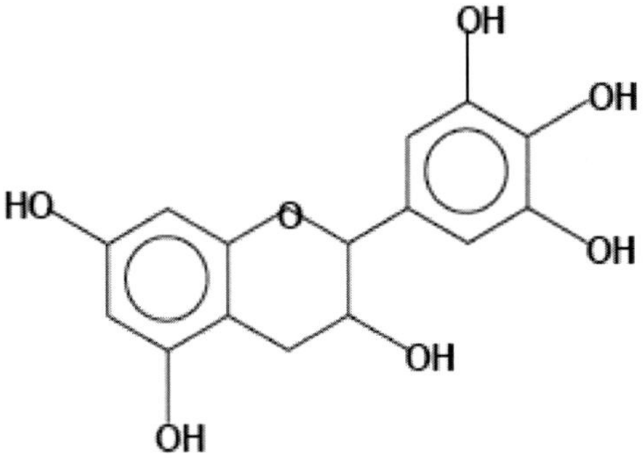

C

The correct equation to calculate the different possibilities does then become $M+Na^+ = 23(Na) + 2$ (endgroups, 2xH) + 272A + 288B + 304C (Table 2). Table 2 indicates that many valid combinations of different repeating units are possible. There are however some cases in which unequivocal assignement of the structure can indeed be done.

Table 2. MALDI fragmentation peaks for industrial mimosa tannin extract. Note that the predominant repeat units in this tannin is 288 Da, indicating that this tannin is predominantly a prorobinetinidin

M+Na+	M+Na+		Unit type			
(exp.)	(calc.)		A	B	C	
Dimers						
602	601		--	2	--	
Trimers						
858	857		2	1	--	
874	873		1	2	--	
		or	2	--	1	angular tannin
*890	889		1	1	1	
		or	--	3	--	
*906	905		--	2	1	angular tannin
		or	1	--	2	angular tannin
922	921		--	1	2	a “diangular” structure
Tetramers						
1147	1145		2	2	--	
		or	3	--	1	
1163	1161		1	3	--	
		or	2	1	1	
*1179	1177		--	4	--	
		or	1	2	1	
		or	2	--	2	
1195	1193		--	3	1	angular tannin
		or	1	1	2	
1211	1209		--	2	2	angular tannin
		or	1	--	3	a "diangular" structure
Pentamers						
1467	1465					
Hexamers						
1756	1753					
Heptamers						
2045	2041					
Octamers						
2333	2329					

*Dominant fragment.

This is the case of angular tannins, namely oligomers in which a repeating unit of type C is bound through both its 6 and its 8 A-ring sites to A and B type units, with its C4 sites equally bound and unbound.

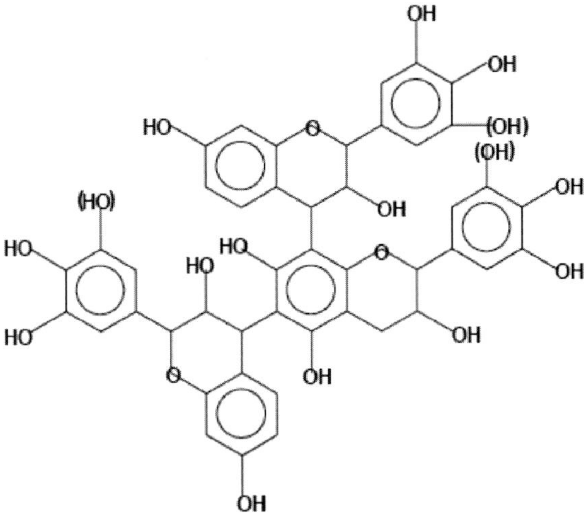

These structures were discovered by high temperature ^{1}H NMR on rotational isomers [1,21,22]. The MALDI-TOF analysis also shows clearly the existence of fragments of angular tannins by the presence of definite peaks at 906, 1195 and 1211 Da. Their presence in mimosa tannin extract, where it is known that angular tannins exist, underlines their total absence in the otherwise similar quebracho tannin extract. It is not possible to say with the data available if angular tannins are naturally absent in quebracho tannin extract or if their absence is the result of the fairly heavy sulphitation this tannin has always to undergo for solubility reasons. The high relative intensity of the very marked peaks of the angular trimer at 906 Da and of the angular tetramer at 1195 Da in Figure 3 indicate that the frequence of angular structures in mimosa tannin extract is rather high. The lower viscosity of solutions of mimosa extract, much lower than solutions of quebracho tannin extract at equal concentration and under the same conditions, is not only due then to mimosa tannin lower number average degree of polymerization [19,20] but also to its more "branched" structure as opposed to the fundamentally "linear" structure of quebracho tannin. The susceptibility to hydrolysis of the interflavonoid bond of quebracho tannin remarked about above, in relation to the well-known total lack of it in mimosa tannin [2,18] , could then be ascribed also to this conformational difference between the two otherwise similar profisetinidin/prorobinetinidin tannins. This observation is of importance indicating for the first time that the difference in spacial structure is one of the main contributing reasons why two tannins of fundamentally very similar chemical composition (they are both profisetinidins/prorobinetinidins) do behave rather differently under several aspects. In the case of mimosa tannin of even greater interest is the the existence of a well definite and clear peak at 1211 Da: this is formed by 4 flavonoid repeating units two of which are of type C. If the sample was just a dimer one could claim that this was a procyanidin fragment, namely two C-type units linked 4,8 and conclude that a certain number of separate procyanidin units exists in mimosa tannin. That the fragment is instead a tetramer first of all negates that the phloroglucinol A-ring units can exist in mimosa tannin as separate procyanidins, but confirms that in this tannin such units are exclusively present reacted as an "angular" within the profisetinidin/prorobinetinidin predominant structures. Second, this fragment is clearly then a di-"angular" unit never observed or isolated before, again confirming the high frequence of angular structures in mimosa tannin.

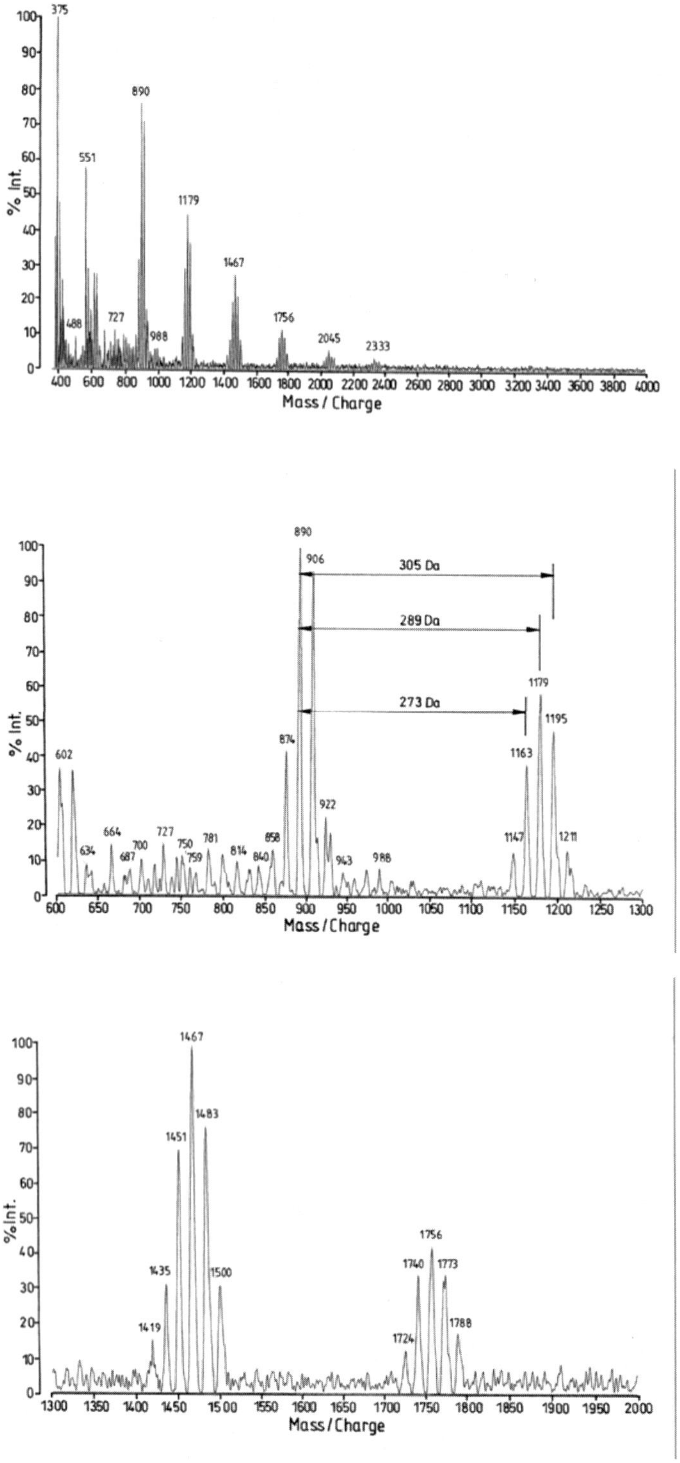

Figure 3. MALDI mass spectrum of (a) natural mimosa tannin extract. (b) details of the 600-1300 Da range with indication of the relevant 288 Da repeat unit. (c) details of the 1300-2000 Da range.

A further interesting difference between mimosa and quebracho tannins can be observed by comparing the results in Figures 1 and 3 and Tables 1 and 2. In quebracho the predominant repeat unit has 272 Da (a type A unit), while in mimosa the predominant repeating unit is of 288 Da (a type B unit). This is particularly evident in the higher oligomers for the two tannins. Based on this, on the dominant fragments for different oligomers and on the relative intensities for the different peaks in Figures 1 and 3 it is possible to conclude that quebracho tannin is composed of between 20% and 30% of B units and of between 70% and 80% of A-type units. Quebracho is then predominantly a profisetinidin. Mimosa tannin instead is composed predominantly of between 50% and 70% of type B units and only of between 15% and 25% of type A units. Mimosa tannin is then predominantly a prorobinetinidin. It is also interesting to note that the number average degree of polymerization obtained from the MALDI-derived oligomer distributions yield values of 6.25 and 5.4 for quebracho and mimosa tannins respectively. Considering the variability of such natural materials, these values compare well with the DP_n values of 6.74 and 4.9 for the same tannins obtained by ^{13}C NMR and other techniques [19,20].

It must be born in mind that in some mainly prorobinetinidin/profisetinidin tannins the structure of the oligomers present is not fixed and immutable. There are almost pure procyanidin oligomers present mixed with pure prorobitenidin oligomers, mixed with hybrid prorobinetinidin/profisetinidin oligomers and with hybrid prorobinetinidin/ profisetinidin/procyanidin oligomers. An example of this is the case of the flavonoids from the bark of *Acacia mangium*, a species now extensively cultivated in Brazil and in South East Asia (Figure 4). This tannin presents two main "mixed" patterns of oligomers overimposed one on the other. As an example (Figure 4):

(1) Starting from the 1210 peak if one adds 289 Da the series 1210-1499-1788-2076.7-2365.4 etc up to the 3535 peak (that is very small) is observed in Figure 4, thus a pure prorobinetinidin pattern of trimers, tetramers, pentamers etc., up to oligomers comprised of 13 repeating units (although their proportion is quite low). This indicates that pure prorobinetidin oligomers , thus pure B type units linked together with perhaps one or two C units but without any A units linked to them do indeed exist.

(2) Starting again from the 1210 Da peak also a pattern adding 272-273 Da is present, namely 1210 - 1483 - 1756 Da but this stops there and the intensity of the peaks is lower, thus they are less abundant. This is hence a mixed prorobinetinidin/profisetinidin series of oligomers. The fisetinidin repeating unit is less abundant, as also indicated by the intensity of these peaks. Adding a 289 Da B unit then one passes to the 2044.9 mass oligomer. Another 289 unit will bring to the 2334 oligomer. Equally, starting from the 1499 peak adding 272-273 Da one also gets the sequence 1499 - 1772 - 2044.9 and again it stops there. Adding a 289 Da unit to the 2044.9 peak and oligomer one gets the peak at 2334 Da, indicating clearly that fisetinidins and robinetinidins mixed oligomers, where both units of type A and B are linked together exist (still with a majority of B units). It also indicates that some peaks such as the 2044.9 Da, for example ,are the superposition of two different types of oligomers.

(3) In Figure 4 there is also a very interesting, clearly identifiable, very low intensity pattern 752 - 1041 - 1330 - 1635 - 1924 - 2217 - 2506 where all the peaks are

separated by a 288-290 repeating motive except for the 1330 - 1635 one that is separated by a 304 Da C unit. This is a definite series of angular oligomers up to at least a 7 repeating units one. Thus, a series of angular tannins of 3+1, 3+2 and 3+3 robinetinidin units linked to a branching C unit. (an angular tannin means there is a C branching unit). It is angular if there are two flavonoid units linked both to the A ring of the C unit, it is branched if on top of this there is another flavonoid series attached to the C4 of the C unit. The pattern indicated is almost certainly a series of angular or branched oligomers of a length never determined before. By the way, whenever there is a C unit linked to A and B units one could have an angular tannin. However in cases where several C-units linked to each other are present, then one has definetely a prodelphinidin or procyanidin oligomer. Furthermore the 289 Da unit can equally be a prorobinetinidin but also a catechin unit, hence one could also have angular tannins with the 289 B unit if one of the -OHs is situated on the A ring rather than the B-ring.

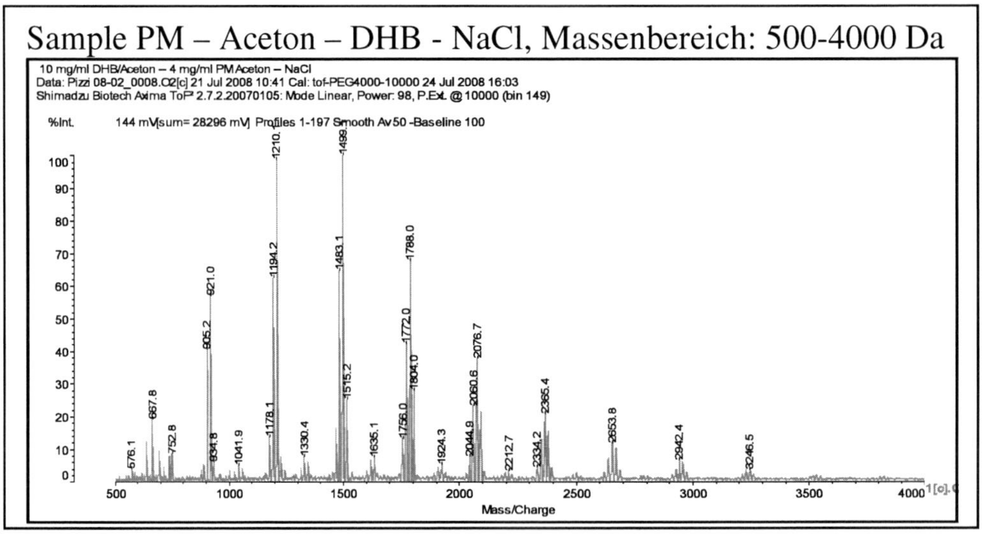

Figure 4. MALDI mass spectrum of ***Acacia mangium*** tannin extract.

Procyanidin and Prodelphinidin Type Polyflavonoids

An example of procyanidin type tannins, in which the great majority, almost the totality of the flavonoid units are linked C4 to C8 are pine tannin and mangrove polyflavonoid tannins. The greater majority of all polyflavonoids fall into this category. They are a class very diffuse, present in many foodstuffs, apple skins, fruit juices etc. Mangrove polyflavonoids are the one that have been examined most in depth as regards their oligomeric structure.

Mangrove tannins can come from a variety of different *Rhizophora* species. In the case of *Rhizophora apiculata* the tannins found are of the procyanidin type [23,24]. These are the most common tannins existing in nature. *Rhizophora apiculata* mangrove tannin most common monomer constituents are catechin, epicatechin, epigallocatechin and epicatechin gallate with molecular weights (MW) respectively of 290.3 Da, 290.3 Da, 306.3 Da and 442.4 Da.

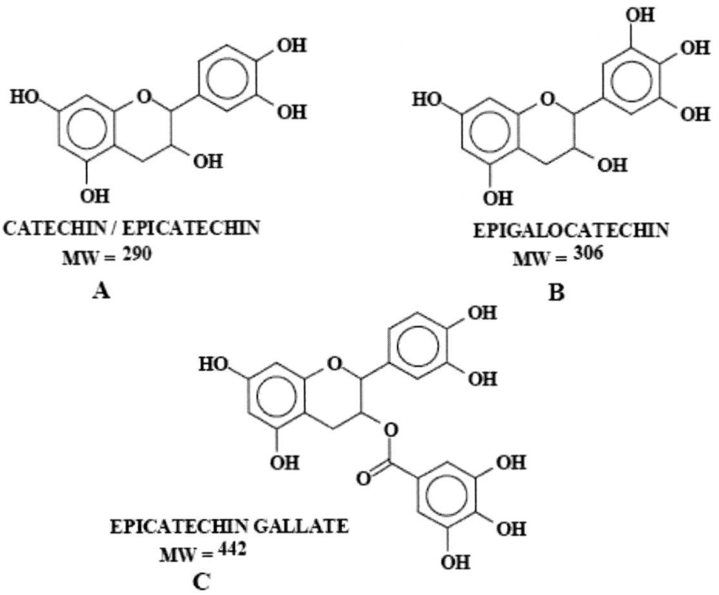

For *Rhizophora apiculata* mangrove tannins, the MALDI –TOF spectra in Figure 5a,b,c indicates clearly that alternate repeating units with mass increments of 264-264.9 Da occur. These have not been identified by previous analysis by other methods [23-26] in mangrove tannins indicating possibly the presence also of other monomers than those shown in Figure 1 and/or different combinations of various structures. Combination of the masses of the catechinin monomers shown in Figure 5 can be used to calculate the masses of the oligomer peaks in the spectra according to the expression M+Na+ = 23(Na) + 2 (endgroups, 2xH) + 290.3 (-2H)A + 306.3 (-2H)B + 442.4 (-2H)C (Table 3). The only problem about this is the presence of a repeating structure the MW of which is regular at 264.0 – 264.9 Da.

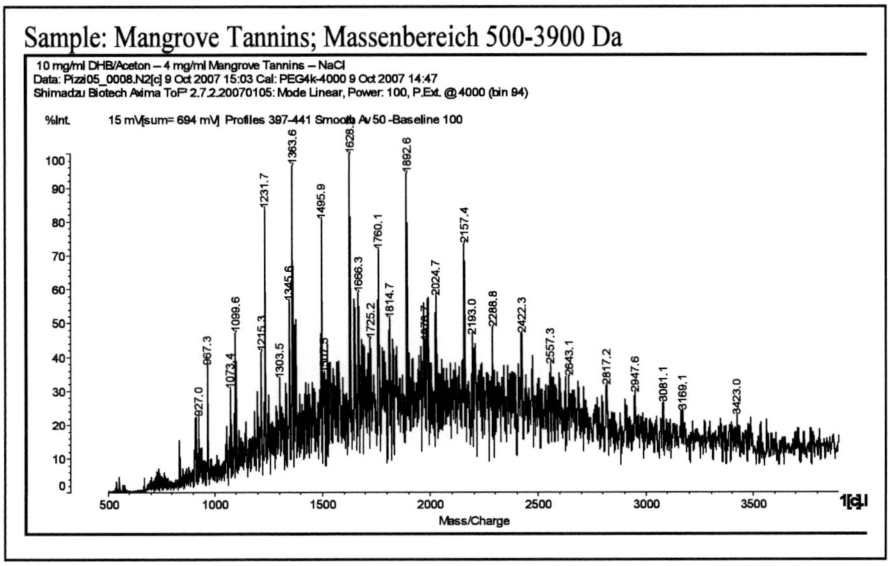

Figure 5. (Continued).

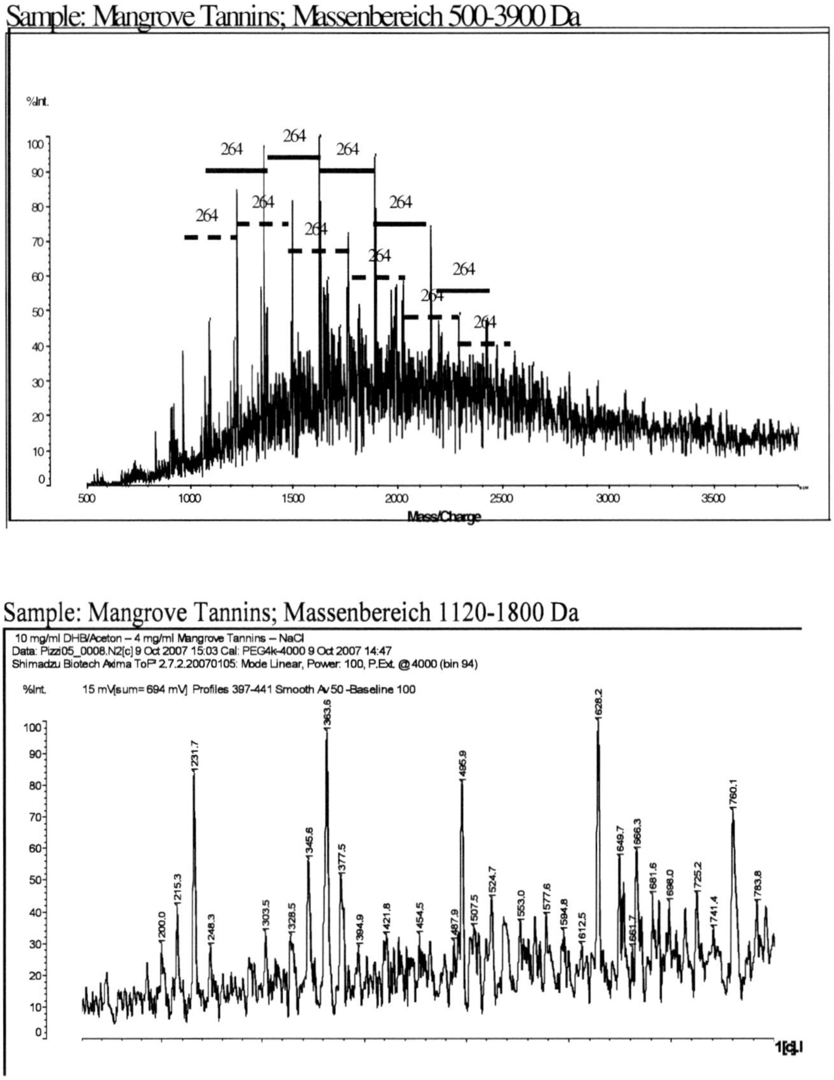

Figure 5. MALDI mass spectrum of (a) mixed *Rhizophora apiculata* mangrove tannin extract, 500-3900 Da range. (b) indication of the relevant 264 Da repeat unit.. (c) details of the 1120-1800 Da range.

This unit has not been identified before, and we will call it here structure D. Calculation of the MALDI masses indicate that certain peaks can only be explained by the presence of epicatechin gallate units in which the gallic acid residue has being removed of 274.3 Da (structure E), these being related to the unknown structure. The equation than becomes M+Na+ = 23(Na) + 2 (endgroups, 2xH) + 290.3 (-2H)A + 306.3 (-2H)B + 442.4 (-2H)C + 274.3 (-2H)E. In Table 3 are shown the results of the combination of monomer units forming the different oligomers observed by MALDI-TOF. It must be noticed that only very few of the dominant peaks (Figure 5a) can be explained only on the basis of the catechinic structures A, B and C. Some mass peaks however are not easily explained without the use of structure D. The majority of the dominant peaks are shown in Tables 4 and 5.

Table 3. MALDI fragmentation peaks for mixed *Rhizophora spp* mangrove tannin extract. Note that the predominant repeat unit in this tannin indicate that it is predominantly a procyanidin

M+Na+	M+Na+				Unit type	
(exp.)	(calc.)	A	B	C	D	E (C-gallic)
Da		290.3	306.3	442.4	264/265	274.3
835	841.9	--	--	--	--	3
927	921.9	1	2	--	--	--
967*	see Table 3					
1073.4	1074	--	2	1	--	--
1099.6*	1094.1	1	--	2	--	--
or	1098.6	--	--	--	2	2
1200	1200		3		1	
1215.3	1210.2	--	3	--	--	1
or	1210.1	--	1	--2		
or	1210.2	2	2			
1231.7*	1226.2	1	3	--	--	--
or						
1248.3	1242.2	--	4			
1328.5	1330.3	1	1	1	--	1
1345.6	1346.2	--	--	3		
or	1346.3	2	1	1		
or	1346.3	--	2	1	--	1
1363*	1362.3	1	2	1		
1377.5	1378.3	--	3	1		
1454.5	1450.5	4	--	--	--	1
1487.9	1482.5	--	3	--	--	2
1507.5	1507.2	--	4	--	1	
1649.7	1650.5	--	1	3		
or	1650.6	2	2	1		
1666.3	1666.3	1	3	1		
1681.6	1682.6	--	4	1		
1725.2	1722.8	4	--	--	--	2
1741.4	1738.8	5	--	--	--	1
or	1738.7	1	--	2	--	2
	1738.8	3	1	--	--	2
1892.6*	1890.9	4	--	1	--	1
2193	2195.2	6	--	1		
2557.3	2556.2	--	6	1	1	
2817.2	2819.7	3	2	3		
or	2819.6	1	1	5		
2947.6	2940.0	--	6	--	--	4
or	2940.0	2	5	--	--	3
	2939.9	--	4	2	--	3
3081	3076.1	4	3	1	--	2
or	3076.0	2	2	3	--	2
	3076.0	--	3	3	--	3
3169.1	3164.2	5	--	2	--	3
or	3164.3	7	1	--	--	3

*Dominant fragment.

Table 4. MALDI fragmentation peaks for mixed *Rhizophora spp* mangrove tannin extract. Note that the predominant repeat units in this tannin is 528-530 Da, indicating that in its main series of peaks this tannin may present pure profisetinidin oligomers as predominant components

$M+Na^+$ (exp.) *Da*	$M+Na^+$ (calc.)	Unit type A *290.3*	B *306.3*	C *442.4*	E *274.3*	D *264-264.9*
835	841.9	--	--	--	3	--
1099.6*	1105.6	--	--	--	3	1
1363.6*	1362.3	1	2	1		
1628.2*	1628.2	1	2	1	--	1
1892.6*	1892.6	1	2	1	--	2
2157.4*	2157.4	1	2	1	--	3
2422.3*	2422.3	1	2	1	--	4

*Dominant fragment.

Table 5. MALDI fragmentation peaks for mixed *Rhizophora spp* mangrove tannin extract. Note that the predominant repeat units in this tannin is still 528-530 Da, indicating that in this MALDI series of peaks this tannin may present predominantly a profisetinidin component but linked to procyanidins units too

$M+Na^+$ (exp.) Da	$M+Na^+$ (calc.)	Unit type A 290.3	B 306.3	C 442.4	E (C-gallic) 274.3	D 264-264.9	DPn Tot	DPn E unit
967.3	967.7			1	1	1 (-2xO)	3	1
1231.7*	1226.2	1	3				4	-
1495.9*	1497.7			1	1	3 (-2xO)	5	3
1760.1*	1756	1	3			2	6	2
2024.7*	2025.7			1	1	5 (-2xO)	7	5
2288.8*	2285.8	1	3			4	8	4
2557.3	2553.7			1	1	7 (-2xO)	9	7

*Dominant fragment.

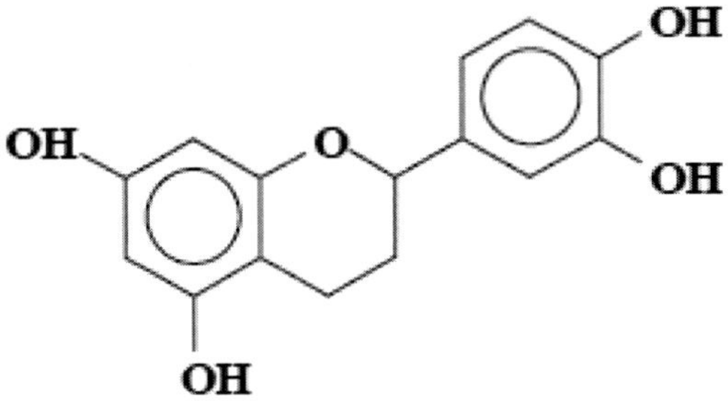

E

274·3

Structure D cannot be inserted in the equation simply because no known flavonoid structure could be found with such a molecular weight. However, this structure partecipates markedly, from peak intensities in Figure 5a its partecipation being predominant to the formation of the mangrove tannin oligomers. Two series of the most intense MALDI mass peaks rely on the repetition of this 264 Da structure. Thus, the oligomers of the series of peaks at 835 Da, 1099 Da, 1363 Da, 1628 Da, 1892 Da, 2157 Da, 2422 Da are separated by the 264 Da motive recurring six times. Equally, the oligomers of the series of peaks at 967 Da, 1231 Da, 1495 Da, 1760 Da, 2024 Da, 2288 Da, 2557 Da are separated by the 264 Da motive again recurring six times. Which means that attached to the starting oligomer to an hexamer of the 264 Da unit is progressively linked to the starting oligomer, whatever this may be. Tables 4 and 5 show the interpretation of the two predominant series present.

It is of interest to find out what structure corresponds to 264 Da. No known monoflavonoid corresponds to such a structure. If one takes structure E however, for a E repeating unit at 272.3 Da, the difference with 264 Da is always of 8 Da, that does not correspond to the mass of any leaving functional group. However, if one considers that there is an –OH group less in a dimer formed by two joined E structures this will give the loss of 16 Da, hence of an oxygen. It means that the repeating unit of the system is not 264 Da but appears to be 264x2 = 528 Da. Thus, the repeating unit is a dimer of structure E whith a –OH group missing. The unit has a single phenolic –OH group which has been lost, as shown below, the alcoholic –OH groups in C3 having already been lost at the separation of the gallic acid.

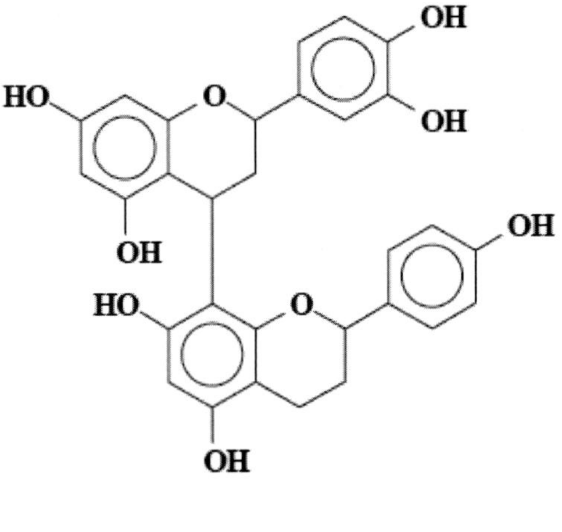

Thus, in Table 4 is shown the main series of dominant MALDI masses indicating that oligomers of this unit appear to occur in *apiculata* mangrove tannins. This is the most likely case seeing the regular progression from trimer to octamer in Table 4.Thus, mixed oligomers where a procyanidin oligomer formed by structures of type A, B and C (1363.6 Da) is linked to progressively increasing number of D structure oligomers are possible. The results in Table 3 of the second more important series of recurrent MALDI peaks clearly confirms that mixed procyanidin and D oligomers covalently linked do exist in such mangrove tannins because none of the masses of the series 835 Da, 1099 Da, 1363 Da, 1628 Da, 1892 Da, 2157 Da, 2422 Da can be explain without having units of structures A, B and C linked to the D oligomers. It appears most likely then that both pure oligomers of the two types as well as linked mixed oligomers do coexist in this tannin.

A mainly prodelphinidin tannin, namely pecan nut tannin extract was also examined (Figure 6) [33]. The main prodelphinidin repeat unit has a molar mass of 306 Da and the main fragments found arrived only up to trimers (304+304+288+2+23 = 921 Da). This unusual result leads to two consequences. In pecan nut tannin extract robinetinidin units are linked within the prodelphinidin main oligomers, and that the interflavonoid bond of prodelphinidins is particularly prone to cleavage (this is known to be so). It means that the finding of trimers only , when the number average degree of polymeryzation of this tannin is known to be of 5.50 [19,20] , indicates that the cleavage of the interflavonoid bond here is mainly a fabrication of the method of analysis used and if MALDI-TOF has to be used in this case much milder conditions needed to be used.

In conclusion MALDI-TOF is a suitable method for examining polyflavonoid tannin oligomers and one that is able to determine through this technique facts on polyflavonoid tannins which are already known by using other approaches. It also appears capable however to determine aspects of the structure and characteristics of the tannins which are too difficult to determine by other techniques.

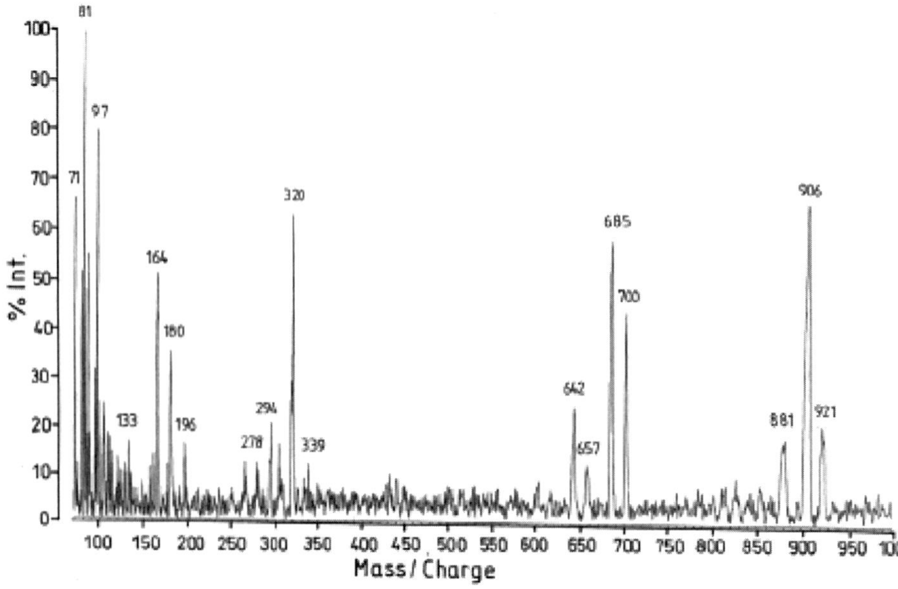

Figure 6. MALDI mass spectrum of natural pecan nut tannin extract.

In the present investigation of the two major commercial polyflavonoid tannins it has been possible to determine by MALDI-TOF that: (i) mimosa tannin is predominantly composed of prorobinetinidins while quebracho is predominantly composed of profisetinidins, that (ii) mimosa tannin is heavily branched due to the presence of considerable proportions of "angular" units in its structure while quebracho tannin is almost completely linear. These structural differences also contribute to the considerable differences in viscoity of water solutions of the two tannins. (iii) the interflavonoid link is more easily hydrolysable, and does appear to sometime hydrolyse in quebracho tannin and profisetinidins, partly due to the linear structure of this tannin, and confirming NMR findings that this tannin is subject to polymerisation / depolymerisation equilibrium. This is not the case for mimosa tannin in which the interflavonoid link is completely stable to hydrolysis. (iv) Sulphitation has been shown to influence the detachment of catechol B-rings much more than pyrogallol-type B-rings. (v) The distribution of tannin oligomers, and the tannins number average degree of polymerisation obtained by MALDI-TOF appear to compare well with the results obtained by other techniques.

Colloidal State of Polyflavonoid Extracts

Raw polyflavonoid extracts present colloidal behaviour. Of importance is the presence in the polyflavonoid extracts of consistent amounts of polymeric carbohydrates (in general hemicellulose fragments, sometime called hydrocolloid gums) extracted together with the tannins. These are always present unless the tannin has undergone special purification, such as the case of their use for medical and pharmaceutical use. These polymeric carbohydrates contribute to maintain the water solutions of polyflavonoid tannin extracts in colloidal state, rendering sometime possible reactions on the tannin that otherwise are not or are less likely to occur in just a water solution. The reactions that can occur under these conditions appear to rely on the surfactant-like action of the hydrocolloid gums and also on the tannin oligomers themselves, hence on their capability to form micelles in water. The ζ -potential of a solution is correlated to the extent of its colloidal state. In Table 6 are reported the The ζ -potentials of water solutions of four industrial polyflavonoid tannin extracts, of a monomer model compound, catechin, and of catechin in gum arabic to imitate the solution of a tannin extract. These show that the colloidal state of a water solution of polyflavonoid tannin is quite definite, but very variable according to the tannin type. Thus, pecan nut pith tannin extract which is known to contain a very small proportion of hydrocolloid gums, around 4%, is clearly much less colloidal than mimosa or quebracho tannin extracts where the amount of hydrocolloid gums is much higher between 10 and 20%. Thus, it must be pointed out that both reactions and structural modifications of the tannins that occur independently of the colloidal state of the solution, as well as reactions that are dependent on their colloidal state , may greatly contribute to the performance of the polyflavonoid extracts. This area has been explored only for application to wood adhesives [27], but no work on this appears to have been carried out in the neutraceutical or pharmaceutical fields where it may be also of importance.

Table 6. Comparative ζ-potentials measurements in mV of natural tannin extracts

Mimosa tannin extract 40% water solution	11.3
Quebracho tannin extract 40% water solution	14.5
Pine tannin extract 40% water solution	2.4
Pecan nut tannin extract 40% water solution	4.9
Catechin water solution	0
Gum arabic 23% water solution	5.2
Catechin/gum arabic mix 23% warter solution	5.2

RHEOLOGY OF INDUSTRIAL POLYFLAVONOIDS

Polyflavonoid tannin extracts have been produced and used industrially for many applications since the end of the 19th century [1,28]. Among these uses are the early one as dyes for silk, and their predominat use to-day as tanning agents for the manufacture of leather [28] as well as their use as wood adhesives [1] plus the growing proportion of food, medical, pharmaceutical and nutracetical applications. Considering the relevance of their rheological characteristics on their main fields of industrial application the literature is almost completely devoid of rheological studies on these materials. It is for this reason that what is known of their rheology is worthwhile to know. Some early rheology work has concentrated on tannins extracted in non-traditional manner, different from industrial practice [29-31] while more recent work investigated the rheology of the major commercially avalaible polyflavonoid tannin extracts [32] extracted by standard industrial practice.

Figures 7-10 show plots of elastic modulus G' and viscous modulus G" over various concentrations (20% -50%) of water solutions of four natural polyflavonoid extracts, namely mimosa, quebracho, pine and pecan nut tannin extracts [32]. Dynamic oscillatory measurements were carried out in order to examine the shear sensitive associations of molecules and clusters at low deformations. Dynamic moduli (storage modulus G' and loss modulus G") of the different extracts were measured as a function of strain amplitude at a fixed frequency to obtain the linear viscoelastic region. The strain sweep for the four natural extracts at various concentrations (20%, 30%, 40%, 50%) measured at 1 rad s^{-1} frequency are shown in Figures 7-10. These figures show that in general G" > G' for the solutions of all the tannin and hence that the solutions of industrial polyflavonoid tannin extracts behave as viscous liquids even at the higher (50%) concentration. This indicates that commercial tannin extracts are primarily composed of relatively short oligomers which do not appear to show the entanglement and elasticity of higher molecular weight polymers. This is supported by measures of number and weight average molecular masses for the four tannins obtained by different techniques [19,20] which show that typical number average degree of polymerization (DP_n) of mimosa, quebracho, pine and pecan industrial tannin extracts [19,20] are respectively of 4.9, 6.7, 5.9 and 5.5. A level of entanglement is however possible for the higher molecular mass fractions of the tannins if one considers that typical values of the weight average degree of polymerization (DP_w) are of respectively 8.8, 12.3, 10.9, 9.5 for mimosa, quebracho, pine and pecan tannins, and the great number of polar hydroxy groups present on these molecules [19,20,33].

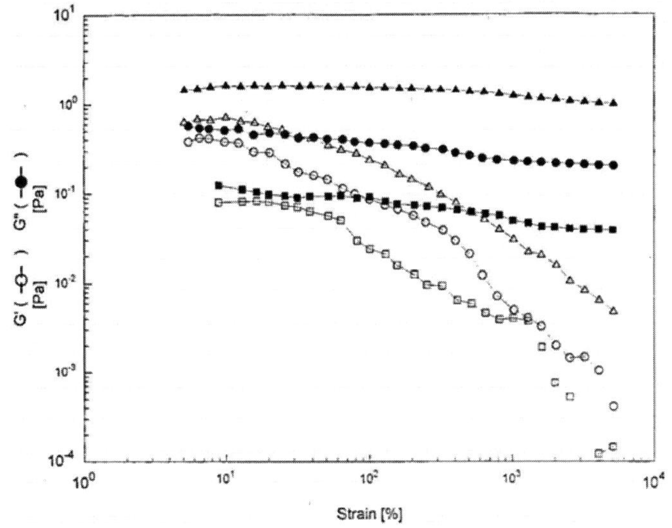

Figure 7. Strain sweeps at ω = 1 rad s^{-1} for mimosa tannin extract solutions at different concentrations: (□) 30%, (o) 40%, (Δ) 50% concentration. (o) G′ curves; (•) G″ curves.

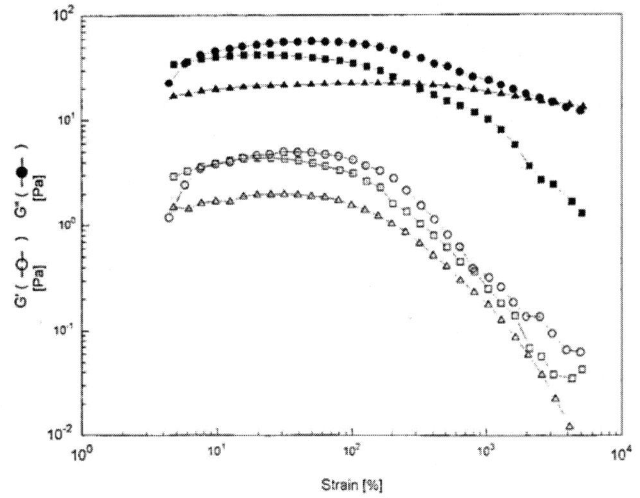

Figure 8. Strain sweeps at ω = 1 rad s^{-1} for quebracho tannin extract solutions at different concentrations: (□) 30%, (o) 40%, (Δ) 50% concentration. (o) G′ curves; (•) G″ curves.

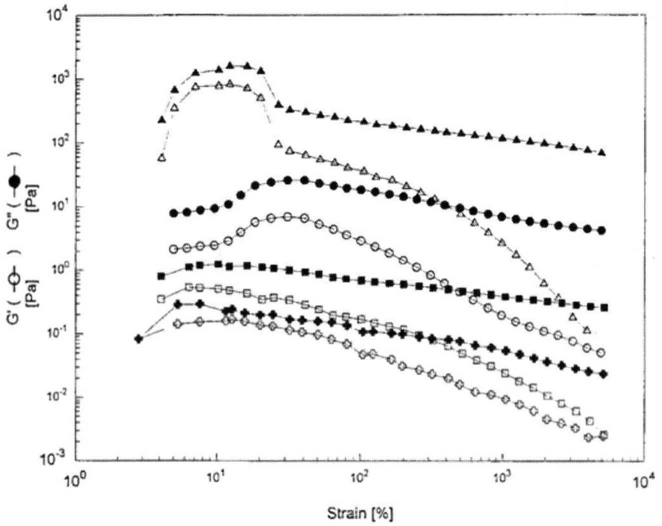

Figure 9. Strain sweeps at ω = 1 rad s^{-1} for pine tannin extract solutions at different concentrations: (♣) 20% ; (□) 30%, (o) 40%, (Δ) 50% concentration. (o) G′ curves; (•) G″ curves.

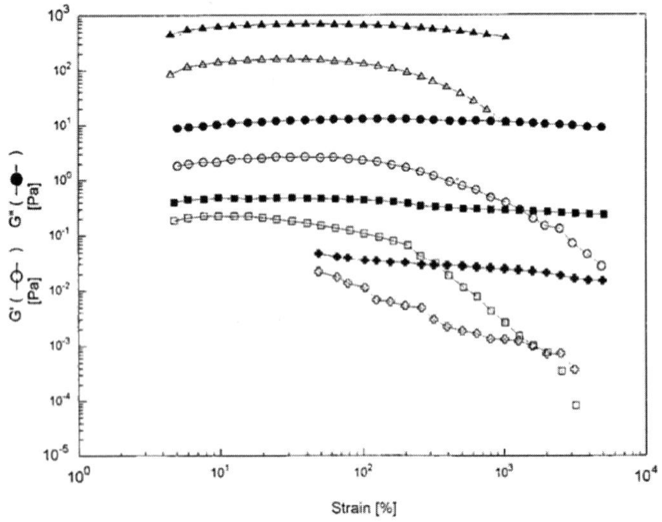

Figure 10. Strain sweeps at ω = 1 rad s^{-1} for pecan tannin extract solutions at different concentrations: (♣) 20% ; (□) 30%, (o) 40%, (Δ) 50% concentration. (o) G′ curves; (•) G″ curves.

These figures also indicate that in the low percentage strain region both moduli appear to be fairly independent of the applied strain amplitude as shown from the almost parallel trend of the two moduli curves. However, when the percentage strain increases the value of G’ starts to decrease significantly in relation to the value of G”, a trend which becomes slightly more evident the lower is the concentration studied. Furthermore, the G### linearity limit appears to decrease somewhat with increasing concentration. This indicates that, notwithstanding the purely viscous liquid behaviour of these tannin extract solutions, (i) microstructures exists for these extracts in solution , a fact supported by the known colloidal interactions for these materials already reported [27,29-32,34-39], and (ii) that such microstructures are labile as they are significantly broken with applied shear, leading to a critical strain after which a significant decline in the elastic modulus results, a fact supported by the well known thixotropic behaviour of concentrated, commercial polyflavonoid tannin extracts water solutions [1,27,30,34,36]. For the two higher concentrations used, and also for the 30% concentration, with only one exception, as the extracts where used at their natural pH which is in the 4.2-5.1 range there was no case where G’ > G” and no concentration occurred at which G’ = G”, as this behaviour has been associated with much higher alkalinity ranges [30].

While these are general trends for all the four polyflavonoid tannins, some important difference between the tannins also exists, mainly based on their differences in viscosity. Firstly, G′ starts decreasing according to the different typical molecular masses of each tannin: to a higher molecular mass corresponds a later start in the decrease of G′. The main difference occurs for pine tannin extract solutions where two plateau for G’ and G” occurs with this becoming more evident the higher is the tannin solution concentration. The existence of another transition at lower percentage strain also indicates the presence of another type of labile microstructure. Secondary forces associations between tannin oligomers and oligomeric sugars, derived from degraded hemicelluloses which are always present in consistant proportions in these extracts, are well known [1,19,20,30]. They have often caused in the past the incorrect determination of absurdly high molecular masses for tannin oligomers due to the formation of ionic polymers between tannins and carbohydrate oligomers. This transition is particularly evident in Figure 9 for the pine tannin extract. It is not possible to conclude from the available data if this is the cause of the additional transition in pine tannin, or rather if the affinity of carbohydrates for tannins is the transition that occurs for all the four tannins. The decrease of these secondary forces associations at higher percentage strains will cause the system to appear to behave as composed of species of lower average molecular mass with the consequent trend observed for G’ in Figures 7-10.

Figures 11-14 show the variation of G’ and G” with frequency for the four tannins each at four different concentrations. The lower the slope of the curves the closer to a newtonian behaviour is the behaviour of the tannin extract solution. For all the tannins and for all the concentrations examined G’ values are smaller than G” and all G” values are relatively low and increase progressively with increasing frequency: the tannin extracts are behaving essentially as a viscous liquid as discussed earlier, the only exceptions being the tannin extract solutions at 20% concentration where G’ and G” cross-over points do indeed occur. For concentrations higher than 20% this appears to suggest that the tannin oligomers are well separated and that, once the interactions with the carbohydrate are eliminated or minimized, there is little possibility of molecular interaction and entanglement, even at the higher concentration.

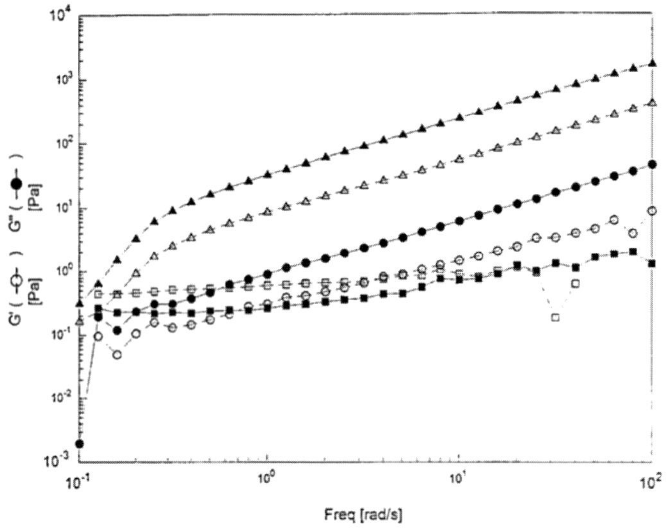

Figure 11. Elastic modulus (G′) and viscous modulus (G″) as a function of frequency (ω) for mimosa tannin extract solutions at different concentrations: (□) 30%, (o) 40%, (Δ) 50% concentration. (o) G′ curves; (•) G″ curves.

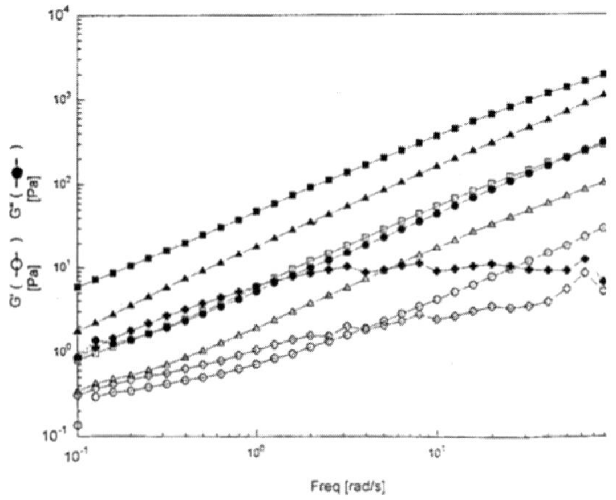

Figure 12. Elastic modulus (G′) and viscous modulus (G″) as a function of frequency (ω) for quebracho tannin extract solutions at different concentrations: (♣) 20% ; (□) 30%,(o) 40%, (Δ) 50% concentration. (o) G′ curves; (•) G″ curves.

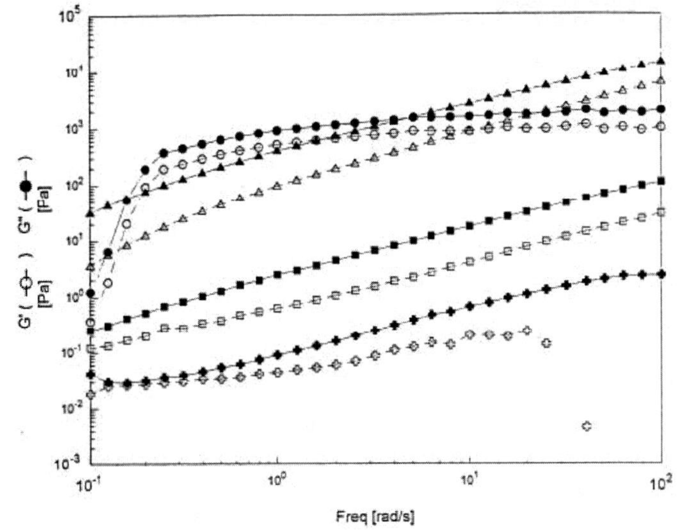

Figure 13. Elastic modulus (G′) and viscous modulus (G″) as a function of frequency (ω) for pine tannin extract solutions at different concentrations: (♣) 20% ; (□) 30%, (o) 40%, (Δ) 50% concentration. (o) G′ curves; (•) G″ curves.

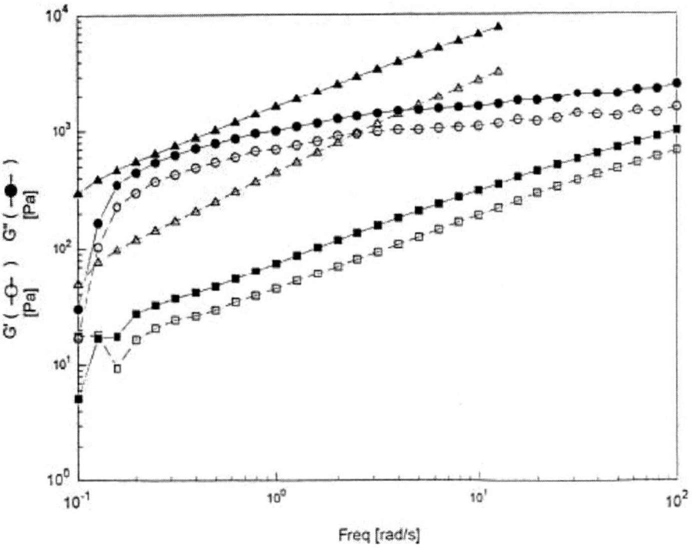

Figure 14. Elastic modulus (G′) and viscous modulus (G″) as a function of frequency (ω) for pecan tannin extract solutions at different concentrations: (♣) 20% ; (□) 30%, (o) 40%, (Δ) 50% concentration. (o) G′ curves; (•) G″ curves.

Thus, is there little interaction in the tannin extracts, resulting in smaller elastic contributions, or must one consider also other parameters? In this respect there are some differences in the curves of the four natural extracts. Considering the differences in percentage strain which had to be used for the different tannin solutions it can be noticed that the value of the two moduli are quite different passing from one tannin to the other (mimosa and quebracho appear for example to have have similar G' and G" values; in reality this is not the case as the two figures are respectively at 100% and 10% strain respectively (Figures 11, 12). This partly reflects the level of molecular association occurring in each different extract. However, (Figure 13) in the pine tannin extract solutions the differences in value between G' and G", at the same imposed frequency, are smaller than for the other three tannins, and the value of both moduli is higher (Figure 13). This means that at parity of conditions the elastic component of a pine tannin extract solutions is both in absolute and proportionally greater than in the solutions of the other tannin extracts. This indicates that the determining parameters as regards the elastic response of a tannin extract solution are both (i) the greater average molecular mass of the tannin as well as (ii) the intensity of the tannin interaction with the carbohydrate oligomers present in the extract, which is related to both the amount of carbohydrate oligomers present and to their average molecular mass as well as to (i) above, however feeble such interactions might be. The first of these two parameters would lead to pine and quebracho tannin solutions having the higher moduli values, followed by pecan tannin extract and mimosa tannin extract (which is indeed the case if one considers the differences in percentage strain which had to be used, and the average molecular masses reported above [19,20]). The second of these two parameters would place the elastic response of the tannin as highest for pine and quebracho (the first mainly but not only for the higher proportion of carbohydrates, and the second for their and their carbohydrates higher molecular mass), followed by pecan (the carbohydrates content of which is very low) and last mimosa. In Figures 11-14 pine tannins and quebracho are the ones with higher numerical values of elastic response (if one considers the differences in percentage strain which had to be used) and pine also presenting the higher proportional value, followed by pecan and by mimosa.

Figures 11-14 also indicate that G' and G" present a pronounced frequency dependence for mimosa and quebracho tannin extracts, as indicated by the sharper slope of the moduli curves. The same figures indicate that G' and G" present instead little or no frequency dependence for pine and pecan tannin extracts.

A case apart appears to be the 20% concentration case for the three tannins for which such a concentration was also used (mimosa was not used at 20% concentration). A G' and G" cross-over point (G' = G", and then at increasing frequency G' > G") occurs for all the three tannin extracts, as it also occurs for mimosa tannin solutions at 30% concentration, in all four cases at the extreme range of the frequency used (Figures 11-14). This again confirms that on top of the effect of the pH [30] , the viscoelastic response of the tannin extracts obtained in these cases is due to intermolecular associations. It is a very clear indication that molecular associations between tannin molecules, and particularly between tannin molecules and carbohydrates to form labile structures of greater apparent molecular mass by either colloidal or other interactions, do indeed occur. An example of the behaviour of a solution of a polymeric carbohydrate, such as gum arabic, at the same four concentrations used for the tannins (Figure 15) indicates both a clear rubbery plateau at the two higher concentrations, but also that G' = G" cross-over points occur. At the two lower concentrations (20%-30%), at the extreme of the frequency range used, it is is indeed the value of G' which becomes higher than the value of G", imitating what seen for the tannin extracts at the same concentration, again confirming the partecipation of carbohydrate oligomers in imparting under certain conditions viscoelastic behaviour to tannin extract solutions, a purified tannin without any carbohydrates rather behaving as a viscous liquid only [37-39].

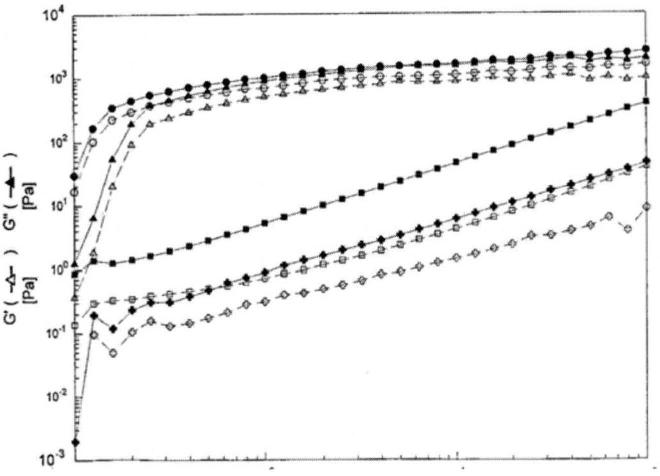

Figure 15. Elastic modulus (G′) and viscous modulus (G″) as a function of frequency (ω) for gum arabic solutions at different concentrations: (♣) 20% ; (□) 30%, (o) 40%, (Δ) 50% concentration. (o) G′ curves; (•) G″ curves.

In conclusion commercial, industrially produced mimosa, quebracho, pine and pecan nut polyflavonoid tannin extracts water solutions of different concentrations were examined by rheometry by measuring dynamic moduli both as a function of strain amplitude and at varying frequency. The water solutions of these materials have been found to behave in general mainly as viscous liquids at the concentrations which are generally used for their main industrial applications [1,27,40]. Clear indications of viscoelastic response are also noticeable, among these the cross-over of the elastic and viscous moduli curves at the lower concentrations of the range investigated, with some differences being noticeable between each tannin and the others, pine and quebracho tannin extracts showing the more marked viscoelastic behaviour. Other than pH dependence (and related structural considerations), the parameters which were found to be of interest as regards the noticeable viscoelastic behaviour of the tannin extracts were the existence in the solutions of labile microstructures which can be broken by applied shear. This is supported by the well known thixotropic behaviour of concentrated, commercial polyflavonoid tannin extracts water solution [1,30,34,36]. Such microstructures appear to be due or (i) to the known colloidal interactions of these materials already reported [1,30,34,35,37-39,41], or (ii) to other types of secondary interactions [35,37-39] between tannin oligomers and particularly between tannin and carbohydrate oligomers present in the extracts. The latter is supported by the dependence of this effect from both the average molecular masses of the tannin and of the carbohydrate oligomers.

ANTI-OXYDANT CAPABILITY OF POLYFLAVONOIDS

The capability of phenols to produce rather stable phenoxyl radicals, capable by their presence of retarding or even inhibiting the progress of radical addition polymerisation is well known [42,43]. In the ambit of research on the improvement of antioxidant capabilities, natural phenolic and polyphenolic materials such as hydrolysable and polyflavonoid tannins, and their model compounds, have been shown by the use of stopped-flow techniques to be capable of similar, but rather more intense effects [44,45]. However, both a simpler to handle and more rapid technique to measure tannins antioxidant capabilities, as well as a screening of the antioxidant capabilities of a variety of different hydrolysable and polyflavonoid tannins has been developed.

Polyflavonoids contain an elevated number of phenolic hydroxyls and their characteristic structure lends itself to the stabilisation of radicals not only by mechanisms characteristic of all phenols but also by the existance of side reactions such as heterocycle pyran ring opening and others.

Electron spin resonance (ESR), among other techniques has been used with good results to study the reactions of radical formation and decay induced by bases and weak Lewis acids in polyflavonoid tannins [37-39,46] and their model compounds [38,45-47]. It is for this reason that ESR has been used as rapid technique for the determination of the antioxidant properties of polyflavonoids [45].

What has been studied is how (i) the structure of different tannins influences the rate of radical transfer from the stable 2,2-diphenyl-1-picrylhydrazyl (DPPH) radical to a tannin and the subsequent rate of radical decay of the phenoxyl radical formed; (ii) the effect of the presence or absence of solvent, and of the type of solvent; but it was mainly aimed at (iii) studying the rate of increase in phenoxyl radical concentration by light irradiation in different tannins, and the subsequent radical decay rate once the inducing light is removed. All these aspect refer to their antioxydanrt capacity.

The tannins used were commercial mimosa (*Acacia mearnsii* formerly *mollissima,* de Wildt) bark tannin extract, a mainly prorobinetinidin tannin; commercial quebracho (*Schinopsis balansae*, variety chaqueno) wood tannin extract, also a mainly prorobinetinidin tannin but with greater percentages od fisetinedin units in it; commercial pecan (*Carya illinoensis*) nut pith tannin extract, a almost totally prodelphinidin tannin; commercial gambier (*Uncaria gambir*) shoots tannin extract, commercial pine (*Pinus radiata*) bark tannin extract, both being mainly procyanidin type tannins. All these are polyflavonoid tannins, plus for comparison commercial oak (*Quercus spp.*) tannin extract, an hydrolysable tannin. Also the tannin extract of chestnut (*Castanea sativa*) wood, an hydrolysable tannin, was tested but far too variable results were obtained and thus the results for this tannin were not reported in the study [45].

One of the more necessary steps to take at the start of such a type of study is to define what is intended for antioxidant capabilities of a tannin. In relation to light-induced degradation of a material, to measure the antioxidant capabilities of any surface finish could be defined as the measurement of two different parameters. These are:

(i) The rate at which the tannin is able to form a radical; this is determined either by the rate of radical transfer from a pre-existing radical species to the tannin to form a more stable phenoxyl radical, or by the rate of radical formation on light irradiation of the tannin, and
(ii) The rate of radical decay of tannin phenoxyl radicals formed.

The first parameter defines the ease and readiness of the tannin in subtracting a radical from, for instance, the substrate; the easier and the more rapid this transfer is, the greater are the antioxidant capabilities of the tannin. The second parameter defines how stable is the tannin phenoxyl radical. Here two interpretations are possible: (i) in general the more stable is the radical, hence the slower is the rate of radical decay, the more marked is the inhibition of radical degradation of the substrate and hence the better are the antioxidant properties of the tannin, but (ii) in the case of tannin radicals considerably more reactive than the substrate, hence where radical termination reactions between two tannin radicals are favourite, the faster the rate of radical decay, hence the faster the quenching between themselves of the tannin radicals formed, the better are the antioxidant properties of the tannin. Cases (i) and (ii) define two different effects: while case (i) has general applicability in all cases, case (ii) might assume disproportionate importance in the case of experiments, like those reported here, in which the substrate is not present. This discussion is then limited at evaluating the importance of the radical decay reaction only from the point of view of case (ii): the slower the radical decay rate, the greater is the antioxidant power of the tannin. An example of the type of cumulative curve obtained is shown in Figures 16 and 17.

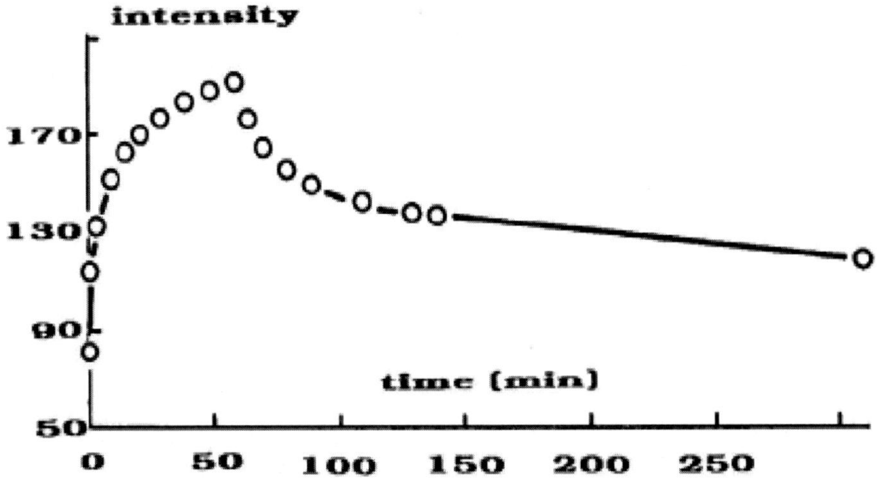

Figure 16. Intensity increase and decrease of the average of the two opposite symmetrical peaks representing the ESR signal during UV irradiation experiments of Quebracho flavonoid tannin extract powder without vacuum, in air, and in a quartz sample-holder. The initial part of the curve up to the maximum of intensity describes the increase in radical concentration as a function of time during irradiation while the decreasing intensity section describes the radical decay reaction from the moment the UV lamp has been switched off.

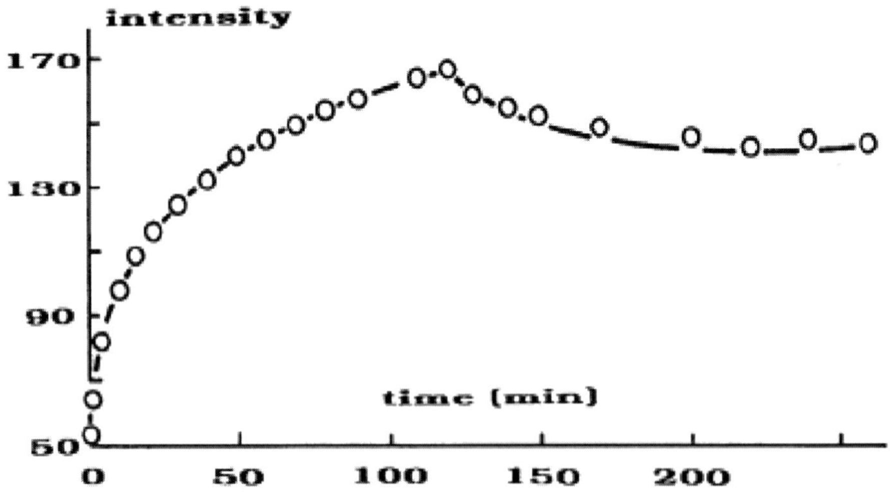

Figure 17. Intensity increase and decrease of the average of the two symmetrical, opposite peaks representing the ESR signal during UV irradiation experiments of Mimosa flavonoid tannin extract powder under vacuum and in a glass sample-holder. The initial part of the curve up to the maximum of intensity describes the increase in radical concentration as a function of time during irradiation while the decreasing intensity section describes the radical decay reaction from the moment the UV lamp has been switched off.

The increase in intensity of the ESR signal, which corresponds to the reaction of radical formation due to the irradiation of the three flavonoid and one hydrolysable tannins examined, can be modelled by a first order kinetic law of the type $I/I_o=ae^{kt}$ (Table 7).

Comparison of the rate constants or of the semitransformation times $t_{1/2}$ allows a few deductions, namely

1. In absence of vacuum, thus in presence of singlet oxygen, mimosa and quebracho tannins present the faster radical formation reaction, while pecan and oak tannins are somewhat slower.
2. In vacuum, thus in absence of singlet oxygen, mimosa tannin shows the more rapid rate of formation, followed by quebracho and pecan tannins which are almost comparable, finally followed by oak tannin which is the slowest of them all.
3. With a few exceptions, the results in quartz and glass cells are comparable.

Thus, in air, the above results (Table 7) indicate that mimosa and quebracho should present the best antioxidant characteristics, with the results of mimosa under vacuum indicating a greater consistency, while pecan and oak tannin appears to have poorer antioxidant characteristics.

Equally, the decrease in intensity as a function of time of the ESR signal after stopping the irradiation of the specimen, hence the radical decay reaction itself, is correctly described by first order kinetics of the form $I/I_0=a'e^{-k't}$ and shown in Table 8 and indicates that

1. In general without vacuum, oak and pecan mantain the radical for much longer than quebracho and even longer than mimosa tannin.

2. In general with vacuum, quebracho presents the slowest radical decay reaction, followed by oak, then pecan and last by mimosa tannin.
3. Differences in the behaviour between quartz and glass cells are noticeable. With vacuum for instance, pecan in a glass cell appears to have the slowest radical decay rate, an unexpected occurrence considering all the other results.

Table 7. Radical formation (= First reaction step) kinetics according to a first order kinetic law derived from electron spin resonance experiments. (I/I_o=a e^{kt})

Tannin	Vacuum Conditions	Cell Material	Parameters			
			a	$k(s^{-1})$	r	$t_{1/2}(s)$
Mimosa	Without	quartz	1.4974	$1.549x10^{-4}$	0.809	4474
	Vacuum	glass	1.5069	$1.510x10^{-4}$	0.786	4604
	With	quartz	1.7192	$1.120x10^{-4}$	0.838	6187
	Vacuum	glass	1.6806	$1.148x10^{-4}$	0.839	6038
Quebracho	Without	quartz	1.5546	$1.513x10^{-4}$	0.785	4580
	Vacuum	glass	1.6545	$1.605x10^{-4}$	0.770	4316
	With	quartz	1.4770	$0.580x10^{-4}$	0.832	11939
	Vacuum	glass	1.8611	$0.744x10^{-4}$	0.806	9319
Pecan	Without	quartz	1.1835	$0.442x10^{-4}$	0.668	15671
	Vacuum	glass	1.2018	$0.463x10^{-4}$	0.672	14968
	With	quartz	1.6345	$0.652x10^{-4}$	0.827	10634
	Vacuum	glass	1.6595	$0.558x10^{-4}$	0.823	12424
Oak	Without	quartz	1.1748	$0.610x10^{-4}$	0.792	11360
	Vacuum	glass	1.2057	$0.581x10^{-4}$	0.742	11927
	With	quartz	1.1050	$0.383x10^{-4}$	0.898	18079
	Vacuum	glass	1.2253	$0.496x10^{-4}$	0.902	13962

Thus, in radical formation the order of faster to slower rate remains the same with just differences in relative rates determined by the conditions used (vacuum or not, quartz or glass), and is

mimosa=quebracho>>pecan>/=oak

In the radical decay reaction instead the slower to faster rate changes quite considerably according to the conditions, particularly but not only according to the presence or absence of vacuum. Thus, without vacuum and the air singlet oxygen present the rate of radical decay is

mimosa>quebracho>>pecan=oak (> faster than)

while under vacuum

mimosa>pecan>/=oak>>quebracho

In air then, the balance of the two reactions indicate that the differences between the various tannins should not be major. As, however, radicals have to form before they can decay, the rapidity of radical assumption or formation is the most likely important factor, and thus mimosa and quebracho should be considerably better as antioxidants than the other two tannins. If it is considered that quebracho is as rapid as mimosa to form radicals but that its radicals definitely present a slower radical decay rate, the first conclusion which could be drawn is that quebracho appears to have a slightly better overall antioxidant behaviour than mimosa, but that such a difference is not likely to be very marked. All three flavonoid tannins appear to have considerably better behaviour as antioxidants than the hydrolysable tannin.

The general behaviour of tannins described above can also be seen however from a point of view of relative intensity of the ESR signals, thus total radicals formed, rather than just from a purely kinetic rate point of view (table 8). Table 9 puts in perspective the relative quantities of radicals formed, directly related to the surge in intensity during a fixed period of time of 60 minutes (which in all the cases without vacuum corresponds to the peak of maximum radical concentration obtained at which the inducing light was switched off).

From Table 9 it is easy to see that differences in ESR intensity units, hence in radical concentration, is much higher for quebracho (111, 101, Table 9) than for all the other three tannins. The results for the other three tannins are comparable to each other, presenting only minor differences.

Table 8. Radical decay (=second reaction step) kinetics according to a first order kinetic law derived from electron spin resonance experiments. ($I/I_o=a'e^{-k't}$).

Tannin	Vacuum Conditions	Cell Material	Parameters			
			a	$k(s^{-1})$	r	$t_{1/2}(s)$
Mimosa	Without	quartz	0.909	$0.874x10^{-4}$	0.92	7931
	Vacuum	glass	0.928	$0.639x10^{-4}$	0.90	10839
	With	quartz	0.927	$0.227x10^{-4}$	0.89	30586
	Vacuum	glass	0.951	$0.148x10^{-4}$	0.87	46896
Quebracho	Without	quartz	0.901	$0.559x10^{-4}$	0.91	11571
	Vacuum	glass	0.846	$0.379x10^{-4}$	0.81	18294
	With	quartz	0.950	$0.024x10^{-4}$	0.92	289665
	Vacuum	glass	0.920	$0.028x10^{-4}$	0.92	249264
Pecan	Without	quartz	0.886	$0.163x10^{-4}$	0.71	42402
	Vacuum	glass	0.886	$0.076x10^{-4}$	0.61	91184
	With	quartz	0.951	$0.147x10^{-4}$	0.86	47185
	Vacuum	glass	0.936	$0.020x10^{-4}$	0.75	344069
Oak	Without	quartz	0.931	$0.102x10^{-4}$	0.74	68177
	Vacuum	glass	0.934	$0.197x10^{-4}$	0.71	35102
	With	quartz	0.987	$0.043x10^{-4}$	0.80	160107
	Vacuum	glass	0.997	$0.055x10^{-4}$	0.93	127249

Table 9. Radical formation reaction. Maximum intensity (10^{-5}) and starting intensity (10^{-5}) in intensity units of ESR signal and of relative radical concentration

Tannin	Vacuum Conditions	Cell Material	Peak intensity (relative radical concentration)			
			Maximum (at 60 min.)	Starting (at 0 min.)	difference	
					units	%
Mimosa	Without	quartz	95	41	54	132
	Vacuum	glass	67	29	38	131
	With	quartz	179	65	114	177
	Vacuum	glass	145	53	92	174
Quebracho	Without	quartz	191	80	111	139
	Vacuum	glass	164	63	101	160
	With	quartz	450	230	220	96
	Vacuum	glass	311	115	196	170
Pecan	Without	quartz	182	137	45	33
	Vacuum	glass	147	109	38	35
	With	quartz	471	207	264	128
	Vacuum	glass	343	153	190	124
Oak	Without	quartz	222	160	62	39
	Vacuum	glass	182	128	54	42
	With	quartz	651	511	140	27
	Vacuum	glass	349	229	120	52

Expressing the same results (Table 9) in percentages show mimosa to give comparable results to those of quebracho: this gives a faulse idea of the situation because it is the difference in units which is directly related to the increase in radical concentration on the tannin, and thus the percentage should not be considered. The percentages are shown in Table 9 to warn about this error in interpretation. These results confirm again that quebracho has the best antioxidant characteristics, but also show that there is not much difference between the other tannins.

In the cases with vacuum in which the role of the singlet oxygen is minimized (radical formation in flavonoids is generally considerably easier in presence rather than absence of air, hence of singlet oxygen as shown by both more rapid radical formation and decay without rather than with vacuum in Tables 7, 8 and 9) the real dependence of radical formation from just the characteristic structure of the tannin can be deduced. Here the difference in units follows the order

pecan>/=quebracho>>oak>mimosa

It is interesting to relate such a scale to the structural and chemical characteristics of the three flavonoid tannins in question. Formation of radicals on the flavonoid B-rings generally leads to heterocycle ring opening, and pyran ring opening is much favourite in prodelphinidins (pecan) because of their pyrogallol B-ring/phloroglucinol A-ring structure which ensures better stabilization by delocalisation of the radical on a greater number of possible sites. For this reason mimosa (a 70% prorobinetinidin) should then be better than quebracho (mainly a profistinidin) which is not the case. There must then be at least another major structural reaction influencing the above scale. The other frequent bond cleavage reaction characteristic of flavonoid polymers is the cleavage of the interflavonoid linkage. Radical formation is also likely to be stabilised through this reaction. Interflavonoid bond cleavage is relatively easy in pecan and quebracho tannins and notoriously difficult in mimosa tannin [18,48]. It appears that it is the ease of this reaction superimposed onto the ease of pyran ring opening which is likely to lead to the scale shown above.

ease of pyran ring opening =	pecan=mimosa>quebracho
	+
ease of interflavonoid bond cleavage=	pecan=quebracho>>mimosa

This appears to indicate that in general the higher is the number of -OHs on the flavonoid B-rings, but particularly the higher is the number of -OHs on the flavonoids A-rings the greater appears to be the antioxidant behaviour of the flavonoid tannin, although this characteristic is again overcome by the ease of interflavonoid bond cleavage. The fact that interflavonoid bond cleavage appear to be strongly related to antioxidant behaviour under vacuum might not mean that this reaction determines radical formation or stability. It might only mean that the stereochemistry of tannins which present easier bond cleavage is such, for instance the structure is more open, that radical formation and uptake are facilitated.

The structural parameters which influence the antioxidant properties of the tannins change of importance in presence of air, hence in presence of singlet oxygen. The total scale is mimosa=quebracho>>pecan>/=oak. Here it appears that there is a clear inverse relationship between the number of A-rings -OHs and of ease of interflavonoid bond cleavage with the rates of radical formation and decay, namely: in presence of air the greater the number of A-rings -OHs and the easier the interflavonoid links cleavage the lesser is the antioxidant activity of the tannin. Thus, the parameters of importance are the same in presence or absence of air, but the effect is exactly opposite in the two cases. This indicates that another tannin property might also have a bearing on the antioxidant capability of the tannin, namely its colloidal state. Flavonoid tannins present decreasing colloidal state according to the scale mimosa=quebracho>pecan [27]. In presence of singlet oxygen the effect of migration of such a radical species within the colloidal micelles will afford much more rapid radical formation or uptake by the tannin, thus improve its radical uptake characteristics (and at the same time possibly also accelerate radical decay within the micelles). This is indeed the case from the results in Tables 1 and 2. If the singlet oxygen is not present, hence in absence of air, the effect of the colloidal state is non-existent for the radical formation reaction and radical formation is much slower. The effect might have very little bearing on the radical decay reaction, although with the data available it is impossible to say.

In conclusion the four parameters the combination of which appears to have a bearing on the antioxidant capabilities of a tannin are (i) the extent of its colloidal state, (ii) the ease of interflavonoid bond cleavage (or better its stereochemical structure), (iii) the ease of pyran ring opening and (iv) the relative numbers of A- and B-rings -OH groups. It is the combination of these four factors which will determine the behaviour as an antioxidant of a particular tannin under each set of particular application conditions. With the data presently available it is impossible to quantify the relative extent of the four effects as a function of application conditions.

Table 10. First order kinetics of radical decay reaction after radical transfer to tannin from DPPH, in methanol

Tannin	Radical decay reaction					Radical formation
	a'	k'(s^{-1})	r	$t_{1/2}$(s^{-1})	Max peak Intensity ($x10^5$)	
Quebracho	1.092	-8.3x10-5	0.978	8349	38	15 int. units in 1200 s
Mimosa	0.972	-1.7x10-5	0.952	40765	5	too fast to measure
Pecan	0.932	-5.5x10-5	0.988	12600	19	too fast to measure
Pine	0.977	-1.03x10-5	0.848	67282	55	44 int. units in 1200 s
Gambier	0.999	-0.14x10-5	0.945	498561	117	105 int.units/13000 s
Oak	0.934	-1.96x10-5	0.708	35357	21	too fast to measure

* In dioxane only two radical decay rates could be reliably measured:
Quebracho (a'=0.900, k'=$4.24x10^{-5}$ s^{-1}, r=0.960) and Gambier (a'=1.053, k'=$6.7x10^{-5}$ s^{-1}, r=0.953).

The experiments of radical transfer from DPPH to a tannin in solution also gave some interesting results. Three solvents were tried: tetrahydrofurane was discarded because did not dissolve the tannins. Dioxane dissolved the tannin but presented problems of radical transfer between DPPH and tannin: some of the few reliable results in dioxane are reported in Table 10. Solutions of tannin and DPPH in methanol instead gave reliable results: these are also shown in Table 10. These show that as regards the radical decay reaction mimosa is slower, thus has better antioxidant power than quebracho, this result closely matching and supporting what already obtained by radical transfer in solvent with the stopped-flow apparatus experiments [44]. This result supports again the use of ESR techniques for this type of determination. As regards the other tannins the increasing order of the rate of the radical decay reaction (thus passing from the slowest to the fastest radical decay rate) (Table 10) is as follows

gambier<pine=/<mimosa=/<oak<pecan<quebracho

which presents quite a different order from the experiments done without solvent and simply by light irradiation. The order of quebracho, pecan and oak in the above scale reproduces what obtained without vacuum in the experiments without solvent, except for the relative position of mimosa tannin in the scale which is now completely different. It is clear then, that solvation parameters also appear to play an important role under certain conditions. This goes to shaw the complexity of the interrelation of parameters in tannins radical reactions. As regards the radical formation reaction the results obtained can be calculated only in a very few cases, the reaction in the other cases being either too fast or too unreliable (Table 10).

ANTIVIRAL ACTIVITY OF POLYFLAVONOIDS

Tannins are well known to have antimicrobial activity. This is logical as their capability to tan proteins means that they will complex irreversibly also with the protein in bacterial membranes, inhibiting any activity they might have. Thus, pharmaceutical containing tannins and aimed at curing bacterial intestinal infections have been around already for some time. Some studies on their anticaries effectiveness have also been conducted [49]. Independently from these, almost obvious, pharmaceutical applications of tannins several experimental studies on their use for other pharmaceutical/medical applications have been reported. Particularly well reported are the studies on their antitumor and anticancer activity [50-53]. More recently, work on their antiviral effectiveness has been investigated [54,55]. The data which follow in Tables 11-18 are the preliminary results obtained on the the antiviral activity of 12 different flavonoid and hydrolysable tannins which were carried out by the medical dept. of Leuven university [54,55].

Table 11. Tannins concentration required to protect CEM cells against the cytopathogenicity of HIV by 50 %

Anti-HIV-1 and -HIV-2 activity of the compounds		
in human T-lymphocyte (CEM) cells		
	EC_{50} (μg/ml)	EC_{50} (μg/ml)
Compound	HIV-1	HIV-2
1. Mimosa tannin	6.0 ± 0.0	>20
2. Mimosa tanin intermediate[33,56]	5.0 ± 1.4	>20
3. Chestnut tannin	1.4 ± 0.5	>20
4. Tara+Chestnut mix	5.0 ± 1.4	>20
5. Quebracho standard	6.5 ± 0.7	>20
6. Quebracho highly purified	7.5 ± 0.7	>20
7. Quebracho highly sulphited	7.0 ± 1.4	>20
8. Pecan nut tannin	5.0 ± 1.4	>20
9. Cube Gambier	9.0 ± 1.4	>20
10. Radiata Pine Tannin	7.0 ± 1.4	>20
11. Maritime Pine Tannin	7.5 ± 0.7	>20
12. Sumach Tannin	11.0 ± 1.4	>20
13. Spruce Tannin	>100	>100
EC_{50} = effective concentration or concentration required to protect CEM cells against the cytopathogenicity of HIV by 50 %		

Table 12. Cytotoxicity and antiviral activity of compounds in HEL cell cultures, Herpes and vesicular stomatitis viruses. Tannins added before virus administration

Cytotoxicity and antiviral activity of compounds in E_6SM cell cultures						
Compound	Minimum cytotoxic concentration[a] (µg/ml)	Minimum inhibitory concentration[b] (µg/ml)				
		Herpes simplex virus-1 (KOS)	Herpes simplex virus-2 (G)	Vaccinia virus	Vesicular stomatitis virus	Herpes simplex virus-1 TK⁻ KOS ACV[r]
1	200	40	16	16	>80	40
2	≥40	40	16	16	>80	40
3	≥40	40	16	16	>80	47
4	≥40	40	48	16	>80	47
5	40	47	36	16	>80	47
6	40	80	36	16	>80	47
7	≥40	40	40	16	>80	36
8	40	16	16	16	>80	36
9	8	>80	>80	>80	>80	>80
10	40	40	>80	16	>80	40
11	40	>80	>80	80	>80	47
12	40	36	36	16	>80	36
13	40	>16	>16	>16	>16	>16
Brivudin	>400	0.128	400	16	>400	>400
Ribavirin	>400	>400	>400	400	>400	>400
Acyclovir	>400	0.384	0.128	>400	>400	48
Ganciclovir	>100	0.0064	0.0064	100	>100	2.4

[a]Required to cause a microscopically detectable alteration of normal cell morphology.
[b]Required to reduce virus-induced cytopathogenicity by 50 %.

The results in Tables 11-18 evaluate both the effectiveness of 12 different tannins as measured by the Minimum Inhibitory Concentration (MIC) of the tannin required to reduce virus-induced cytopathogenicity by 50 %. The lower is the MIC value the better is the compound as an antiviral substance.

Equally important, the results in the tables measure the Minimum Cytotoxic Concentration (MCC) required to cause a microscopically detectable alteration of normal cell morphology. The higher the MCC the less toxic to the patient's cells is the compound and the better is the compound as an antiviral substance.

Table13. Cytotoxicity and antiviral activity of compounds in HEL cell cultures, vesicular stomatitis, Coxsackie and respiratory syncytial viruses

Cytotoxicity and antiviral activity of compounds in HeLa cell cultures				
Compound	Minimum cytotoxic concentration[a] (μg/ml)	Minimum inhibitory concentration[b] (μg/ml)		
		Vesicular Stomatitis virus	Coxsackie virus B4	Respiratory syncytial virus
1	400	>80	>80	12 +/-5
2	400	>80	>80	12 +/-5
3	400	>80	>80	43 +/-4
4	400	43.4 +/-4	>80	35 +/-7
5	400	>80	>80	40 +/-0.2
6	400	>80	>80	40 +/-0.2
7	400	>80	>80	43 +/-5
8	400	>80	>80	9 +/-1
9	400	>80	>80	>80
10	400	>80	>80	40 +/-0.2
11	400	>80	>80	40 +/-0.2
12	80	>16	>16	>16
13	≥80	>80	>80	>80
Brivudin	>400	>400	>400	>400
(S)-DHPA	>400	400	>400	>400
Ribavirin	>400	48	240	9.4

[a]Required to cause a microscopically detectable alteration of normal cell morphology.
[b]Required to reduce virus-induced cytopathogenicity by 50 %.

Thus, what is looked for is the lowest possible MIC and the highest possible MCC. These results are in vitro screening tests. A good results must be still translated into being effective by the carrier used to deliver it and the way the substance is delivered to the relevant site where it is needed. Nonetheless as these are very advanced results and they should be recorded , they are reported in full here. It is evident that different tannins can be very effective against different viruses, polyphenolic grouping being the cause of this behaviour. Most likely, they tan the proteins and they associate with the carbohydrates of the virus membrane. In all an effect similar to their well known association with hide proteins to give leather and with carbohydrates.

Table 14. Inhibitory effects of tannins on the proliferation of murine leukemia cells (L1210/0), murine mammary carcinoma cells (FM3A) and human T-lymphocyte cells (Molt4/C8, CEM/0)

Compound	IC50 (μg/ml)			
	L1210/0	FM3A/0	Molt4/C8	CEM/0
1	18 ± 0	153 ± 66	74 ± 18	58 ± 0
2	16 ± 1	148 ± 74	66 ± 27	61 ± 1
3	17 ± 0	141 ± 7	98 ± 22	65 ± 2
4	17 ± 0	114 ± 1	75 ± 57	56 ± 0
5	12 ± 4	76 ± 16	20 ± 1	51 ± 30
6	15 ± 2	79 ± 27	33 ± 21	45 ± 27
7	14 ± 2	82 ± 26	40 ± 27	55 ± 25
8	21 ± 6	≥ 200	81 ± 7	66 ± 11
9	13 ± 4	80 ± 22	17 ± 2	18 ± 1
10	65 ± 4	≥ 200	65 ± 28	71 ± 9
11	53 ± 23	≥ 200	94 ± 1	111 ± 40
12	17 ± 0	18 ± 1	17 ± 0	18 ± 2
13	49 ± 16	> 200	145 ± 78	83 ± 20

[a]50% inhibitory concentration.

Table 15. Cytotoxicity and antiviral activity of compounds in HEL cell cultures, influenza viruses

Cytotoxicity and antiviral activity of compounds in MDCK cell cultures							
Compound	Minimum cytotoxic concentration[a] (μg/ml)	EC_{50}					
		Influenza A H1N1		Influenza A H3N2		Influenza B	
			MTS		MTS		MTS
1	100		3.3 +/-1.2		1.7 +/-1.3		2.3 +/-1.9
2	100		2.2 +/-0.1		1.7 +/-0.6		2.3 +/-1.5
3	100		4.0 +/-2.8		2.0 +/-0		1.4 +/-0.8
4	33.3		4.1 +/-2.8		2.2 +/-0.8		1.4 +/-0.9
5	100		1.7 +/-0.1		2.1 +/-0.4		3.5 +/-3.2
6	100		5.4 +/-3.8		3.7 +/-1.6		3.6 +/-3.0
7	100		4.4 +/-2.8		1.9 +/-0.4		3.4 +/-3.0
8	33.3		2.1 +/-0.1		3.0 +/-1.5		1.8 +/-1.1
9	100		5.5 +/-4.6		4.4 +/-3.6		2.7 +/-2.6
10	100		4.2 +/-3.1		2.7 +/-1.0		2.7 +/-2.7
11	100		2.9 +/-1.2		2.2 +/-0.3		1.5 +/-1.1
12	20		2.0 +/-1.6		0.9 +/-0.2		2.6 +/-1.9
13	100		9.9 +/-5.7		9.5 +/-4.8		1.9 +/-1.9
Oseltamivir carboxylate (μM)	>100		0.05		0.65		10.65
Ribavirin (μM)	60		4.55		6.32		9.07
Amantadin (μM)	>100		21.39		0.78		>100
Rimantadin (μM)	>100		18.45		0.05		>100

[a]Required to cause a microscopically detectable alteration of normal cell morphology.

Compounds added prior to virus administration.

Table 16. Cytotoxicity and antiviral activity of compounds in HEL cell cultures, Corona viruses

	Feline CORONA virus (FIPV)		*Human Corona (SARS) virus*	
	EC50 (μg/ml)	CC50 (μg/ml)	EC50 (μg/ml)	CC50 (μg/ml)
1	52 ± 19	> 100	> 100	> 100
2	67 ± 47	> 100	> 100	> 100
3	49 ± 17	> 100	> 100	> 100
4	43 ± 2	> 100	> 100	> 100
5	49 ± 10	≥ 100	44 ± 10	> 100
6	55 ± 19	> 100	49 ± 21	> 100
7	32 ± 1	> 100	40 ± 1	> 100
8	72 ± 40	> 100	> 100	> 100
9	≥ 100	> 100	> 100	> 100
10	20 ± 21	> 100	> 100	> 100
11	44 ± 5	> 100	56 ± 13	> 100
12	7.8 ± 8.0	81 ± 13	> 100	> 100
13	63 ± 32	> 100	> 100	> 100

Table 17. Cytotoxicity and antiviral activity of compounds in HEL cell cultures, Herpes and Vaccinia viruses. Tannins added after virus administration

Cytotoxicity and antiviral activity of compounds in HEL cell cultures						
Compound	Minimum cytotoxic concentration[a] (μg/ml)	Minimum inhibitory concentration[b] (μg/ml)				
		Herpes simplex virus-1 (KOS)	Herpes simplex virus-2 (G)	Vaccinia virus	Vesicular stomatitis virus	Herpes simplex virus-1 TK⁻ KOS ACV[r]
1	200	6 +/-2	1.8 +/-0.2	>40	>40	6 +/-2
2	200	4 +/-0	2 +/-1	8 +/-0	>40	4 +/-0
3	200	15 +/-1	3 +/-1	24 +/-1	>40	17 +/-3
4	200	15 +/-1	8 +/-0	24 +/-1	>40	20 +/-2
5	≥40	>40	>40	20 +/-2	>40	>40
6	≥40	>40	8 +/-0	>40	>40	>40
7	≥40	8 +/-0	>40	20 +/-2	>40	>40
8	40	4 +/-0	4 +/-0	8 +/-0	>8	4 +/-0
9	≥40	>40	>40	>40	>40	>40
10	40	8 +/-0	4 +/-0	8 +/-0	>8	>8
11	40	>8	8 +/-0	>8	>8	>8
12	40	>8	8 +/-0	>8	>8	>8
13	200	>40	>40	>40	>40	>40
Brivudin (μM)*	>250	0.016	10	6	>250	50
Ribavirin (μM)*	>250	250	50	30	50	250
Acyclovir (μM)*	>250	0.08	0.08	>250	>250	50
Ganciclovir (μM)*	>100	0.0064	0.032	>100	>100	12

Compounds added prior to virus administration.

[a]Required to cause a microscopically detectable alteration of normal cell morphology.

[b]Required to reduce virus-induced c ytopathogenicity by 50 %.

* Controls.

REFERENCES

[1] Pizzi A. Wood Adhesives Chemistry and Technology, Vol. 1. New York: Dekker, 1983.
[2] Meikleham N, Pizzi A, Stephanou A. *J. Appl. Polymer Sci*. 1994; 54: 1827.
[3] Pizzi A, Meikleham N, Stephanou A. *J. Appl. Polymer Sci*. 1995; 55: 929.
[4] Pizzi A., Meikleham N. *J. Appl. Polymer Sci.* 1995; 55: 1265.
[5] Merlin A, Pizzi A. J. Appl. Polymer Sci.. 1996; 59: 945.
[6] Masson E, Merlin A, Pizzi A. *J. Appl. Polymer Sci*.. 1996; 60: 263.
[7] Masson E, Pizzi A, Merlin A. *J. Appl. Polymer Sci*..1996; 60: 1655.
[8] Masson E, Pizzi A, Merlin A. *J. Appl. Polymer Sci*..1997; 64: 243.
[9] Pizzi A, Meikleham N, Dombo B, Roll W. Holz Roh Werkstoff 1995; 53: 201.
[10] Pizzi A. Advanced Wood Adhesives Technology. New York: Dekker, 1994.
[11] Karas M, Bachmann D, Bahr U, Hillenkamp F. *Int. J. Mass Spectrom Ion. Proc.* 1987; 78: 53.
[12] Bahr U, Deppe A, Karas M, Hillenkamp F, Giessmann U. *Anal. Chem*. 1992; 64: 2866.
[13] Ehring H, Karas M, Hillenkamp F, *Org. Mass Spectrom*.1992; 27: 472.
[14] Danis PO, Karr DE, Mayer F, Holle A, Watson CH. *Org. Mass Spectrom*. 1992; 27: 843.
[15] Danis PO, Karr DE. *Org. Mass Spectrom*. 1993; 28: 923.
[16] Pasch H, Resch M. *GIT Fachz Lab*. 1996; 40: 90.
[17] Pasch H, Gores F. *Polymer* 1995; 36: 1999.
[18] Pizzi A, Stephanou A. *J. Appl. Polymer Sci*.. 1994; 51: 2109.
[19] Thompson D, Pizzi A. *J. Appl. Polymer Sci.*.1995; 55: 107.
[20] Fechtal M, Riedl B. *Holzforschung* 1993; 47: 349.
[21] Botha JJ, Ferreira D, Roux DG. J Chem Soc, *Chem. Commun*. 1978: 700.
[22] Pizzi A, Cameron FA, Eaton NJ. *J. Macromol Sci. Chem. Ed*. 1986; A23(4): 515.
[23] Rahim, AA. PhD thesis, University Sains Malaysia, Penang, Malaysia 2005.
[24] Oo CW, Pizzi A, Pasch H, Kassim MJ, *J.Appl.Polymer Sci.,* 2008, 109(2): 963-967.
[25] Oo, CW PhD thesis, University of sains Malaysia, Penang, Malaysia 2008.
[26] Rahim, AA, Rocca E, Steinmetz J, Kassim M J, Adnan R, Sani Ibrahim M. *Corrosion Science* 2007, 49, 402.
[27] Pizzi A and Stephanou A, *J.Appl.Polymer Sci*., 1994, 51: 2125-2130.
[28] Colleri L. Le Fabbriche Italiane di Estratto di Castagno; Milanostampa S.p.A.: Farigliano (CN), Italy, 1989.
[29] Kim, S.R.; Saratchandra, D.; Mainwaring, D.E. *J. Appl. Polym Sci.* 1995, 56, 905.
[30] Kim, S.R.; Saratchandra, D.; Mainwaring, D.E. *J. Appl. Polym Sci.* 1995, 56, 915.
[31] Kim, S.R.; Mainwaring, D.E. *Holzforschung* 1996, 50, 42.
[32] Garnier, S.; Pizzi, A.; Vorster, O.C.; Halasz, L. J.Appl.Polymer Sci., 2001, 81(7): 1634-1642.
[33] Pasch, H.; Pizzi, A.; Rode, K. Polymer, 2001, 42, 7531.
[34] Pizzi, A. *Forest Prod. J.* 1978, 28(12), 42.
[35] Pizzi, A.; Meikleham, N.; Stephanou, A. *J. Appl. Polym Sci.* 1995, 55, 929.
[36] Pizzi, A.; Vogel, M.C. *J. Macromol. Sci. Chem. Ed* 1983, A19(2), 369.
[37] Masson, E.; Merlin, A.; Pizzi, A. *J. Appl. Polym Sci.* 1996, 60, 263.

[38] Masson, E.; Pizzi, A.; Merlin, A. *J. Appl. Polym Sci.* 1996, 60, 1655.
[39] Masson, E.; Pizzi, A.; Merlin, A. *J. Appl. Polym Sci.* 1997, 64, 243.
[40] Roux, D.G. in Mimosa Extract, LIRI Leather Industries Research Inst.: Grahamstown, South Africa, 1965, pages 33-51.
[41] Pizzi, A. Advanced Wood Adhesives Technology, Marcel Dekker: New York, 1994.
[42] Allcock, H.R. and Lampe, F.W., 1990, Contemporary Polymer Chemistry, Prentice Hall,New Jersey.
[43] Seymour; R.B. and Carraher, C.E., 1992, Polymer Chemistry, an introduction, Dekker, New York.
[44] Martin, F., 1995, Ph.D. thesis, University of Nancy 1, Vandoeuvre, France.
[45] Noferi, M.; Masson, E.; Merlin, A.; Pizzi, A. and Deglise, X. *J. Appl. Polymer Sci.*, 1997, 63, 475-482.
[46] Merlin, A. and Pizzi, A., *J. Appl. Polymer Sci.*, 1996, 59: 945-952.
[47] Jensen, O.H. and Pedersen, J.A., *Tetrahedron,* 1983, 39, 1609.
[48] Pizzi, A. and Stephanou, A., *J. Appl. Polymer Sci.*, 1993, 50, 2105.
[49] Mitsunaga, T. in Plant Polyphenols 2 – (G.G.Gross, R.W.Hemingway, T.Yoshida Eds.), Kluwer Academic/Plenum Publishers, New York, pp. 555-574, 1999.
[50] L.-L.Yang, L.-L., Wang, C.-C., Yen, K.-Y., Yoshida, T., Hatano, T., Okuda, T., in Plant Polyphenols 2 – (G.G.Gross, R.W.Hemingway, T.Yoshida Eds.), Kluwer Academic/Plenum Publishers, New York, pp. 615-628, 1999.
[51] Nakamura, Y., Matsuda, M., Honma, T., Tomita, I., Shibata, N., Warashina, T., Noro, T., Hara, Y. in Plant Polyphenols 2 – (G.G.Gross, R.W.Hemingway, T.Yoshida Eds.), Kluwer Academic/Plenum Publishers, New York, pp. 629-642, 1999.
[52] Miyamoto, K., Murayama, T., Hatano, T., Yoshida, T., Okuda, T. in Plant Polyphenols 2 – (G.G.Gross, R.W.Hemingway, T.Yoshida Eds.), Kluwer Academic/Plenum Publishers, New York, pp. 643-664, 1999.
[53] Noro, T., Ohki, T., Noda, Y., Warashina, T., Noro, K., Tomita, I., Nakamura, Y. in Plant Polyphenols 2 – (G.G.Gross, R.W.Hemingway, T.Yoshida Eds.), Kluwer Academic/Plenum Publishers, New York, pp. 665-674, 1999.
[54] Balzarini, J., Persoons, L., Absillis, A., Van Berckelaer, L., Pizzi, A. Rijk Universiteit Leuven, Belgium and University of Nancy 1, France, unpublished results (2006).
[55] Pizzi, A., Tannins: major sources, properties and applications, Chapter 8 in Monomers, Polymers and Composites from Renewable Resources (M.N.Belgacem and A.Gandini Eds.), Elsevier, Amsterdam (2008), pp179 – 199.
[56] Pizzi, A., Stephanou, A. ***Holzforschung Holzverwertung***, 1992, 44(4): 62-68

In: Flavonoids: Biosynthesis, Biological Effects…
Editor: Raymond B. Keller
ISBN: 978-1-60741-622-7

Chapter 4

GRAPEFRUIT FLAVONOIDS: NARINGIN AND NARINGININ

Ricky W. K. Wong*[*] and A. Bakr M. Rabie
Biomedical and Tissue Engineering, the University of Hong Kong

ABSTRACT

Naringin is the flavonoid compound found in grapefruit that gives grapefruit its characteristic bitter flavor. Grapefruit processors attempt to select fruits with a low naringin content, and often blend juices obtained from different grapefruit varieties to obtain the desired degree of bitterness. Naringin is believed to enhance our perception of taste by stimulating the taste buds; some people consume a small amount of grapefruit juice before a meal for this reason.

Naringin and its aglycone naringinin are commonly used health supplements; they exert a variety of biological actions. This article attempts to review their pharmacokinetics and pharmacological actions from scientific publications up to November 2008 including effects on the cardiovascular system, on the skeletal system, on smooth muscle, on the gastric intestinal system, on the endocrine system, also effects against tumours, protection against toxins in chemotherapy drugs and the environment, antioxidant effects, drug interactions, anti-inflammatory effects, and the newly discovered osteogenic and antibacterial actions.

Keywords: Naringin, Narginenin, antioxidant effect, drug interactions, osteogenic effect, antibacterial effect, anti-inflammatory effect.

INTRODUCTION

Naringin is the flavonoid compound found in grapefruit that gives grapefruit its characteristic bitter flavor. Grapefruit processors attempt to select fruits with a low naringin content, and often blend juices obtained from different grapefruit varieties to obtain the desired degree of bitterness. Naringin is believed to enhance our perception of taste by stimulating the taste buds (some people consume a small amount of grapefruit juice before a meal for this reason). Naringin may be instrumental in inhibiting cancer-causing compounds and thus may have potential chemotherapeutic value. Studies have also shown that naringin interferes with enzymatic activity in the intestines and, thus, with the breakdown of certain drugs, resulting in higher blood levels of the drug. A number of drugs that are known to be affected by the naringin in grapefruit include calcium channel blockers, estrogen, sedatives, medications for high blood pressure, allergies, AIDS, and cholesterol-lowering drugs. Caffeine levels and effects of caffeine may also be extended by consuming grapefruit or grapefruit juice. While the effect of naringin on the metabolism of a drug can increase the drug's effectiveness, it can also result in dosages that are inadvertently too high. Therefore, it's best not to take any drugs with grapefruit juice unless the interaction with the drug is known. In addition, the effects of drinking grapefruit juice is cumulative, which means that if you drank a glass of grapefruit juice daily with your medication for a week, the drug interaction would be stronger at the end of the week than at the beginning.

Research on naringin and naringinin shows the following effects:

(A) Effects on cardiovascular system

Reference	Robbins et al., 1988
Study	The effect on hematocrits of adding grapefruit to the daily diet was determined using 36 human subjects (12 F, 24 M) over a 42-day study.
Results	The effect on hematocrits of adding grapefruit to the daily diet was determined using 36 human subjects (12 F, 24 M) over a 42-day study.
Conclusion	Ingestion of grapefruit lowers elevated hematocrits in human subjects.

Reference	Bok et al., 1999
Study	The cholesterol-lowering effects of tangerine peel extract and a mixture of two citrus flavonoids were tested.
Results	The inhibition of HMG-CoA reductase and ACAT activities resulting from either tangerine-peel extract or its bioflavonoids could account for the decrease in fecal neutral sterol.
Conclusion	Plasma and hepatic cholesterol and hepatic activities of 3-hydroxy-3-methyl-glutaryl-CoA (HMG-CoA) reductase and acyl CoA: cholesterol transferase (ACAT) are lower in rats fed citrus peel extract or a mixture of citrus bioflavonoids.

Reference	Shin et al., 1999
Study	The effects of the citrus bioflavonoid naringin were tested by using it as a supplement in a high-cholesterol diet.
Results	The combination of the inhibited HMG-CoA reductase (-24.4%) and ACAT (-20.2%) activities as a result of naringin supplementation could account for the decrease of fecal neutral sterols.

* Tel: 852-28590554; Fax: 852-25593803; E-mail: fyoung@hkucc.hku.hk

Conclusion	Hypocholesterolemic effect of naringin associated with hepatic cholesterol regulating enzyme changes in rats.
Reference	Lee et al., 2001
Study	The anti-atherogenic effects of the citrus flavonoids, naringin and naringenin, were evaluated in high cholesterol-fed rabbits.
Results	The anti-atherogenic effect of the citrus flavonoids, naringin and naringenin, is involved with a decreased hepatic ACAT activity and with the downregulation of VCAM-1 and MCP-1 gene expression.
Conclusion	Anti-atherogenic effect of citrus flavonoids, naringin and naringenin.

Reference	Choi et al., 2001
Study	The interactive effect of naringin and vitamin E was studied with respect to cholesterol metabolism and antioxidant status in high-cholesterol-fed rats.
Results	Naringin lowers the plasma lipid concentrations when the dietary vitamin E level is low. The HMG-CoA reductase-inhibitory effect of naringin was more potent when dietary vitamin E was at a normal level.
Conclusion	Interactive effect of naringin and vitamin E on cholesterol biosynthesis.

Reference	Choe et al., 2001
Study	This study evaluated the effect of naringin on blood lipid levels and aortic fatty streaks, and its action mechanism in hypercholesterolemic rabbits.
Results	Naringin treatment inhibited hypercholesterolemia-induced intercellular adhesion molecule-1 (ICAM-1) expression on endothelial cells. Hypercholesterolemia caused fatty liver and elevation of liver enzymes, which was prevented by naringin but not by lovastatin.
Conclusion	Naringin has an antiatherogenic effect with the inhibition of intercellular adhesion molecule-1 in hypercholesterolemic rabbits.

Reference	da Silva et al., 2001
Study	The effect of naringin and rutin on the metabolism lipidic of chicks hypercholesterolemic was evaluated.
Results	Naringin and rutin reduced the levels of total cholesterol significantly, cholesterol-LDL, cholesterol-VLDL and triglycerols, not presenting, however, reductions in the levels of cholesterol-HDL.
Conclusion	Hypocholesterolemic effect of naringin and rutin flavonoids

Reference	Naderi et al., 2003
Study	The susceptibility of LDL to in vitro oxidation was assessed. LDL oxidation were monitored by change in 234-absorbance in the presence and absence of pure flavonoids.
Results	Genistein, morin and naringin have stronger inhibitory activity against LDL oxidation than biochanin A or apigenin.
Conclusion	Flavonoids prevent in vitro LDL oxidation and probably would be important to prevent atherosclerosis.

Reference	Jung et al., 2003
Study	The effect of naringin on hypercholesterolemic subjects was studied. A hypercholesterolemic group (n=30) and healthy control group (n=30) were established.
Results	Naringin supplementation was found to lower the plasma total cholesterol by 14% and low-density lipoprotein cholesterol concentrations by 17%, apolipoprotein B levels were significantly lowered, erythrocyte superoxide dismutase and catalase activities were significantly increased.
Conclusion	Naringin may play an important role in lowering plasma cholesterol and regulating the antioxidant capacity in hypercholesterolemic subjects.

Reference	Kim et al., 2004
Study	The lipid lowering and antioxidant capacity of naringin was evaluated in LDL receptor knockout (LDLR-KO) mice fed a cholesterol (0.1 g/100 g) diet.
Results	The hepatic HMG-CoA reductase activity was significantly lower in the naringin and lovastatin supplemented groups than in the control group, the superoxide dismutase, catalase, and glutathione reductase activities were all significantly higher in the naringin-supplemented group than in the control group.
Conclusion	Naringin lowers the plasma cholesterol level via the inhibition of hepatic HMG-CoA reductase activity and improve the activities of hepatic antioxidant enzymes against oxidative stress.
Reference	Chiou and Xu, 2004
Study	Effects of flavonoids to improve retinal function recovery after ischemic insult were studied. Electroretinography was used to measure the b-wave recovery as an indication of retinal function recovery.
Results	Naringenin, hesperetin, and rutin were found to produce marked positive effects on b-wave recovery, whereas naringin, hesperidin, and quercetin showed poor recovery of b-wave after ischemic insult of the retina.
Conclusion	Flavonoids that showed strong increase of ocular blood flow also showed marked increase of retinal function recovery.

Reference	Singh and Chopra, 2004
Study	The protective effect of naringin against the damage inflicted by ROS during renal I/R was investigated in Sprague-Dawley rats using histopathological and biochemical parameters.
Results	Pretreatment of animals with naringin markedly attenuated renal dysfunction, morphological alterations, reduced elevated TBARS levels and restored the depleted renal antioxidant enzymes.
Conclusion	Reactive oxygen species (ROS) play a causal role in renal ischemia/reperfusion (I/R) induced renal injury and naringin exert renoprotective effects probably by the radical scavenging and antioxidant activities.

Reference	Jeon et al., 2004
Study	To confirm the hypocholesterolemic role of naringin, male rabbits were fed 0.5% high-cholesterol diet or high-cholesterol diet supplemented with either 0.05% naringin or 0.03% lovastatin for 8 weeks.
Results	The naringin and lovastatin supplements significantly lowered plasma total- and LDL-cholesterol and hepatic lipids levels, while significantly increasing HDL-C/total-C ratio compared to the control group.
Conclusion	Both naringin and lovastatin contributed to hypocholesterolemic action. Naringin seemed to preserve tissue morphology from damages induced by high cholesterol diet.
Reference	Orallo et al., 2005
Study	The potential vasorelaxant, antioxidant and cyclic nucleotide PDE inhibitory effects of the citrus-fruit flavonoids naringin and (+/-)-naringenin were comparatively studied.
Results	(+/-)-naringenin relaxed, in a concentration-dependent manner, the contractions elicited by phenylephrine (PHE, 1 microM) or by a high extracellular KCl concentration (60 mM) in intact rat aortic rings.
Conclusion	The vasorelaxant effects of (+/-)-naringenin seem to be basically related to the inhibition of phosphodiesterase (PDE)1, PDE4 and PDE5 activities.

Reference	Reshef et al., 2005
Study	Patients with stage I hypertension, the antihypertensive effect of juice of the so-called sweetie fruit (a hybrid between grapefruit and pummelo) with and without high flavonoid content were studied.
Results	The high-flavonoid (HF) sweetie juice was more effective than LF sweetie juice in reducing diastolic blood pressure.
Conclusion	The active ingredients associated with the antihypertensive effect of sweetie juice are the flavonoids naringin and narirutin.

Reference	Jung et al., 2006
Study	The effect of the flavonoids hesperidin and naringin on glucose and lipid regulation in C57BL/KsJ-db/db mice was studied.
Results	Hesperidin and naringin effectively lowered the plasma free fatty acid and plasma and hepatic triglyceride levels, and simultaneously reduced the hepatic fatty acid oxidation and carnitine palmitoyl transferase activity.
Conclusion	Hesperidin and naringin are beneficial for improving hyperlipidemia and hyperglycemia in type-2 diabetic animals.

Reference	Rajadurai and Prince, 2006
Study	The preventive effect of naringin in isoproterenol (ISO)-induced myocardial infarction (MI) in rats was studied.
Results	Pretreatment with naringin significantly decreased the levels of total, ester, and free cholesterol, triglycerides, and free fatty acids in serum and heart and increased phospholipids in heart.
Conclusion	Naringin has a lipid-lowering effect in ISO-induced MI rats.

Reference	Rajadurai and Prince, 2006
Study	The cardioprotective potential of naringin on lipid peroxides, enzymatic and nonenzymatic antioxidants and histopathological findings in isoproterenol (ISO)-induced myocardial infarction (MI) in rats were evaluated.
Results	Oral administration of naringin to ISO-induced rats showed a significant decrease in the levels of lipid peroxidative products and improved the antioxidant status. Histopathological findings of the myocardial tissue showed the protective role of naringin in ISO-induced rats.
Conclusion	Naringin possess anti-lipoperoxidative and antioxidant activity in experimentally induced cardiac toxicity.

Reference	Rajadurai and Prince, 2007
Study	The preventive role of naringin on cardiac troponin T (cTnT), lactate dehydrogenase (LDH)-isoenzyme, cardiac marker enzymes, electrocardiographic (ECG)-patterns and lysosomal enzymes in isoproterenol (ISO)-induced myocardial infarction (MI) in male Wistar rats were investigated.
Results	Pretreatment with naringin positively altered the levels of cTnT, intensity of the bands of the LDH1 and LDH2-isoenzyme and the activities of cardiac marker enzymes, ECG-patterns and lysosomal hydrolases in ISO-induced rats.
Conclusion	Naringin possess cardioprotective effect in ISO-induced MI in rats.

Reference	Kim et al., 2006
Study	Naringin was investigated for its differential effects on hepatic cholesterol regulation when supplemented for 3 weeks and 6 weeks in Sprague-Dawley rats.
Results	Supplementation with naringin did not exhibit a hypolipidemic effect when given with a HFHC diet. Naringin can, however, be beneficial for lowering hepatic cholesterol biosynthesis and levels of plasma lipids in this animal model.
Conclusion	Naringin time-dependently lowers hepatic cholesterol biosynthesis and plasma cholesterol in rats fed high-fat and high-cholesterol diet.

Reference	Rajadurai and Prince, 2007
Study	The preventive role of naringin on heart weight, blood glucose, total proteins, albumin/globulin (A/G) ratio, serum uric acid, serum iron, plasma iron binding capacity and membrane bound enzymes and glycoproteins such as hexose, hexosamine, fucose and sialic acid in isoproterenol (ISO)-induced myocardial infarction (MI) in rats and in vitro free radical scavenging assay were studied. The preventive role of naringin on mitochondrial enzymes in isoproterenol (ISO)-induced myocardial infarction in male albino Wistar rats was studied.
Results	Pretreatment with naringin exhibited a significant effect and altered these biochemical parameters positively in ISO-induced rats. Naringin also scavenges. 1,1-diphenyl-2-picrylhydrazyl,2,2'-azinobis-(3-ethyl-benzothiazoline-6-sulfonic acid) and nitric oxide radicals in vitro. Oral pretreatment with naringin to ISO-induced rats daily for a period of 56 days significantly minimized the alterations in all the biochemical parameters and restored the normal mitochondrial function. Transmission electron microscopic observations also correlated with these biochemical findings.
Conclusion	Naringin has cardioprotective role in ISO-induced MI in rats

Reference	Morikawa et al., 2008
Study	The effect of some flavanones on the adipocytic conversion of the human preadipocyte cell line, AML-I.
Results	Among four structure-related flavanones including naringenin, naringenin-7-rhamnoglucoside (naringin), hesperetin, and hesperetin-7-rhamnoglucoside (hesperidin), the aglycones such as naringenin and hesperetin exhibited the growth arrest of AML-I cells.
Conclusion	Apoptosis by flavanones does not inhibit the adipocytic conversion of AML-I preadipocytes.

Reference	Lee et al., 2008
Study	The exact molecular mechanisms underlying the roles of integrated cell cycle regulation and MAPK signaling pathways in the regulation of naringin-induced inhibition of cell proliferation in vascular smooth muscle cells (VSMCs)
Results	Naringin treatment resulted in significant growth inhibition and G(1)-phase cell cycle arrest mediated by induction of p53-independent p21WAF1 expression; expression of cyclins and CDKs in VSMCs was also down-regulated.
Conclusion	The Ras/Raf/ERK pathway participates in p21WAF1 induction, leading to a decrease in cyclin D1/CDK4 and cyclin E/CDK2 complexes and in naringin-dependent inhibition of cell growth. These novel and unexpected findings provide a theoretical basis for preventive use of flavonoids to the atherosclerosis disease.

Reference	Rajadurai and Prince, 2008
Study	To evaluate the preventive role of naringin on mitochondrial lipid peroxides, antioxidants and lipids in isoproterenol (ISO)-induced myocardial infarction (MI) in male Wistar rats.
Results	Oral pretreatment with naringin (10, 20 and 40 mg/kg) to ISO-induced rats daily for a period of 56 days significantly decreased the levels of mitochondrial lipid peroxides with a significant increase in the activities/levels of mitochondrial antioxidants and significantly minimized the alterations in the mitochondrial lipid levels in ISO-induced rats.
Conclusion	Naringin prevents alterations in mitochondrial lipid peroxides, antioxidants and lipids in ISO-induced MI in rats.

(B) Effects on skeletal system

Reference	Wood, 2004
Study	The influence of dietary bioflavonoid (rutin [R], quercetin [Q], and naringin [N]) supplementation on physiological molar crestal alveolar bone(CAB)-cemento-enamel junction (CEJ) distances in young male albino rats was studied.
Results	The N group demonstrated the lowest CAB-CEJ distance, followed by the R and Q groups ($P < .001$-.05), except in the mandibular lingual region, where the Q group had a lower CAB-CEJ distance than the N and R groups ($P < .05$). The control group showed the largest CAB-CEJ distances.
Conclusion	Rutin, quercetin, and naringin supplementation reduce molar crestal alveolar bone-cemento-enamel junction distance in young rats.

Reference	Wong and Rabie, 2006
Study	The amount of new bone produced by naringin in collagen matrix to that produced by bone grafts and collagen matrix in rabbits was compared.
Results	A total of 284% and 490% more new bone was present in defects grafted with naringin in collagen matrix than those grafted with bone and collagen, respectively.
Conclusion	Naringin in collagen matrix have the effect of increasing new bone formation locally and can be used as a bone graft material.

Reference	Wong and Rabie, 2006
Study	The effect of naringin, which was also a HMG-CoA reductase inhibitor, was studied in UMR 106 osteoblastic cell line in vitro.
Results	Naringin significantly increased bone cell activities in vitro.
Conclusion	Besides statin, this provided another example of HMG-CoA reductase inhibition that increases the bone cell activities

Reference	Li et al., 2006
Study	The osteoblastic activity of extracts of Drynaria fortunei (Kunze) J. Sm. rhizome was assayed in the UMR106 cell line cultured in vitro.
Results	The ethanol extract, and its ethyl acetate and n-butanol fractions exhibited stimulating activity.
Conclusion	Two active constituents were isolated and identified as naringin and neoeriocitrin.

Reference	Wei et al., 2007
Study	A retinoic acid-induced osteoporosis model of rats was used to assess whether naringin has similar bioactivity against osteoporosis in vitro.
Results	A blood test showed that naringin-treated rats experienced significantly lower activity of serum alkaline phosphatase and had higher femur bone mineral density, compared to untreated rats.
Conclusion	These outcomes suggest that naringin offer a potential in the management of osteoporosis in vitro.

Reference	Mandadi et al., 2008
Study	Effects of feeding citrus bioactive compounds and crude extract on bone quality in orchidectomized rats were evaluated.
Results	The citrus crude extract or the purified bioactive compounds increased ($p<0.05$) the plasma antioxidant status, plasma IGF-I, and bone density, preserved ($p<0.05$) the concentration of calcium in the femur and in the 5th lumbar, and numerically improved bone strength.
Conclusion	Potential benefit of the citrus crude extract and its bioactive compounds on bone quality appears to preserve bone calcium concentration and increase antioxidant status.

Reference	Wu et al., 2008
Study	Naringin was shown to enhance alkaline phosphatase activity, osteocalcin level, osteopontin synthesis and cell proliferation in primary cultured osteoblasts.
Results	Naringin increased mRNA and protein levels of BMP-2 using Western blot, ELISA and RT-PCR assay, also prevented the decreasing of BMP-2 and bone loss inducing by ovariectomy in vivo.
Conclusion	Naringin increase BMP-2 expression and enhance osteogenic response via the phosphoinositide 3-kinase (PI3K), Akt, c-Fos/c-Jun and AP-1-dependent signaling pathway.

(C) Effects on smooth muscle

Reference	Herrera and Marhuenda, 1993
Study	Effect of naringin and naringenin on contractions induced by noradrenaline in rat vas deferens was studied.
Results	Naringin significantly increased contractions induced by noradrenaline in rat vas deferens. Naringenin increased the contractile effect of noradrenaline and was dose dependent.
Conclusion	Naringin and naringinin increased contractions induced by noradrenaline in rat vas deferens.

Reference	
Study	The potency, structure-activity relationship, and mechanism of vasorelaxation of flavonols: fisetin, rutin, quercetin; flavones: chrysin, flavone, baicalein; flavanones: naringenin, naringin; isoflavones: diadzein and flavanes: epigallo catechin gallate, were examined in the isolated rat aorta.
Results	Most of the flavonoids tested showed concentration dependent relaxant effects against K+ (80 mM) and phenylephrine (PE, 0.1 microM)-induced contractions with a greater inhibition of the responses to the alpha1-adrenoceptor agonist.
Conclusion	Relaxant effects of flavonoids on vascular smooth muscle of the isolated rat thoracic aorta.

Reference	Saponara et al., 2006
Study	The mechanical and electrophysiological effects of (+/-)-naringenin were investigated In vascular smooth muscle cells.
Results	(+/-)-Naringenin induced concentration-dependent relaxation in endothelium-denuded rat aortic rings.
Conclusion	The vasorelaxant effect of the naturally-occurring flavonoid (+/-)-naringenin on endothelium-denuded vessels was due to the activation of BK (Ca) channels in myocytes.

(D) Effects on gastric intestinal system

Reference	Parmar, 1983
Study	The gastric anti-ulcer activity of a specific histidine decarboxylase inhibitor naringenin, has been studied on the various types of ulcers experimentally induced in rats, viz., pylorus-ligated (Shay method) and restraint ulcers, and on the gastric mucosal damage induced by aspirin, phenylbutazone or reserpine.
Results	Naringenin possessed significant anti-ulcer activity in all these models, manifesting a dose-dependent anti-ulcer effect.
Conclusion	Naringenin, a specific histidine decarboxylase inhibitor, has gastric anti-ulcer activity.

Reference	Martín et al., 1994
Study	To determine the gastroprotective properties of naringin on and the involvement of endogenous prostaglandins in mucosal injury produced by absolute ethanol.
Results	Oral pretreatment with the highest dose of naringin (400 mg/kg), 60 min before absolute ethanol was the most effective antiulcer treatment.
Conclusion	Naringin has a 'cytoprotective' effect against ethanol injury in the rat, but this property appears to be mediated by non-prostaglandin-dependent mechanisms.

Reference	Fenton and Hord, 2004
Study	Whether specific flavonoids induce cell migration in colon epithelial cells either wild type or heterozygous for Apc genotype was studied.
Results	Naringin and hesperidin induced the greatest migratory response in IMCE cells at 1 microM and induced migration greater than untreated control cells.
Conclusion	Flavonoids promote cell migration in nontumorigenic colon epithelial cells differing in Apc genotype.

(E) Effects on endocrine system

Reference	Divi and Doerge, 1996
Study	A structure-activity study of 13 commonly consumed flavonoids was conducted to evaluate inhibition of thyroid peroxidase (TPO), the enzyme that catalyzes thyroid hormone biosynthesis.
Results	Inhibition by the more potent fisetin, kaempferol, naringenin, and quercetin, was consistent with mechanism-based inactivation of TPO as previously observed for resorcinol and derivatives. Myricetin and naringin inhibited TPO by different mechanisms.
Conclusion	Dietary flavonoids inhibit thyroid peroxidase.

Reference	Déchaud et al., 1999
Study	This study reports on some environmental chemicals with estrogenic activity (xenoestrogens) and their binding interaction for human plasma sex-hormone binding globulin (hSHBG).
Results	The flavonoid phytoestrogens genistein and naringenin were also identified as hSHBG ligands, whereas their glucoside derivatives, genistin and naringin, had no binding activity for hSHBG.
Conclusion	Naringinin interacts with human sex hormone-binding globulin.

Reference	Asgary et al., 2002
Study	Several flavonoids, such as rutin, kaempferol, quercetin, apigenin, naringin, morin and biochanin A were selected to determine their antioxidant effects on in vitro insulin, hemoglobin and albumin glycosylation.
Results	Biochanin A, the best inhibitor of insulin and hemoglobin glycosylation, inhibits their glycosylation 100% and 60%, respectively. Glycosylation of albumin was inhibited 100% by both biochanin A and apigenin.
Conclusion	Plants containing flavonoids may have preventive effects in diabetic complications.

Reference	Jung et al., 2004
Study	The effect of citrus bioflavonoids on blood glucose level, hepatic glucose-regulating enzymes activities, hepatic glycogen concentration, and plasma insulin levels was studied, and assessed the relations between plasma leptin and body weight, blood glucose, and plasma insulin.
Results	Hesperidin and naringin supplementation significantly reduced blood glucose compared with the control group. Naringin also markedly lowered the activity of hepatic glucose-6-phosphatase and phosphoenolpyruvate carboxykinase compared with the control group.
Conclusion	Hesperidin and naringin prevent the progression of hyperglycemia, by increasing hepatic glycolysis and glycogen concentration and/or by lowering hepatic gluconeogenesis.

Reference	Ali and El Kader, 2004
Study	The effect of various doses of naringin was studied on streptozotocin (STZ)-induced hyperglycaemic rats to evaluate the possible hypoglycaemic and antioxidant activity of naringin in diabetes.
Results	Exogenous administration of naringin to hyperglycaemic rats causes a dose-dependent decrease of the glucose level, an increase of the insulin concentration, a decrease of the H_2O_2 and TBARS levels, as well as the increase of the total antioxidant status.
Conclusion	Naringin provided a significant amelioration of hypoglycaemic and antioxidant activity in STZ-induced diabetic rats.

Reference	Li et al., 2006
Study	Using purified intestinal brush border membrane vesicles and everted intestinal sleeves, glucose uptake in intestine was studied with naringinin and naringin.
Results	Naringenin, but not naringin, significantly inhibited glucose uptake in the intestine.
Conclusion	Inhibition of intestinal glucose uptake and renal glucose reabsorption explains, the antihyperglycemic action of naringenin and its derivatives.

Reference	Punithavathi et al., 2008
Study	The combined protective role of low dose of naringin (15 mg kg(-1)) and vitamin C (25 mg kg(-1)) and high dose of naringin (30 mg kg(-1)) and vitamin C (50 mg kg(-1)) on streptozotocin (STZ)-induced toxicity was studied in male Wistar rats.
Results	Oral administration of high doses of naringin (30 mg kg(-1)) and vitamin C (50 mg kg(-1)) to diabetic rats for a period of 21 days normalized all the above-mentioned biochemical parameters.
Conclusion	The antihyperglycemic and antioxidant effects of naringin and vitamin C in STZ-induced type II diabetes mellitus in rats.

(F) Effects against tumour

Reference	So et al., 1996
Study	Two citrus flavonoids, hesperetin and naringenin, and four noncitrus flavonoids, baicalein, galangin, genistein, and quercetin, were tested singly and in one-to-one combinations for their effects on proliferation and growth of a human breast carcinoma cell line, MDA-MB-435. These compounds, were tested for their ability to inhibit development of mammary tumors in female Sprague-Dawley rats.
Results	IC50 values for the one-to-one combinations ranged from 4.7 micrograms/ml (quercetin + hesperetin, quercetin + naringenin) to 22.5 micrograms/ml (naringenin + hesperetin). Rats given orange juice had a smaller tumor burden than controls, although they grew better than any of the other groups.
Conclusion	Citrus flavonoids are effective inhibitors of human breast cancer cell proliferation in vitro, especially when paired with quercetin.

Reference	Calomme et al., 1996
Study	The antimutagenicity of the Citrus flavonoids naringin, hesperidin, nobiletin, and tangeretin against the mutagens benzo[a]pyrene, 2-aminofluorene, quercetin, and nitroquinoline N-oxide was investigated in the Salmonella/microsome assay.
Results	Naringin and hesperidin showed a weak antimutagenic activity against benzo[a]pyrene.
Conclusion	The antimutagenic properties the Citrus flavonoids, especially tangeretin and nobiletin, might prevent cancer.

Reference	Le Marchand et al., 2000
Study	To investigate the possible relationship between intake of flavonoids-powerful dietary antioxidants that may also inhibit P450 enzymes-and lung cancer risk, we conducted a population-based, case-control study in Hawaii.
Results	Authors found statistically significant inverse associations between lung cancer risk and the main food sources of the flavonoids quercetin (onions and apples) and naringin (white grapefruit).
Conclusion	Foods rich in certain flavonoids may protect against certain forms of lung cancer. Decreased bioactivation of carcinogens by inhibition of CYP1A1 should be explored.

Reference	Russo et al., 2000
Study	Authors investigated the free-radical scavenging capacity of bioflavonoids (rutin, catechin, and naringin) and the effects of these polyphenols on xanthine oxidase activity, spontaneous lipid peroxidation, and DNA cleavage.
Results	The bioflavonoids under examination showed a dose-dependent free-radical scavenging effect, a significant inhibition of xanthine oxidase activity, and an antilipoperoxidative capacity. In addition, they showed a protective effect on DNA cleavage.
Conclusion	Bioflavonoids as antiradicals, antioxidants and DNA cleavage protectors.

Reference	Kanno et al., 2005
Study	The effect of naringenin on tumor growth in various human cancer cell lines and sarcoma S-180-implanted mice was studied.
Results	Naringenin inhibited tumor growth in sarcoma S-180-implanted mice, following intraperitoneal or peroral injection once a day for 5 d. Naringin also inhibited tumor growth by peroral injection but not intraperitoneal injection.
Conclusion	Inhibitory effects of naringenin on tumor growth in human cancer cell lines and sarcoma S-180-implanted mice.

Reference	Ugocsai et al., 2005
Study	The effects of various flavonoids and carotenoids on Rhodamine 123 accumulation in MDR Colo 320 human colon cancer cells expressing MDR1/LRP were studied. The Colo 205 cell line was used as a drug-sensitive control.
Results	Catechin, Neohesperidin, Naringin, Robinin, Phloridzin, Dihydrobinetin and Sakuranetin, had only marginal effects on Rhodamine 123 accumulation.
Conclusion	The tested flavonoids were weak apoptosis inducers on multidrug-resistant (MDR) and parent cells.

Reference	Vanamala et al., 2006
Study	The hypothesis that untreated and irradiated grapefruit as well as the isolated citrus compounds naringin and limonin would protect against azoxymethane (AOM)-induced aberrant crypt foci (ACF) by suppressing proliferation and elevating apoptosis through anti-inflammatory activities was examined.
Results	Lower levels of iNOS and COX-2 are associated with suppression of proliferation and upregulation of apoptosis, which may have contributed to a decrease in the number of high multiplicity ACF in rats provided with untreated grapefruit and limonin.
Conclusion	Consumption of grapefruit or limonin may help to suppress colon cancer development.

Reference	Schindler and Mentlein, 2006
Study	Whether secondary plant constituents, i.e., flavonoids, tocopherols, curcumin, and other substances regulate VEGF in human tumor cells in vitro was studied by measuring VEGF release by ELISA from MDA human breast cancer cells and, for comparison, U-343 and U-118 glioma cells.
Results	The rank order of VEGF inhibitory potency was naringin > rutin > alpha-tocopheryl succinate > lovastatin > apigenin > genistein > alpha-tocopherol >or= kaempferol > gamma-tocopherol; chrysin and curcumin were inactive except at a concentration of 100 micromol/L. Glioma cells were similarly sensitive, with U343 more than U118, especially for alpha-TOS and tocopherols.
Conclusion	Glycosylated flavonoids (i.e., naringin, a constituent of citrus fruits, and rutin, a constituent of cranberries) induced the greatest response to treatment at the lowest concentration in MDA human breast cancer cells.

Reference	Luo et al., 2008
Study	the effects of 12 different flavonoids and other substances on cell proliferation and VEGF expression in human ovarian cancer cells, OVCAR-3 were studied.
Results	The rank order of VEGF protein secretion inhibitory potency was genistein > kaempferol > apigenin > quercetin > tocopherol > luteolin > cisplatin > rutin > naringin > taxifolin.
Conclusion	Genistein, quercetin, and luteolin have shown strong inhibition to cell proliferation and VEGF expression of human ovarian cancer cells, and they show promising in the prevention of ovarian cancers.

Reference	Miller et al., 2008
Study	Six citrus flavonoids were tested for antineoplastic activity. The hamster cheek pouch model was utilized, and the solutions of the flavonoids (2.0-2.5%) and the solution of the carcinogen, 7,12-dimethylbenz[a]anthracene (0.5%), were applied topically to the pouches.
Results	The results with naringin and naringenin show that both of these flavonoids significantly lowered tumor number [5.00 (control group), 2.53 (naringin group), and 3.25 (naringenin group)]. Naringin also significantly reduced tumor burden [269 mm(3)(control group) and 77.1 mm(3)(naringin group)].
Conclusion	Naringin and naringenin, 2 flavonoids found in high concentrations in grapefruit, may be able to inhibit the development of cancer.

Reference	Kim et al., 2008
Study	Identified a novel mechanism of the anticancer effects of naringin in urinary bladder cancer cells.
Results	Naringin treatment resulted in significant dose-dependent growth inhibition together with G(1)-phase cell-cycle arrest at a dose of 100 microM (the half maximal inhibitory concentration) in 5637 cells. Naringin treatment strongly induced p21WAF1 expression, independent of the p53 pathway, and downregulated expression of cyclins and cyclin dependent kinases (CDKs).
Conclusion	The Ras/Raf/ERK pathway participates in p21WAF1 induction, subsequently leading to a decrease in the levels of cyclin D1/CDK4 and cyclin E-CDK2 complexes and naringin-dependent inhibition of cell growth. These provide a theoretical basis for the therapeutic use of flavonoids to treat malignancies.

(G) Protections against toxins in chemotherapy drugs and the environment

Reference	Gordon et al., 1995
Study	55 different flavonoids were tested for their effect on okadaic acid-inhibited autophagy, measured as the sequestration of electroinjected [3H] raffinose.
Results	Naringin (naringenin 7-hesperidoside) and several other flavanone and flavone glycosides (prunin, neoeriocitrin, neohesperidin, apiin, rhoifolin, kaempferol 3-rutinoside) offered virtually complete protection against the autophagy-inhibitory effect of okadaic acid.
Conclusion	Naringin and other okadaic acid-antagonistic flavonoids could have potential therapeutic value as protectants against pathological hyperphosphorylations, environmental toxins, or side effects of chemotherapeutic drugs.

Reference	Kawaguchi et al., 1999
Study	Suppressive effects of naringin on lipopolysaccharide-induced tumor necrosis factor (TNF) release followed by liver injury were investigated.
Results	Treatment with naringin 3 h prior to lipopolysaccharide challenge resulted in complete protection from lipopolysaccharide lethality in D-galactosamine-sensitized mice.
Conclusion	Action of naringin is mediated through suppression of lipopolysaccharide-induced TNF production.

Reference	Blankson et al., 2000
Study	The protein phosphatase-inhibitory algal toxins, okadaic acid and microcystin-LR, induced overphosphorylation of keratin and disruption of the keratin cytoskeleton in freshly isolated rat hepatocytes. In hepatocyte cultures, the toxins elicited DNA fragmentation and apoptotic cell death within 24 h.
Results	All these toxin effects could be prevented by the grapefruit flavonoid, naringin. The cytoprotective effect of naringin was apparently limited to normal hepatocytes, since the toxin-induced apoptosis of hepatoma cells, rat or human, was not prevented by the flavonoid.
Conclusion	Prevention of toxin-induced cytoskeletal disruption and apoptotic liver cell death by the grapefruit flavonoid, naringin.

Reference	Bear and Teel, 2000a
Study	Authors investigated the effects of five citrus phytochemicals on the in vitro metabolism of the tobacco-specific nitrosamine NNK and on the dealkylation of methoxyresorufin (MROD) and pentoxyresorufin (PROD) in liver and lung microsomes of the Syrian golden hamster.
Results	Results suggest that naringenin and quercetin from citrus fruits inhibit the activity of cytochrome P450 (CYP) isoforms that activate NNK and may afford protection against NNK-induced carcinogenesis.
Conclusion	Naringenin inhibits the activity of cytochrome P450 (CYP) isoforms that activate NNK

Reference	Bear and Teel, 2000b
Study	Using Aroclor 1254 induced rat liver S9, four citrus flavonoids: diosmin, naringenin, naringin and rutin were tested for their effects on the mutagenicity of HCA's MeIQx, Glu-P-1*, IQ and PhIP in Salmonella typhimurium TA98.
Results	MeIQx induced mutagenesis and PhIP induced mutagenesis in S. typhimurium were significantly inhibited by all four flavonoids. Glu-P-1 induced mutagenesis was inhibited by rutin and naringenin. IQ induced mutagenesis was significantly inhibited by each flavonoid except diosmin.
Conclusion	Diosmin, naringin, naringenin and rutin are chemoprotective towards CYPIA2 mediated mutagenesis of heterocyclic amines (HCA's)

Reference	Jagetia and Reddy, 2002
Study	The effect of various doses of naringin was studied on the alteration in the radiation-induced micronucleated polychromatic (MPCE) and normochromatic (MNCE) erythrocytes in mouse bone marrow exposed to 2 Gy of 60Co gamma-radiation.
Results	naringin is able to protect mouse bone marrow cells against the radiation-induced DNA damage and decline in the cell proliferation as observed by a reduction in the micronucleus frequency and an increase in PCE/NCE ratio, respectively, in the naringin-pretreated irradiated group.
Conclusion	Naringin protects against the radiation-induced genomic instability in the mice bone marrow.

Reference	Seo et al., 2003
Study	The effect of naringin supplements on the alcohol, lipid, and antioxidant metabolism in ethanol-treated rats was investigated.
Results	Naringin would appear to contribute to alleviating the adverse effect of ethanol ingestion by enhancing the ethanol and lipid metabolism as well as the hepatic antioxidant defense system.
Conclusion	Naringin supplement regulate lipid and ethanol metabolism

Reference	Kanno et al., 2003
Study	The effects of naringin on H_2O_2-induced cytotoxicity and apoptosis in mouse leukemia P388 cells were investigated.
Results	H_2O_2-induced cytotoxicity was significantly attenuated by naringin or the reduced form of glutathione, a typical intracellular antioxidant. Naringin suppressed chromatin condensation and DNA damage induced by H_2O_2.
Conclusion	Naringin from natural products is a useful drug having antioxidant and anti-apoptopic properties.

Reference	Jagetia et al., 2003
Study	The radioprotective action of 2 mg/kg naringin in the bone marrow of mice exposed to different doses of (60)Co gamma-radiation was studied by scoring the frequency of asymmetrical chromosomal aberrations.
Results	Naringin at 5 μM scavenged the 2,2-azino-bis-3-ethyl benzothiazoline-6-sulphonic acid cation radical very efficiently, where a 90% scavenging was observed.
Conclusion	Naringin can protect mouse bone marrow cells against radiation-induced chromosomal damage.

Reference	Kumar et al., 2003
Study	The effect of naringin and naringenin protect hemoglobin from nitrite-induced oxidation to methemoglobin was studied.
Results	Naringenin was more effective than naringin, probably because of the extra phenolic group in the aglycone.
Conclusion	Naringin and naringenin inhibit nitrite-induced methemoglobin formation.

Reference	Kawaguchi et al., 2004
Study	The protective effect of the naringin was studied in an endotoxin shock model based on Salmonella infection. Intraperitoneal (i. p.) infection with 10 (8) CFU Salmonella typhimurium aroA caused lethal shock in lipopolysaccharide (LPS) -responder but not LPS-non-responder mice.
Results	Administration of 1 mg naringin 3 h before infection resulted in protection from lethal shock, similar to LPS-non-responder mice. Also resulted not only in a significant decrease in bacterial numbers in spleens and livers, but also in a decrease in plasma LPS levels.
Conclusion	Suppression of infection-induced endotoxin shock in mice by naringin.

Reference	Kanno et al., 2004
Study	The effect of naringin on the cytotoxicity and apoptosis in mouse leukemia P388 cells treated with Ara-C. Ara-C caused cytotoxicity in a concentration and time-dependent manner in the cells was examined.
Results	Naringin remarkably attenuated the Ara-C-induced apoptosis and completely blocked the DNA damage caused by Ara-C treatment at 6 h using the Comet assay.
Conclusion	Naringin blocked apoptosis caused by Ara-C-induced oxidative stress, resulting in the inhibition of the cytotoxicity of Ara-C.

Reference	Singh et al., 2004a
Study	The effect of naringin, a bioflavonoid with anti-oxidant potential, was studied on Fe-NTA-induced nephrotoxicity in rats.
Results	Pre-treatment of animals with naringin, 60 min before Fe-NTA administration, markedly attenuated renal dysfunction, morphological alterations, reduced elevated TBARS, and restored the depleted renal anti-oxidant enzymes.
Conclusion	There is a protective effect of naringin on Fe-NTA-induced nephrotoxicity in rats.

Reference	Singh et al., 2004b
Study	The effect of naringin, a bioflavonoid with anti-oxidant potential, was studied in glycerol-induced ARF in rats.
Results	Pretreatment of animals with naringin 60 min prior to glycerol injection markedly attenuated renal dysfunction, morphological alterations, reduced elevated thiobarbituric acid reacting substances (TBARS), and restored the depleted renal antioxidant enzymes.
Conclusion	There is a protective effect of naringin in glycerol-induced renal failure in rats.

Reference	Jagetia et al., 2004
Study	Whether naringin treatment may help to overcome the iron-induced toxic effects in vitro was studied.
Results	Pretreatment of HepG2 cells with naringin resulted in an elevation in all the antioxidant enzymes.
Conclusion	Enhanced antioxidant status by naringin could compensate the oxidative stress and may facilitate an early recovery from iron-induced genomic insult in vitro.

Reference	Jagetia and Reddy, 2005
Study	The alteration in the antioxidant status and lipid peroxidation was investigated in Swiss albino mice treated with 2 mg/kg b.wt. naringin, a citrus flavoglycoside, before exposure to 0.5, 1, 2, 3, and 4 Gy gamma radiation.
Results	The alteration in the antioxidant status and lipid peroxidation was investigated in Swiss albino mice treated with 2 mg/kg b.wt. naringin, a citrus flavoglycoside, before exposure to 0.5, 1, 2, 3, and 4 Gy gamma radiation.
Conclusion	Naringin protects mouse liver and intestine against the radiation-induced damage by elevating the antioxidant status and reducing the lipid peroxidation

Reference	Yeh et al., 2005
Study	The interaction of beta-carotene with three flavonoids-naringin, rutin and quercetin-on DNA damage induced by ultraviolet A (UVA) in C3H10T1/2 cells was studied.
Results	All three flavonoids had some absorption at the UVA range, but the effects were opposite to those on DNA damage and beta-carotene oxidation.
Conclusion	A combination of beta-carotene with naringin, rutin or quercetin may increase the safety of beta-carotene.

Reference	Shiratori et al., 2005
Study	The efficacy of naringin and naringenin on endotoxin- induced uveitis (EIU) in rats was studied. EIU was induced in male Lewis rats by a footpad injection of lipopolysaccharide (LPS).
Results	40 microM/kg of naringin and naringenin suppressed increases in cell count owing to LPS treatment by 31% and 38%, respectively.
Conclusion	Possible mechanism for the antiocular inflammatory effect may be the suppression of PGE_2 and NO by naringin and naringenin.

Reference	Kanno et al., 2006)
Study	The effect of naringin, on LPS-induced endotoxin shock in mice and NO production in RAW 264.7 macrophages was studied.
Results	Naringin suppressed LPS -induced production of NO and the expression of inflammatory gene products such as iNOS, TNF-alpha, COX-2 and IL-6 as determined by RT-PCR assay.
Conclusion	Suppression of the LPS-induced mortality and production of NO by NG is due to inhibition of the activation of NF-kappaβ

Reference	Jagetia et al., 2005
Study	The effect of naringin, a grapefruit flavonone was studied on bleomycin-induced genomic damage and alteration in the survival of cultured V79 cells.
Results	Treatment of cells with naringin before exposure to different concentrations of bleomycin arrested the bleomycin-induced decline in the cell survival accompanied by a significant reduction in the frequency of micronuclei when compared with bleomycin treatment alone.
Conclusion	Naringin reduced the genotoxic effects of bleomycin and consequently increased the cell survival and therefore may act as a chemoprotective agent in clinical situations.

Reference	Hori et al., 2007
Study	A diversity of antioxidants and plant ingredients were examined for their protective effect in cultured Balb/c 3T3 cells against ultraviolet A (UVA)-induced cytotoxicities of extracted air pollutants and benz[a]pyrene (B[a]P).
Results	The B[a]P phototoxicity was not eliminated by well-known antioxidants but was markedly diminished by diversity of plant ingredients.
Conclusion	Among the plant ingredients tested in the current study, morin, naringin, and quercetin were found to be desirable protectors against B[a]P phototoxicity.

Reference	Attia, 2008
Study	Anti-mutagenic effects of naringin, against lomefloxacin-induced genomic instability in vivo were evaluated in mouse bone marrow cells by chromosomal aberration and micronucleus (MN) assays.
Results	Naringin was neither genotoxic nor cytotoxic in mice at doses equivalent to 5 or 50 mg/kg. Pre-treatment of mice with naringin significantly reduced lomefloxacin-induced chromosomal aberrations and the MN formation in bone marrow.
Conclusion	Naringin has a protective role in the abatement of lomefloxacin-induced genomic instability that resides, at least in part, in its anti-radical effects.

Reference	Benković et a., 2008
Study	The radioprotective effects of water-soluble derivate of propolis (WSDP) collected in Croatia, and single flavonoids, caffeic acid, chrysin and naringin in the whole-body irradiated CBA mice were investigated.
Results	Possible genotoxic effects of all test components were assessed on non-irradiated animals. The higher efficiency of test components was observed when given preventively.
Conclusion	Propolis and related flavonoids given to mice before irradiation protected mice from lethal effects of whole-body irradiation and diminish primary DNA damage in their white blood cells as detected by the alkaline comet assay.

(H) Antioxidant effects

Reference	Younes and Siegers, 1981
Study	Depletion of hepatic glutathione in phenobarbital-induced rats by phorone (diisopropylidene acetone) led to an enhancement of spontaneous lipid peroxidation in vitro. Addition of exogenous glutathione, dithiocarb or one of the flavonoids (+)-catechin, (-)-epicatechin, 3-O-methylcatechin, quercetin, taxifolin, rutin, naringin or naringenin led in every case to a dose-dependent inhibition of this peroxidative activity.
Results	The concentration values yielding 50% inhibition (I (50)) varied from 1.0 x 10 (-6) M for glutathione to 1.9 x 10 (-5) M for naringenin.
Conclusion	Some flavonoids have inhibitory action on enhanced spontaneous lipid peroxidation following glutathione depletion.

Reference	Kroyer, 1986
Study	The antioxidant properties of freeze-dried citrus fruit peels (orange, lemon, grapefruit) and methanolic extracts from the peel were studied.
Results	Freeze-dried orange peel showed the highest, lemon peel somewhat less and grapefruit peel the lowest but still remarkable antioxidant activity.
Conclusion	Citrus fruit peels have antioxidant activity.

Reference	Affany et al., 1987
Study	Cumene hydroperoxide induces in vitro the peroxidation of erythrocyte membrane. The protective effect of various flavonoids was compared to that of butylated hydroxytoluene (BHT). Protective effect was evaluated by the inhibition of peroxidation product formation.
Results	Quercetin and catechin showed a protective effect against lipid peroxidation as high as that of BHT. Morin, rutin, trihydroxyethylrutin, and naringin were active but to a lesser degree.
Conclusion	Flavonoids have protective effect against lipid peroxidation of erythrocyte membranes.

Reference	Ratty and Das, 1988
Study	The in vitro effects of several flavonoids on nonenzymatic lipid peroxidation in the rat brain mitochondria was studied. The lipid peroxidation was indexed by using the 2-thiobarbituric acid test.
Results	The flavonoids, apigenin, flavone, flavanone, hesperidin, naringin, and tangeretin promoted the ascorbic acid-induced lipid peroxidation.
Conclusion	Polyhydroxylated substitutions on rings A and B, a 2,3-double bond, a free 3-hydroxyl substitution and a 4-keto moiety confer antiperoxidative properties.

Reference	Chen et al., 1990
Study	The superoxide anions scavenging activity and antioxidation of seven flavonoids were studied. The superoxide anions were generated in a phenazin methosulphate-NADH system and were assayed by reduction of nitroblue tetrazolium.
Results	The scavenging activity ranked: rutin was the strongest, and quercetin and naringin the second, while morin and hispidulin were very weak.
Conclusion	Flavonoids are superoxide scavengers and antioxidants.

Reference	Ng et al., 2000
Study	A variety of flavonoids, lignans, an alkaloid, a bisbenzyl, coumarins and terpenes isolated from Chinese herbs was tested for antioxidant activity as reflected in the ability to inhibit lipid peroxidation in rat brain and kidney homogenates and rat erythrocyte hemolysis. The pro-oxidant activities of the aforementioned compounds were assessed by their effects on bleomycin-induced DNA damage.
Results	The flavonoid rutin and the terpene tanshinone I manifested potent antioxidative activity in the lipid peroxidation assay but no inhibitory activity in the hemolysis assay. The lignan deoxypodophyllotoxin, the flavonoid naringin and the coumarins columbianetin, bergapten and angelicin slightly inhibited lipid peroxidation in brain and kidney homogenates.
Conclusion	Aromatic hydroxyl group is very important for antioxidative effects of the compounds. None of the compounds tested exerted an obvious pro-oxidant effect.

Reference	Jeon et al., 2001
Study	To determine the antioxidative effects of the citrus bioflavonoid, naringin, a potent cholesterol-lowering agent, compared to the cholesterol-lowering drug, lovastatin, in rabbits fed a high cholesterol diet.
Results	Naringin regulate antioxidative capacities by increasing the SOD and catalase activities, up-regulating the gene expressions of SOD, catalase, and GSH-Px, and protecting the plasma vitamin E. Lovastatin exhibited an inhibitory effect on the plasma and hepatic lipid peroxidation and increased the hepatic catalase activity.
Conclusion	Antioxidative activity of naringin and lovastatin in high cholesterol-fed rabbits.

Reference	Jeon et al., 2002
Study	Twenty male rabbits were served a high-cholesterol diet or high-cholesterol diet supplemented with naringin or probucol for 8 weeks to compare the antioxidative effects of the naringin and antioxidative cholesterol-lowering drug (probucol).
Results	The probucol supplement was very potent in the antioxidative defense system, whereas naringin exhibited a comparable antioxidant capacity based on increasing the gene expressions in the antioxidant enzymes, increasing the hepatic SOD and CAT activities, sparing plasma vitamin E, and decreasing the hepatic mitochondrial H_2O_2 content.
Conclusion	Antioxidant effects of naringin and probucol in cholesterol-fed rabbits

Reference	Yu et al., 2005
Study	A variety of in vitro models such as beta-carotene-linoleic acid, 1,1-diphenyl-2-picryl hydrazyl (DPPH), superoxide, and hamster low-density lipoprotein (LDL) were used to measure the antioxidant activity of 11 citrus bioactive compounds.
Results	Flavonoids, which contain a chromanol ring system, had stronger antioxidant activity as compared to limonoids and bergapten, which lack the hydroxy groups.
Conclusion	Several structural features were linked to the strong antioxidant activity of flavonoids.

Reference	Gorinstein et al., 2005
Study	The influence of naringin versus red grapefruit juice on plasma lipid levels and plasma antioxidant activity in rats fed cholesterol-containing and cholesterol-free diets was compared.
Results	After 30 days of different feeding, it was found that diets supplemented with red grapefruit juice and to a lesser degree with naringin improved the plasma lipid levels mainly in rats fed cholesterol and increased the plasma antioxidant activity.
Conclusion	Naringin is a powerful plasma lipid lowering and plasma antioxidant activity increasing flavonone. However, fresh red grapefruit is preferable than naringin.

Reference	Hsu and Yen 2006
Study	The relationship between the influence of flavonoids on cell population growth and their antioxidant activity was studied.
Results	The inhibition of flavonoids (naringenin, rutin, hesperidin, resveratrol, naringin and quercetin) on 3T3-L1 pre-adipocytes was 28.3, 8.1, 11.1, 33.2, 5.6 and 71.5%, respectively.
Conclusion	Induction of cell apoptosis in 3T3-L1 pre-adipocytes by flavonoids is associated with their antioxidant activity.

Reference	Pereira et al., 2007
Study	In order to understand the contribution of the metal coordination and the type of interaction between a flavonoid and the metal ion, in this study a new metal complex of Cu (II) with naringin was synthesized and characterized by FT-IR, UV-VIS, mass spectrometry (ESI-MS/MS), elemental analysis and 1H-NMR.
Results	The results of these analyses indicate that the complex has a Cu (II) ion coordinated via positions 4 and 5 of the flavonoid.
Conclusion	The Naringin-Cu (II) complex 1 showed higher antioxidant, anti-inflammatory and tumor cell cytotoxicity activities than free naringin without reducing cell viability. Naringin and naringinin have been identified as prooxidants independent of transition metal catalysed autoxidation reactions.

Reference	Nafisi et al., 2008
Study	To examine the interactions of three flavonoids; morin (Mor), apigenin (Api) and naringin (Nar) with yeast RNA in aqueous solution at physiological conditions
Results	Spectroscopic evidence showed major binding of flavonoids to RNA with overall binding constants of K(morin)=9.150x10(3)M(-1), K(apigenin)=4.967x10(4)M(-1), and K(naringin)=1.144x10(4)M(-1).
Conclusion	The affinity of flavonoid-RNA binding is in the order of apigenin>naringin>morin.

Reference	Zielińska-Przyjemska and Ignatowicz., 2008
Study	Three citrus flavonoids - naringin, naringenin and hesperidin - have been examined for their ability to activate caspase-3, a marker of apoptosis execution, in human polymorphonuclear neutrophils in vitro, stimulated and non-stimulated with phorbol 12-myristate 13-acetate.
Results	Flavonoids inhibited the neutrophil ability to generate superoxide radical and 10-100 microm hesperidin appeared the most active phytochemical.
Conclusion	Reactive oxygen species may inhibit apoptosis via caspase-3 inhibition and the antioxidant action of citrus flavonoids may reverse this process.

Reference	Nafisi et al., 2008
Study	To examine the interactions of morin (Mor), naringin (Nar), and apigenin (Api) with calf thymus DNA in aqueous solution at physiological conditions,
Results	Spectroscopic evidence shows both intercalation and external binding of flavonoids to DNA duplex with overall binding constants of K(morin) = 5.99 x 10(3) M(-1), K(apigenin) = 7.10 x 10(4) M(-1), and K(naringin) = 3.10 x 10(3) M(-1).
Conclusion	The affinity of ligand-DNA binding is in the order of apigenin > morin > naringin. DNA aggregation and a partial B- to A-DNA transition occurs upon morin, apigenin, and naringin complexion.

(I) Antimicrobial effects

Reference	Ng et al., 1996
Study	Coumarins, flavonoids and polysaccharopeptide were tested for antibacterial activity. The bacteria used for this study included clinical isolates of Staphylococcus aureus, Shigella flexneri, Salmonella typhi, Escherichia coli and Pseudomonas aeruginosa.
Results	When tested at the dose of 128 mg/l, the flavonoids (rutin, naringin and baicalin) inhibited 25% or less of P. aeruginosa and only baicalin was active against S. aureus.
Conclusion	Naringin inhibited P. aeruginosa.

Reference	Paredes et al., 2003
Study	The effect of hesperetin, naringenin and its glycoside form on the Sindbis neurovirulent strain (NSV) replication in vitro was studied. All flavanones tested were not cytotoxic on Baby Hamster cells 21 clone 15 (BHK-21).
Results	Hesperetin and naringenin had inhibitory activity on NSV infection. However their glycosides, hesperidin and naringin did not have inhibitory activity. Implying that the presence of rutinose moiety of flavanones blocks the antiviral effect.
Conclusion	Anti-Sindbis activity of flavanones hesperetin and naringenin.

Reference	Cvetnić and Vladimir-Knezević, 2004
Study	Antibacterial and antifungal activity of ethanolic extract of grapefruit (Citrus paradisi Macf., Rutaceae) seed and pulp was examined against 20 bacterial and 10 yeast strains
Results	Ethanolic extract exibited the strongest antimicrobial effect against Salmonella enteritidis (MIC 2.06%, m/V). Other tested bacteria and yeasts were sensitive to extract concentrations ranging from 4.13% to 16.50% (m/V).
Conclusion	There exist antimicrobial activity of grapefruit seed and pulp ethanolic extract.

Reference	Wood, 2007
Study	The present study evaluates two separate, but related, dietary trials-trial 1, dietary naringenin (NAR) supplementation; and trial 2, dietary rutin (R), quercetin (Q), and naringin (N) supplementation-on dental caries formation in 40 different male albino rats, at the expense of dextrose, for periods of 42 days.
Results	An inverse dose-dependent relationship was established among the NAR experimental groups and control group. In dietary trial 2, statistically significant reductions in occlusal caries were observed for R, Q, and N in the maxillary molars and for Q and N in the mandibular molars compared with the control group.
Conclusion	Selected bioflavonoids may show promise as an alternative means of reducing dental caries.

Reference	Tsui et al., 2007
Study	The effects of naringin on the growth of periodontal pathogens such as A. actinomycetemcomitans and P. gingivalis were studied in vitro. For comparison, the effects of naringin on several oral microbes were also studied.
Results	Naringin also had an inhibitory effect against all bacteria and yeasts tested.
Conclusion	Naringin possesses significant antimicrobial properties on periodontal pathogens in vitro. It also has an inhibitory effect on some common oral microorganisms in low concentrations.

(J) Drug interactions

Reference	Fuhr et al., 1993
Study	The effects of grapefruit juice and naringenin on the activity of the human cytochrome P450 isoform CYP1A2 were evaluated using caffeine as a probe substrate.
Results	In vitro naringin was a potent competitive inhibitor of caffeine 3-demethylation by human liver microsomes (Ki = 7-29 microM). In vivo grapefruit juice decreased the oral clearance of caffeine and prolonged its half-life.
Conclusion	Grapefruit juice and naringenin inhibit CYP1A2 activity in man.

Reference	Bailey et al., 1993a
Study	The pharmacokinetics of felodipine and its single primary oxidative metabolite, dehydrofelodipine, were studied after drug administration with 200 ml water, grapefruit juice, or naringin in water at the same concentration as the juice in a randomized crossover trial of nine healthy men.
Results	Grapefruit juice produces a marked and variable increase in felodipine bioavailability. Naringin solution produced much less of an interaction, showing that other factors were important.
Conclusion	Grapefruit juice produces a marked and variable increase in felodipine bioavailability.

Reference	Bailey et al., 1993b
Study	The pharmacokinetics of nisoldipine coat-core tablet were studied in a Latin square-designed trial in which 12 healthy men were administered the drug with water, grapefruit juice, or encapsulated naringin powder at the same amount as that assayed in the juice.
Results	The bioavailability of some dihydropyridine calcium antagonists can be markedly augmented by grapefruit juice. The naringin capsule did not change nisoldipine pharmacokinetics.
Conclusion	The bioavailability of some dihydropyridine calcium antagonists can be augmented by grapefruit juice but does not involve naringin.

Reference	Runkel et al., 1997
Study	To investigate whether the presence of naringin is demanded for the inhibition of the coumarin 7-hydroxylase in man or other compounds are responsible for it.
Results	While increasing amounts of grapefruit juice delay the excretion of 7-hydroxycoumarin by 2 h, increasing doses of naringin in water up to twofold do not cause any alteration in the time course of excretion.
Conclusion	As naringin alone is ineffective, the inhibitory effect of grapefruit juice on the metabolism of coumarin is caused by at least one compound other than naringin.

Reference	Fuhr et al., 1998
Study	A randomized crossover interaction study on the effects of grapefruit juice on the pharmacokinetics of nimodipine and its metabolites.
Results	Grapefruit juice increases oral nimodipine bioavailability.
Conclusion	To avoid the interaction, nimodipine should not be taken with grapefruit juice.

Reference	Bailey et al., 1998
Study	To test whether naringin or 6',7'-dihydroxybergamottin is a major active substance in grapefruit juice-felodipine interaction in humans.
Results	The findings show the importance of in vivo testing to determine the ingredients in grapefruit juice responsible for inhibition of cytochrome P450 3A4 in humans.
Conclusion	Naringin and 6',7'-dihydroxybergamottin are not the major active ingredients, although they may contribute to the grapefruit juice-felodipine interaction.

Reference	Ubeaud et al., 1999
Study	NRG's inhibition of the metabolism of SV in rat hepatocytes (the intrinsic clearance of SV) was studied.
Results	Naringenin present in grapefruit juice inhibits in vitro the metabolism of simvastatin, a HMG-CoA reductase inhibitor.
Conclusion	In vitro inhibition of simvastatin (SV) metabolism in rat and human liver by naringenin (NRG).

Reference	Ueng et al., 1999
Study	In vitro and in vivo effects of naringin on microsomal monooxygenase were studied to evaluate the drug interaction of this flavonoid.
Results	Naringenin is a potent inhibitor of benzo(a)pyrene hydroxylase activity in vitro and naringin reduces the P450 1A2 protein level in vivo.
Conclusion	These effects may indicate a chemopreventive role of naringin against protoxicants activated by P450 1A2.

Reference	Mitsunaga et al., 2000
Study	To see whether grapefruit juice bioflavonoids alter the permeation of vincristine across the blood-brain barrier, we conducted experiments with cultured mouse brain capillary endothelial cells (MBEC4 cells) in vitro and ddY mice in vivo.
Results	The in vivo brain-to-plasma concentration ratio of [3H]vincristine in ddY mice was decreased by coadministration of 0.1 mg/kg quercetin, but increased by 1.0 mg/kg quercetin. Kaempferol had a similar biphasic effect. Cchrysin, flavon, hesperetin, naringenin increased [3H]vincristine uptake in the 10-50 microM range, and glycosides (hesperidin, naringin, rutin) were without effect.
Conclusion	Patients taking drugs which are P-glycoprotein substrates may need to restrict their intake of bioflavonoid-containing foods and beverages, such as grapefruit juice.

Reference	Ho et al., 2001
Study	33 flavonoids, occurring ubiquitously in foods of plant origin, were tested for their ability to alter the transport of the beta-lactam antibiotic cefixime via the H+-coupled intestinal peptide transporter PEPT1 in the human intestinal epithelial cell line Caco-2. To evaluate the inhibition of CYP3A4 activity in human liver microsomes by flavonoids, furanocoumarins and related compounds and investigate possibly more important and potential inhibitors of CYP3A4 in grapefruit juice.
Results	Quercetin, genistein, naringin, diosmin, acacetin, and chrysin increased uptake of [14C] cefixime dose dependently by up to 60%. Bergapten (5-methoxypsoralen) with the lowest IC50 value (19-36 microM) was the most potent CYP3A4 inhibitor.
Conclusion	Flavonoids with EGF-receptor tyrosine kinase inhibitory activities enhance the intestinal absorption of the beta-lactam antibiotic cefixime in Caco-2 cells. Bergapten appears to be a potent inhibitor of CYP3A4, and may therefore be primarily responsible for the effect of grapefruit juice on CYP3A4 activity.

Reference	Choi and Shin, 2005
Study	The effect of naringin on the bioavailability and pharmacokinetics of paclitaxel after oral administration of paclitaxel or its prodrug coadministered with naringin to rats was studied.
Results	The bioavailability of paclitaxel coadministered as a prodrug with or without naringin was remarkably higher than the control.
Conclusion	Enhanced paclitaxel bioavailability after oral coadministration of paclitaxel prodrug with naringin to rats.

Reference	Kim and Choi, 2005
Study	The pharmacokinetics of verapamil and one of its metabolites, norverapamil, were investigated after oral administration of verapamil at a dose of 9 mg/kg without or with oral naringin at a dose of 7.5 mg/kg in rabbits. With naringin, the total area under the plasma concentration-time curve (AUC) of verapamil was significantly greater, the AUC(verapamil)/AUC(norverapamil) ratio was considerably greater.
Results	With naringin, the total area under the plasma concentration-time curve (AUC) of verapamil was significantly greater, the AUC(verapamil)/AUC(norverapamil) ratio was considerably greater.
Conclusion	The metabolism of verapamil and the formation of norverapamil were inhibited by naringin possibly by inhibition of CYP3A in rabbits.

Reference	Choi and Han, 2005
Study	Pharmacokinetic parameters of diltiazem and desacetyldiltiazem were determined in rats following an oral administration of diltiazem to rats in the presence and absence of naringin.
Results	Absolute and relative bioavailability values of diltiazem in the presence of naringin were significantly higher than those from the control group.
Conclusion	The concomitant use of naringin significantly enhanced the oral exposure of diltiazem in rats.

Reference	Yeum and Choi, 2006
Study	The effect of naringin on the pharmacokinetics of verapamil and its major metabolite, norverapamil in rabbits were studied.
Results	Pretreatment of naringin enhanced the oral bioavailability of verapamil.
Conclusion	Verapamil dosage should be adjusted when given with naringin or a naringin-containing dietary supplement.

Reference	Lim and Choi, 2006
Study	The effects of oral naringin on the pharmacokinetics of intravenous paclitaxel in rats were studied.
Results	After intravenous administration of paclitaxel, the AUC was significantly greater, and Cl was significantly slower than controls.
Conclusion	The inhibition of hepatic P-gp by oral naringin could also contribute to the significantly greater AUC of intravenous paclitaxel by oral naringin.

Reference	Bailey et al., 2007
Study	Inhibition of OATP1A2 transport by flavonoids in grapefruit (naringin) and orange (hesperidin) was conducted in vitro. Two randomized, crossover, pharmacokinetic studies were performed clinically.
Results	Naringin most probably directly inhibited enteric OATP1A2 to decrease oral fexofenadine bioavailability. Inactivation of enteric CYP3A4 was probably not involved.
Conclusion	Naringin is a major and selective clinical inhibitor of organic anion-transporting polypeptide 1A2 (OATP1A2) in grapefruit juice.

Reference	Li et al., 2007
Study	The esterase-inhibitory potential of 10 constitutive flavonoids and furanocoumarins toward p-nitrophenylacetate (PNPA) hydrolysis was investigated.
Results	In Caco-2 cells, demonstrated to contain minimal CYP3A activity, the permeability coefficient of the prodrugs lovastatin and enalapril was increased in the presence of the active flavonoids kaempferol and naringenin, consistent with inhibition of esterase activity.
Conclusion	Kaempferol and naringenin are shown to mediate pharmacokinetic drug interaction with the prodrugs lovastatin and enalapril due to their capability of esterase inhibition.

Reference	de Castro et al., 2007
Study	The potential interaction between selected ingredients of grapefruit juice and, the transport of talinolol, a P-gp substrate, across Caco-2 cells monolayers was determined in the absence and presence of distinct concentrations of grapefruit juice, bergamottin, 6',7'-dihydroxybergamottin, 6',7'-epoxybergamottin, naringin, and naringenin.
Results	The flavonoid aglycone naringenin was around 10-fold more potent than its glycoside naringin with IC(50) values of 236 and 2409 microM, respectively.
Conclusion	The in vitro data suggest that compounds present in grapefruit juice are able to inhibit the P-gp activity modifying the disposition of drugs that are P-gp substrates such as talinolol.

Reference	Shim et al., 2007
Study	The cellular uptake of benzoic acid was examined in the presence and the absence of naringin, naringenin, morin, silybin and quercetin in Caco-2 cells.
Results	All the tested flavonoids except naringin significantly inhibited the cellular uptake of [(14)C]-benzoic acid. Particularly, naringenin and silybin exhibited strong inhibition effects.
Conclusion	Some flavonoids appeared to be competitive inhibitors of monocarboxylate transporter 1 (MCT1)

Reference	Shirasaka et al., 2008
Study	The impact of P-gp and Oatp on intestinal absorption of the beta(1)-adrenoceptor antagonist talinolol.
Results	Naringin inhibited talinolol uptake by Oatp1a5 (IC (50) = 12.7 muM).
Conclusion	The absorption behavior of talinolol can be explained by the involvement of both P-gp and Oatp, based on characterization of talinolol transport by Oatp1a5 and P-gp, and the effects of naringin.

Reference	Taur and Rodriguez-Proteau, 2008
Study	To study cimetidine as a substrate of P-glycoprotein (P-gp) and organic cation transport systems and the modulatory effects of eight flavonoid aglycones and glycosides on these transport systems using Caco-2 and LLC-PK1 cells.
Results	Intracellular uptake rate of (14)C-tetraethylammonium (TEA) was reduced in the presence of quercetin, naringenin and genistein in LLC-PK1 cells.
Conclusion	Quercetin, naringenin, genistein, and xanthohumol reduced P-gp-mediated transport and increased the basolateral uptake rate of cimetidine. Quercetin, naringenin, genistein, but not xanthohumol, reduced intracellular uptake rate of TEA in LLC-PK1 cells. These results suggest that flavonoids may have potential to alter the disposition profile of cimetidine and possibly other therapeutics that are mediated by P-gp and/or cation transport systems.

Reference	de Castro et al., 2008
Study	grapefruit juice (white and ruby red) and its selected components (naringin, naringenin, and bergamottin) was investigated on the activity of the P-glycoprotein (P-gp) in male Sprague-Dawley rats.
Results	The flavonoids naringenin (0.7 mg/kg) and naringin (2.4 and 9.4 mg/kg) had a similar effect increasing the talinolol C max and AUC (0-infinity) by 1.5- to 1.8-fold, respectively.
Conclusion	the effect of GFJ on P-gp activity seems to depend on the variety, the concentration of compounds in the juice, and the composition of different ingredients.

(K) Anti-inflammatory effects

Reference	Lambev et al., 1980a
Study	Experiments are carried out on 35 male albino rats. The effect of the flavonoids naringin and rutin on the level of mastocytic and nonmastocytic histamine is studied, as well as on its release induced by compound 48/80 (2 mg/kg i. p.). The histamine content is determined fluorimetrically.
Results	Naringin and rutin have no effect on the levels of mastocytic and nonmastocytic histamine. They prevent the release of mastocytic histamine, induced by compound 48/80.
Conclusion	Flavonoids with antioxidant action (naringin and rutin) prevent the release of mastocytic and nonmastocytic histamine.

Reference	Lambev et al., 1980b
Study	The authors examined antiexudative activity of bioflavonoids naringin and rutin in comparative aspect in two models of acute inflammation. The experiments were carried out on 180 male white rats and 24 guinea pigs.
Results	The two flavonoids manifested marked antiexudative effect in rats with experiments peritonitis.
Conclusion	Naringin has antiexudative effect of in experimental pulmonary edema and peritonitis.

Reference	Middleton and Drzewiecki, 1984
Study	Eleven flavonoids included flavone, quercetin, taxifolin, chalcone, apigenin, fisetin, rutin, phloretin, tangeretin, hesperetin, and naringin were studied for their effects on human basophil histamine release triggered by six different stimuli.
Results	The flavonols, quercetin and fisetin, and the flavone, apigenin, exhibited a predilection to inhibit histamine release stimulated by IgE-dependent ligands (antigen, anti-IgE, and con A). The flavanone derivatives, taxifolin and hesperetin, were inactive, as were the glycosides, rutin and naringin. The open chain congeners, chalcone and phloretin, also possessed inhibitory activity.
Conclusion	Flavonoid inhibited human basophil histamine release stimulated by various agents.

Reference	Park et al., 2005
Study	The passive cutaneous anaphylaxis-inhibitory activity of the flavanones isolated from the pericarp of Citrus unshiu (Family Rutaceae) and the fruit of Poncirus trifoliata (Family Rutaceae) was studied.
Results	Naringenin, hesperetin and ponciretin potently inhibited IgE-induced beta-hexosaminidase release from RBL-2H3 cells and the PCA reaction.
Conclusion	Flavanone glycosides can be activated by intestinal bacteria, and may be effective toward IgE-induced atopic allergies.

Reference	Fujita et al., 2008
Study	The competitive inhibitory effects of extracts from immature citrus fruit on CYP activity.
Results	Extracts having relatively strong inhibitory effects for CYP3A4 tended to contain higher amounts of naringin, bergamottin and 6',7'-dihydroxybergamottin.
Conclusion	Citrus extracts containing high levels of narirutin and hesperidin and lower levels of furanocoumarins such as C. unshiu are favorable as antiallergic functional ingredients.

(L) Other effects

Reference	Chan et al., 1999
Study	Flavonoids containing phenol B rings, e.g. naringenin, naringin, hesperetin and apigenin, were studied if they formed prooxidant metabolites that oxidised NADH upon oxidation by peroxidase/H_2O_2.
Results	Prooxidant phenoxyl radicals formed by these flavonoids cooxidise NADH to form NAD radicals which then activated oxygen.
Conclusion	Naringin and naringinin have been identified as prooxidants independent of transition metal catalysed autoxidation reactions.

REFERENCES

Affany, A., Salvayre, R. and Douste-Blazy, L. (1987). Comparison of the protective effect of various flavonoids against lipid peroxidation of erythrocyte membranes (induced by cumene hydroperoxide). *Fundam. Clin. Pharmacol.,* 1(6): 451-7.

Ajay, M., Gilani, A.U. and Mustafa, M.R. (2003). Effects of flavonoids on vascular smooth muscle of the isolated rat thoracic aorta. *Life Sci.,* 74(5): 603-12.

Ali, M.M. and El Kader, M.A. (2004). The influence of naringin on the oxidative state of rats with streptozotocin-induced acute hyperglycaemia. *Z. Naturforsch. [C],* 59(9-10): 726-33.

Ameer, B., Weintraub, R.A., Johnson, J.V., Yost, R.A. and Rouseff, R.L. (1996). Flavanone absorption after naringin, hesperidin, and citrus administration. *Clin. Pharmacol. Ther.,* 60(1): 34-40.

Asgary, S., Naderi, G.A., Zadegan, N.S. and Vakili, R. (2002). The inhibitory effects of pure flavonoids on in vitro protein glycosylation. *J. Herb. Pharmacother.,* 2(2): 47-55.

Attia, S.M. (2008) Nov. Abatement by naringin of lomefloxacin-induced genomic instability in mice. *Mutagenesis,* 23(6): 515-2. Epub 2008 Aug 28.

Bailey, D.G., Arnold, J.M., Munoz, C. and Spence, J.D. (1993a). Grapefruit juice--felodipine interaction: mechanism, predictability, and effect of naringin. *Clin. Pharmacol. Ther.,* 53(6): 637-42.

Bailey, D.G., Arnold, J.M., Strong, H.A., Munoz, C. and Spence, J.D. (1993b). Effect of grapefruit juice and naringin on nisoldipine pharmacokinetics. *Clin. Pharmacol. Ther.,* 54(6): 589-94.

Bailey, D.G., Dresser, G.K., Leake, B.F. and Kim, R.B. (2007). Naringin is a major and selective clinical inhibitor of organic anion-transporting polypeptide 1A2 (OATP1A2) in grapefruit juice. *Clin. Pharmacol. Ther.,* 81(4): 495-502.

Bailey, D.G., Kreeft, J.H., Munoz, C., Freeman, D.J. and Bend, J.R. (1998). Grapefruit juice-felodipine interaction: effect of naringin and 6', 7' -dihydroxybergamottin in humans. *Clin. Pharmacol. Ther.,* 64(3): 248-56.

Bear, W.L. and Teel, R.W. (2000a.) Effects of citrus phytochemicals on liver and lung cytochrome P450 activity and on the in vitro metabolism of the tobacco-specific nitrosamine NNK. *Anticancer Res.,* 20(5A): 3323-9.

Bear, W.L. and Teel, R.W. (2000b). Effects of citrus flavonoids on the mutagenicity of heterocyclic amines and on cytochrome P450 1A2 activity. *Anticancer Res.,* 20(5B): 3609-14.

Benković, V., Orsolić, N., Knezević, A.H., Ramić, S., Dikić, D., Basić, I. and Kopjar, N. (2008) Jan. Evaluation of the radioprotective effects of propolis and flavonoids in gamma-irradiated mice: the alkaline comet assay study. *Biol. Pharm. Bull,* 31(1): 167-72.

Blankson, H., Grotterød, E.M. and Seglen, P.O. (2000). Prevention of toxin-induced cytoskeletal disruption and apoptotic liver cell death by the grapefruit flavonoid, naringin. *Cell Death Differ.,* 7: 739-746.

Bok, S.H., Lee, S.H., Park, Y.B., Bae, K.H., Son, K.H., Jeong, T.S. and Choi, M.S. (1999). Plasma and hepatic cholesterol and hepatic activities of 3-hydroxy-3-methyl-glutaryl-CoA reductase and acyl CoA: cholesterol transferase are lower in rats fed citrus peel extract or a mixture of citrus bioflavonoids. *J. Nutr.,* 129(6): 1182-5.

Calomme, M., Pieters, L., Vlietinck, A. and Vanden Berghe, D. (1996). Inhibition of bacterial mutagenesis by Citrus flavonoids. *Planta Med.,* 62(3): 222-6.

Chan, T., Galati, G. and O'Brien, P.J. (1999). Oxygen activation during peroxidase catalysed metabolism of flavones or flavanones. *Chem. Biol. Interact.,* 122(1): 15-25.

Chen, Y.T., Zheng, R.L., Jia, Z.J. and Ju, Y. (1990). Flavonoids as superoxide scavengers and antioxidants. *Free Radic. Biol. Med.,* 9(1): 19-21.

Chiou, G.C. and Xu, X.R. (2004). Effects of some natural flavonoids on retinal function recovery after ischemic insult in the rat. *J. Ocul. Pharmacol. Ther.,* 20(2): 107-13.

Choe, S.C., Kim, H.S., Jeong, T.S., Bok, S.H. and Park, Y.B. (2001). Naringin has an antiatherogenic effect with the inhibition of intercellular adhesion molecule-1 in hypercholesterolemic rabbits. *J. Cardiovasc. Pharmacol,* 38(6): 947-55.

Choi, M.S., Do, K.M., Park, Y.S., Jeon, S.M., Jeong, T.S., Lee, Y.K., Lee, M.K. and Bok, S.H. (2001) Effect of naringin supplementation on cholesterol metabolism and antioxidant status in rats fed high cholesterol with different levels of vitamin E. *Ann. Nutr. Metab.,* 45(5): 193-201.

Choi, J.S. and Han, H.K. (2005). Enhanced oral exposure of diltiazem by the concomitant use of naringin in rats. *Int. J. Pharm.,* 305(1-2): 122-8.

Choi, J.S. and Shin, S.C. (2005). Enhanced paclitaxel bioavailability after oral coadministration of paclitaxel prodrug with naringin to rats. *Int. J. Pharm.,* 292(1-2):149-56.

Cvetnić, Z. and Vladimir-Knezević, S. (2004). Antimicrobial activity of grapefruit seed and pulp ethanolic extract. *Acta. Pharm.,* 54(3): 243-50.

da Silva, R.R., de Oliveira, T.T., Nagem, T.J., Pinto, A.S., Albino, L.F., de Almeida, M.R., de Moraes, G.H. and Pinto, J.G. (2001). Hypocholesterolemic effect of naringin and rutin flavonoids. *Arch. Latinoam Nutr.*, 51(3): 258-64.

de Castro, W.V., Mertens-Talcott, S., Derendorf, H. and Butterweck, V. (2007). Grapefruit juice-drug interactions: Grapefruit juice and its components inhibit P-glycoprotein (ABCB1) mediated transport of talinolol in Caco-2 cells. *J. Pharm. Sci.,* 96(10): 2808-17.

Déchaud, H., Ravard, C., Claustrat, F., de la Perrière, A.B. and Pugeat, M. (1999). Xenoestrogen interaction with human sex hormone-binding globulin (hSHBG). *Steroids,* 64(5): 328-34.

Divi, R.L. and Doerge, D.R. (1996). Inhibition of thyroid peroxidase by dietary flavonoids. *Chem. Res. Toxicol.,* 9(1): 16-23.

Fenton, J.I. and Hord, N.G. (2004). Flavonoids promote cell migration in nontumorigenic colon epithelial cells differing in Apc genotype: implications of matrix metalloproteinase activity. *Nutr. Cancer,* 48(2): 182-8.

Fuhr, U., Klittich, K. and Staib, A.H. (1993). Inhibitory effect of grapefruit juice and its bitter principal, naringenin, on CYP1A2 dependent metabolism of caffeine in man. *Br J Clin Pharmacol,* 35(4): 431-6.

Fuhr, U., Maier-Brüggemann, A., Blume, H., Mück, W., Unger, S., Kuhlmann, J., Huschka, C., Zaigler, M., Rietbrock, S. and Staib, A.H. (1998). Grapefruit juice increases oral nimodipine bioavailability. *Int. J. Clin. Pharmacol. Ther.,* 36(3): 126-32.

Fujita, T. Kawase, A. Niwa, T. Tomohiro, N. Masuda, M. Matsuda, H. and Iwaki, M. (2008) May. Biol. Pharm. Bull. *Comparative evaluation of 12 immature citrus fruit extracts for the inhibition of cytochrome P450 isoform activitie, 31(5): 925-30.*

Gordon, P.B., Holen, I. and Seglen, P.O. (1995). Protection by naringin and some other flavonoids of hepatocytic autophagy and endocytosis against inhibition by okadaic acid. *J. Biol. Chem.,* 270(11): 5830-8.

Herrera, M.D. and Marhuenda, E. (1993). Effect of naringin and naringenin on contractions induced by noradrenaline in rat vas deferens--I. Evidence for postsynaptic alpha-2 adrenergic receptor. *Gen. Pharmacol.,* 24(3): 739-42.

Ho, P.C., Saville, D.J. and Wanwimolruk, S. (2001). Inhibition of human CYP3A4 activity by grapefruit flavonoids, furanocoumarins and related compounds. *J. Pharm. Pharm. Sci.,* 4(3): 217-27.

Hori, M., Kojima, H., Nakata, S., Konishi, H., Kitagawa, A. and Kawai, K. (2007). A search for the plant ingredients that protect cells from air pollutants and benz[a]pyrene phototoxicity. *Drug Chem. Toxicol.,* 30(2): 105-16.

Hsiu, S.L., Huang, T.Y., Hou, Y.C., Chin, D.H. and Chao, P.D. (2002). Comparison of metabolic pharmacokinetics of naringin and naringenin in rabbits. *Life Sci.,* 70(13): 1481-9.

Hsu, C.L. and Yen, G.C. (2006). Induction of cell apoptosis in 3T3-L1 pre-adipocytes by flavonoids is associated with their antioxidant activity. *Mol. Nutr. Food Res.,* 50(11): 1072-9.

Jagetia, A., Jagetia, G.C. and Jha, S. (2007). Naringin, a grapefruit flavanone, protects V79 cells against the bleomycin-induced genotoxicity and decline in survival. *J. Appl. Toxicol.,* 27(2): 122-32.

Jagetia, G.C. and Reddy, T.K. (2002). The grapefruit flavanone naringin protects against the radiation-induced genomic instability in the mice bone marrow: a micronucleus study. *Mutat Res,* 519(1-2): 37-48.

Jagetia, G.C. and Reddy, T.K. (2005). Modulation of radiation-induced alteration in the antioxidant status of mice by naringin. *Life Sci.,* 77(7): 780-94.

Jagetia, G.C., Reddy, T.K., Venkatesha, V.A. and Kedlaya, R. (2004). Influence of naringin on ferric iron induced oxidative damage in vitro. *Clin. Chim. Acta,* 347(1-2): 189-97.

Jagetia, G.C., Venkatesha, V.A. and Reddy, T.K. (2003). Naringin, a citrus flavonone, protects against radiation-induced chromosome damage in mouse bone marrow. *Mutagenesis,* 18(4): 337-43.

Jeon, S.M., Bok, S.H., Jang, M.K., Kim, Y.H., Nam, K.T., Jeong, T.S., Park, Y.B. and Choi, M.S. (2002). Comparison of antioxidant effects of naringin and probucol in cholesterol-fed rabbits. *Clin. Chim. Acta,* 317(1-2): 181-90.

Jeon, S.M., Bok, S.H., Jang, M.K., Lee, M.K., Nam, K.T., Park, Y.B., Rhee, S.J. and Choi, M.S. (2001). Antioxidative activity of naringin and lovastatin in high cholesterol-fed rabbits. *Life Sci.,* 69(24): 2855-66.

Jeon, S.M., Park, Y.B. and Choi, M.S. (2004). Antihypercholesterolemic property of naringin alters plasma and tissue lipids, cholesterol-regulating enzymes, fecal sterol and tissue morphology in rabbits. *Clin. Nutr.,* 23(5): 1025-34.

Jung, U.J., Kim, H.J., Lee, J.S., Lee, M.K., Kim, H.O., Park, E.J., Kim, H.K., Jeong, T.S. and Choi, M.S. (2003). Naringin supplementation lowers plasma lipids and enhances erythrocyte antioxidant enzyme activities in hypercholesterolemic subjects. *Clin. Nutr.,* 22(6): 561-8.

Jung, U.J., Lee, M.K., Park, Y.B., Kang, M.A. and Choi, M.S. (2006). Effect of citrus flavonoids on lipid metabolism and glucose-regulating enzyme mRNA levels in type-2 diabetic mice. *Int. J. Biochem. Cell Biol.,* 38(7): 1134-45.

Jung, U.J., Lee, M.K., Jeong, K.S. and Choi, M.S. (2004). The hypoglycemic effects of hesperidin and naringin are partly mediated by hepatic glucose-regulating enzymes in C57BL/KsJ-db/db mice. *J. Nutr.,* 134(10): 2499-503.

Kanaze, F.I., Bounartzi, M.I., Georgarakis, M. and Niopas, I. (2007). Pharmacokinetics of the citrus flavanone aglycones hesperetin and naringenin after single oral administration in human subjects. *Eur. J. Clin. Nutr.,* 61(4): 472-7.

Kanno, S., Shouji, A., Asou, K. and Ishikawa, M. (2003). Effects of naringin on hydrogen peroxide-induced cytotoxicity and apoptosis in P388 cells. *J. Pharmacol. Sci.,* 92(2): 166-70.

Kanno, S., Shouji, A., Hirata, R., Asou, K. and Ishikawa, M. (2004). Effects of naringin on cytosine arabinoside (Ara-C)-induced cytotoxicity and apoptosis in P388 cells. *Life Sci.,* 75(3): 353-65.

Kanno, S., Shouji, A., Tomizawa, A., Hiura, T., Osanai, Y., Ujibe, M., Obara, Y., Nakahata, N. and Ishikawa, M. (2006). Inhibitory effect of naringin on lipopolysaccharide (LPS)-induced endotoxin shock in mice and nitric oxide production in RAW 264.7 macrophages. *Life Sci.,* 78(7): 673-81.

Kanno, S., Tomizawa, A., Hiura, T., Osanai, Y., Shouji, A., Ujibe, M., Ohtake, T., Kimura, K. and Ishikawa, M. (2005). Inhibitory effects of naringenin on tumor growth in human cancer cell lines and sarcoma S-180-implanted mice. *Biol. Pharm. Bull,* 28(3): 527-30.

Kawaguchi, K., Kikuchi, S., Hasegawa, H., Maruyama, H., Morita, H. and Kumazawa, Y. (1999). Suppression of lipopolysaccharide-induced tumor necrosis factor-release and liver injury in mice by naringin. *Eur. J. Pharmacol.,* 368(2-3): 245-50.

Kawaguchi, K., Kikuchi, S., Hasunuma, R., Maruyama, H., Ryll, R. and Kumazawa, Y. (2004). Suppression of infection-induced endotoxin shock in mice by a citrus flavanone naringin. *Planta Med.,* 70(1): 17-22.

Kim, D.I., Lee, S.J., Lee, S.B., Park, K., Kim, W.J. and Moon, S.K. (2008) Sep. Requirement for Ras/Raf/ERK pathway in naringin-induced G1-cell-cycle arrest via p21WAF1 expression. *Carcinogenesis, 29(9): 1701-9.* Epub 2008 Feb 22.

Kim, H.J. and Choi, J.S. (2005). Effects of naringin on the pharmacokinetics of verapamil and one of its metabolites, norverapamil, in rabbits. *Biopharm Drug Dispos,* 26(7): 295-300.

Kim, S.Y., Kim, H.J., Lee, M.K., Jeon, S.M., Do, G.M., Kwon, E.Y., Cho, Y.Y., Kim, D.J., Jeong, K.S., Park, Y.B., Ha, T.Y. and Choi, M.S. (2006). Naringin time-dependently lowers hepatic cholesterol biosynthesis and plasma cholesterol in rats fed high-fat and high-cholesterol diet. *J. Med. Food,* 9(4): 582-6.

Kim, H.J., Oh, G.T., Park, Y.B., Lee, M.K., Seo, H.J. and Choi, M,S. (2004). Naringin alters the cholesterol biosynthesis and antioxidant enzyme activities in LDL receptor-knockout mice under cholesterol fed condition. *Life Sci.,* 74(13): 1621-34.

Kroyer, G. (1986). The antioxidant activity of citrus fruit peels. *Z. Ernahrungswiss.,* 25(1): 63-9.

Kumar, M.S., Unnikrishnan, M.K., Patra, S., Murthy, K. and Srinivasan, K.K. (2003). Naringin and naringenin inhibit nitrite-induced methemoglobin formation. *Pharmazie,* 58(8): 564-6.

Lambev, I., Belcheva, A. and Zhelyazkov, D. (1980a). Flavonoids with antioxidant action (naringin and rutin) and the release of mastocytic and nonmastocytic histamine. *Acta. Physiol. Pharmacol. Bulg.*, 6(2): 70-5.

Lambev, I., Krushkov, I., Zheliazkov, D. and Nikolov, N. (1980b). Antiexudative effect of naringin in experimental pulmonary edema and peritonitis. *Eksp. Med. Morfol.*, 19(4): 207-12.

Le Marchand, L., Murphy, S.P., Hankin, J.H., Wilkens, L.R. and Kolonel, L.N. (2000). Intake of flavonoids and lung cancer. *J. Natl. Cancer Inst.*, 92(2): 154-60.

Lee, C.H., Jeong, T.S., Choi, Y.K., Hyun, B.H., Oh, G.T., Kim, E.H., Kim, J.R., Han, J.I. and Bok, S.H. (2001). Anti-atherogenic effect of citrus flavonoids, naringin and naringenin, associated with hepatic ACAT and aortic VCAM-1 and MCP-1 in high cholesterol-fed rabbits. *Biochem. Biophys. Res. Commun.*, 284(3): 681-8.

Lee, E.J., Moon, G.S., Choi, W.S., Kim, W.J. and Moon, S.K. (2008) Oct 8. Naringin-induced p21WAF1-mediated G(1)-phase cell cycle arrest via activation of the Ras/Raf/ERK signaling pathway in vascular smooth muscle cell. *Food Chem. Toxicol.*, [Epub ahead of print].

Li, P., Callery, P.S., Gan, L.S. and Balani, S.K. (2007). Esterase inhibition by grapefruit juice flavonoids leading to a new drug interaction. *Drug Metab Dispos,* 35(7): 1203-8.

Li, J.M., Che, C.T., Lau, C.B., Leung, P.S. and Cheng, C.H. (2006). Inhibition of intestinal and renal Na+-glucose cotransporter by naringenin. *Int. J. Biochem. Cell Biol.*, 38(5-6): 985-95.

Li, F., Meng, F., Xiong, Z., Li, Y., Liu, R. and Liu, H. (2006). Stimulative activity of Drynaria fortunei (Kunze) J. Sm. extracts and two of its flavonoids on the proliferation of osteoblastic like cells. *Pharmazie,* 61(11): 962-5.

Lim, S.C. and Choi, J.S. (2006). Effects of naringin on the pharmacokinetics of intravenous paclitaxel in rats. *Biopharm Drug Dispos,* 27(9): 443-7.

Luo, H., Jiang, B.H., King, S.M. and Chen, Y.C. (2008). Inhibition of cell growth and VEGF expression in ovarian cancer cells by flavonoids. *Nutr. Cance,* 60(6): 800-9.

Mandadi, K., Ramirez, M., Jayaprakasha, G.K., Faraji, B., Lihono, M., Deyhim, F. and Patil, B.S. (2008) Oct 18. Itrus bioactive compounds improve bone quality and plasma antioxidant activity in orchidectomized rats. *Phytomedicine,* [Epub ahead of print].

Martín, M.J., Marhuenda, E., Pérez-Guerrero, C. and Franco, J.M. (1994). Antiulcer effect of naringin on gastric lesions induced by ethanol in rats. *Pharmacology,* 49(3): 144-50.

Mata-Bilbao Mde, L., Andrés-Lacueva, C., Roura, E., Jáuregui, O., Escribano, E., Torre, C., and Lamuela-Raventós, R.M. (2007). Absorption and pharmacokinetics of grapefruit flavanones in beagles. *Br. J. Nutr.*, 98(1): 86-92.

Middleton, E. Jr. and Drzewiecki, G. (1984). Flavonoid inhibition of human basophil histamine release stimulated by various agents. *Biochem Pharmacol,* 33(21): 3333-8.

Miller, E.G., Peacock, J.J., Bourland, T.C., Taylor, S.E., Wright, J.M. and Patil, B.S. (2008) Jan-Feb. Inhibition of oral carcinogenesis by citrus flavonoids*, Nutr. Cancer,* 60(1): 69-74.

Mitsunaga. Y., Takanaga, H., Matsuo, H,, Naito, M., Tsuruo, T., Ohtani, H. and Sawada, Y. (2000). Effect of bioflavonoids on vincristine transport across blood-brain barrier. *Eur. J. Pharmacol.*, 395(3): 193-201.

Morikawa, K., Nonaka, M., Mochizuki, H., Handa, K., Hanada, H. anf Hirota, K. (2008) Nov 4. Naringenin and Hesperetin Induce Growth Arrest, Apoptosis, and Cytoplasmic Fat Deposit in Human Preadipocytes. *J. Agric. Food Chem.,* [Epub ahead of print].

Naderi, G.A., Asgary, S., Sarraf-Zadegan, N. and Shirvany, H. (2003). Anti-oxidant effect of flavonoids on the susceptibility of LDL oxidation. *Mol. Cell Biochem.,* 246(1-2): 193-6.

Nafisi, S., Shadaloi, A., Feizbakhsh, A. and Tajmir-Riahi, H.A. (2008) Aug 30. RNA binding to antioxidant flavonoids. *J. Photochem. Photobiol. B,* [Epub ahead of print].

Nafisi, S., Hashemi, M., Rajabi, M. and Tajmir-Riahi, H.A. (2008) Aug. DNA Cell Biol. *DNA adducts with antioxidant flavonoids: morin, apigenin, and naringin, 27(8): 433-42.*

Ng, T.B., Ling, J.M., Wang, Z.T., Cai, J.N. and Xu, G.J. (1996). Examination of coumarins, flavonoids and polysaccharopeptide for antibacterial activity. *Gen. Pharmacol.,* 27(7): 1237-40.

Ng, T.B., Liu, F. and Wang, Z.T. (2000). Antioxidative activity of natural products from plants. *Life Sci.,* 66(8): 709-23.

Orallo, F., Camiña, M., Alvarez, E., Basaran, H. and Lugnier, C. (2005). Implication of cyclic nucleotide phosphodiesterase inhibition in the vasorelaxant activity of the citrus-fruits flavonoid (+/-)-naringenin. *Planta Med.,* 71(2): 99-107.

Paredes, A., Alzuru, M., Mendez, J. and Rodríguez-Ortega, M. (2003). Anti-Sindbis activity of flavanones hesperetin and naringenin. *Biol. Pharm. Bull.* 26(1):108-9.

Park, S.H., Park, E.K. and Kim, D.H. (2005). Passive cutaneous anaphylaxis-inhibitory activity of flavanones from Citrus unshiu and Poncirus trifoliata. *Planta Med.,* 71(1): 24-7.

Parmar, N.S. (1983). The gastric anti-ulcer activity of naringenin, a specific histidine decarboxylase inhibitor. *Int. J. Tissue React,* 5(4): 415-20.

Pereira, R.M., Andrades, N.E., Paulino, N., Sawaya, A.C., Eberlin, M.N., Marcucci, M.C., Favero G.M., Novak, E.M. and Bydlowski, S.P. (2007). Synthesis and characterization of a metal complex containing naringin and Cu, and its antioxidant, antimicrobial, antiinflammatory and tumor cell cytotoxicity. *Molecules,* 12(7): 1352-66.

Punithavathi, V.R., Anuthama, R. and Prince, P.S. (2008) Aug. Combined treatment with naringin and vitamin C ameliorates streptozotocin-induced diabetes in male Wistar rats. *J. Appl. Toxicol.*, 28(6): 806-13.

Rajadurai, M. and Stanely Mainzen Prince, P. (2006). Preventive effect of naringin on lipids, lipoproteins and lipid metabolic enzymes in isoproterenol-induced myocardial infarction in Wistar rats. *J. Biochem. Mol. Toxicol.,* 20(4): 191-7.

Rajadurai M., and Stanely Mainzen Prince, P. (2006). Preventive effect of naringin on lipid peroxides and antioxidants in isoproterenol-induced cardiotoxicity in Wistar rats: biochemical and histopathological evidences. *Toxicology,* 228(2-3): 259-68.

Rajadurai, M. and Stanely Mainzen Prince, P. (2007). Preventive effect of naringin on cardiac markers, electrocardiographic patterns and lysosomal hydrolases in normal and isoproterenol-induced myocardial infarction in Wistar rats. *Toxicology,* 230(2-3): 178-88.

Rajadurai, M. and Prince, P.S. (2007). Preventive effect of naringin on isoproterenol-induced cardiotoxicity in Wistar rats: an in vivo and in vitro study. *Toxicology,* 232(3): 216-25.

Rajadurai, M. and Prince, P.S. (2007). Preventive effect of naringin on cardiac mitochondrial enzymes during isoproterenol-induced myocardial infarction in rats: a transmission electron microscopic study. *J. Biochem. Mol. Toxicol.,* 21(6): 354-61.

Rajadurai, M. and Prince, P.S. (2008) Oct 10. Naringin ameliorates mitochondrial lipid peroxides, antioxidants and lipids in isoproterenol-induced myocardial infarction in Wistar rat. *Phytother Res*, [Epub ahead of print].

Ratty, A.K. and Das, N.P. (1988). Effects of flavonoids on nonenzymatic lipid peroxidation: structure-activity relationship. *Biochem Med. Metab. Biol.* 39(1): 69-79.

Reshef. N., Hayari, Y., Goren, C., Boaz, M., Madar, Z. and Knobler, H. (2005). Antihypertensive effect of sweetie fruit in patients with stage I hypertension. *Am. J. Hypertens,* 18(10): 1360-3.

Robbins, R.C., Martin, F.G. and Roe, J.M. (1988). Ingestion of grapefruit lowers elevated hematocrits in human subjects. *Int. J. Vitam Nutr. Res,* 58(4): 414-7.

Runkel, M., Bourian, M., Tegtmeier, M. and Legrum, W. (1997). The character of inhibition of the metabolism of 1,2-benzopyrone (coumarin) by grapefruit juice in human. *Eur. J. Clin. Pharmacol.,* 53(3-4): 265-9.

Russo, A., Acquaviva, R., Campisi, A., Sorrenti, V., Di Giacomo, C., Virgata, G., Barcellona, M.L. and Vanella, A. (2000). Bioflavonoids as antiradicals, antioxidants and DNA cleavage protectors. *Cell Biol. Toxicol.,* 16(2): 91-8.

Sansone, F., Aquino, R.P., Gaudio, P.D., Colombo, P. and Russo, P. (2008) Nov 1. Physical characteristics and aerosol performance of naringin dry powders for pulmonary delivery prepared by spray-drying. *Eur. J. Pharm. Biopharm.,* [Epub ahead of print].

Saponara, S., Testai, L., Iozzi, D., Martinotti, E., Martelli, A., Chericoni, S., Sgaragli, G., Fusi, F. and Calderone, V. (2006). (+/-)-Naringenin as large conductance Ca(2+)-activated K+ (BKCa) channel opener in vascular smooth muscle cells. *Br. J. Pharmacol.,* 149(8): 1013-21.

Schindler, R. and Mentlein, R. (2006). Flavonoids and vitamin E reduce the release of the angiogenic peptide vascular endothelial growth factor from human tumor cells. *J. Nutr.,* 136(6): 1477-82.

Seo, H.J., Jeong, K.S., Lee, M.K., Park, Y.B., Jung, U.J., Kim, H.J. and Choi, M.S. (2003). Role of naringin supplement in regulation of lipid and ethanol metabolism in rats. *Life Sci.,* 73(7): 933-46.

Shim, C.K., Cheon, E.P., Kang, K.W., Seo, K.S. and Han, H.K. (2007). Inhibition effect of flavonoids on monocarboxylate transporter 1 (MCT1) in Caco-2 cells. *J. Pharm. Pharmacol.,* 59(11): 1515-9.

Shin, Y.W., Bok, S.H., Jeong, T.S., Bae, K.H., Jeoung, N.H., Choi, M.S., Lee, S.H. and Park, Y.B. (1999). Hypocholesterolemic effect of naringin associated with hepatic cholesterol regulating enzyme changes in rats. *Int. J. Vitam Nutr. Res.,* 69(5): 341-7.

Shirasaka, Y., Li, Y., Shibue, Y., Kuraoka, E., Spahn-Langguth, H., Kato, Y. Langguth, P. and Tamai, I. (2008). Nov 12. Concentration-Dependent Effect of Naringin on Intestinal Absorption of beta(1)-Adrenoceptor Antagonist Talinolol Mediated by P-Glycoprotein and Organic Anion Transporting Polypeptide (Oatp). *Pharm Res,* [Epub ahead of print].

Shiratori, K., Ohgami, K., Ilieva, I., Jin, X.H., Yoshida, K., Kase, S. and Ohno, S. (2005). The effects of naringin and naringenin on endotoxin-induced uveitis in rats. *J. Ocul. Pharmacol. Ther.,* 21(4): 298-304.

Singh, D., Chander, V. and Chopra, K. (2004a). Protective effect of naringin, a bioflavonoid on ferric nitrilotriacetate-induced oxidative renal damage in rat kidney. *Toxicology,* 201(1-3): 1-8.

Singh, D., Chander, V. and Chopra, K. (2004b). Protective effect of naringin, a bioflavonoid on glycerol-induced acute renal failure in rat kidney. *Toxicology,* 201(1-3): 143-51.

Singh, D. and Chopra, K. (2004). The effect of naringin, a bioflavonoid on ischemia-reperfusion induced renal injury in rats. *Pharmacol Res.,* 50(2): 187-93.

So, F.V., Guthrie, N., Chambers, A.F., Moussa, M. and Carroll, K.K. (1996). Inhibition of human breast cancer cell proliferation and delay of mammary tumorigenesis by flavonoids and citrus juices. *Nutr. Cancer,* 26(2): 167-81.

Taur, J.S. and Rodriguez-Proteau, R. (2008) Oct 24. Effects of dietary flavonoids on the transport of cimetidine via P-glycoprotein and cationic transporters in Caco-2 and LLC-PK1 cell models. *Xenobiotica,* [Epub ahead of print].

Tsui, V.W., Wong, R.W. and Rabie, A.B. (2007). The inhibitory effects of naringin on the growth of periodontal pathogens in vitro. Phytother Res. [Epub ahead of print]

Ubeaud, G., Hagenbach, J., Vandenschrieck, S., Jung, L. and Koffel, J.C. (1999). In vitro inhibition of simvastatin metabolism in rat and human liver by naringenin. *Life Sci.,* 65(13): 1403-12.

Ueng, Y.F., Chang, Y.L., Oda, Y., Park, S.S., Liao, J.F., Lin, M.F. and Chen, C.F. (1999). In vitro and in vivo effects of naringin on cytochrome P450-dependent monooxygenase in mouse liver. *Life Sci.,* 65(24): 2591-602.

Ugocsai, K., Varga, A., Molnár, P., Antus, S. and Molnár, J. (2005). Effects of selected flavonoids and carotenoids on drug accumulation and apoptosis induction in multidrug-resistant colon cancer cells expressing MDR1/LRP. *In:* Vivo. 19(2): 433-8.

Vanamala, J., Leonardi, T., Patil, B.S., Taddeo, S.S., Murphy, M.E., Pike, L.M., Chapkin, R.S., Lupton, J.R. and Turner, N.D. (2006). Suppression of colon carcinogenesis by bioactive compounds in grapefruit. *Carcinogenesis,* 27(6): 1257-65.

Wei, M., Yang, Z., Li,P., Zhang, Y. and Sse, W.C. (2007). Anti-osteoporosis activity of naringin in the retinoic acid-induced osteoporosis model. *Am. J. Chin. Med.,* 35(4): 663-7.

Wenzel, U., Kuntz, S. and Daniel, H. (2001). Flavonoids with epidermal growth factor-receptor tyrosine kinase inhibitory activity stimulate PEPT1-mediated cefixime uptake into human intestinal epithelial cells. *J. Pharmacol. Exp. Ther.,* 299(1): 351-7.

Wong, R.W. and Rabie, A.B. (2006). Effect of naringin collagen graft on bone formation. *Biomaterials,* 27(9): 1824-31.

Wong, R.W. and Rabie, A.B. (2006). Effect of naringin on bone cells. *J. Orthop. Res.,* 24(11): 2045-50.

Wood, N. (2004). The effects of dietary bioflavonoid (rutin, quercetin, and naringin) supplementation on physiological changes in molar crestal alveolar bone-cemento-enamel junction distance in young rats. *J. Med. Food,* 7(2): 192-6.

Wood, N. (2007). The effects of selected dietary bioflavonoid supplementation on dental caries in young rats fed a high-sucrose diet. *J. Med. Food,* 10(4): 694-701.

Wu, J.B., Fong, Y.C., Tsai, H.Y., Chen, Y.F., Tsuzuki, M. and Tang, C.H. (2008) Jul 7. Naringin-induced bone morphogenetic protein-2 expression via PI3K, Akt, c-Fos/c-Jun and AP-1 pathway in osteoblasts. *Eur. J. Pharmacol,* 588(2-3): 333-41. Epub 2008 May 19.

Yeh, S.L., Wang, W.Y., Huang, C.H. and Hu, M.L. (2005). Pro-oxidative effect of beta-carotene and the interaction with flavonoids on UVA-induced DNA strand breaks in mouse fibroblast C3H10T1/2 cells. *J. Nutr. Biochem.,* 16(12): 729-35.

Yeum, C.H. and Choi, J.S. (2006). Effect of naringin pretreatment on bioavailability of verapamil in rabbits. *Arch. Pharm. Res.,* 29(1): 102-7.

Younes, M. and Siegers, C.P. (1981). Inhibitory Action of some Flavonoids on Enhanced Spontaneous Lipid Peroxidation Following Glutathione Depletion. *Planta,* 43(11): 240-4.

Yu, J., Wang, L., Walzem, R.L., Miller, E.G., Pike, L.M. and Patil, B.S. (2005). Antioxidant activity of citrus limonoids, flavonoids, and coumarins. *J. Agric Food Chem.,* 53(6): 2009-14.

Zielińska-Przyjemska, M. and Ignatowicz, E. (2008) Sep 19. Citrus fruit flavonoids influence on neutrophil apoptosis and oxidative metabolism. *Phytother Res.,* [Epub ahead of print].

In: Flavonoids: Biosynthesis, Biological Effects... ISBN: 978-1-60741-622-7
Editor: Raymond B. Keller

Chapter 5

DEVELOPMENT OF PROMISING NATURALLY DERIVED MOLECULES TO IMPROVE THERAPEUTIC STRATEGIES

***Dominique Delmas*[*,1,2], *Frédéric Mazué*[1,2], *Didier Colin*[1,2], *Patrick Dutartre*[1,2] and *Norbert Latruffe*[1,2]**

[1]Inserm U866, Dijon, F-21000, France
[2]Université de Bourgogne, Faculté des Sciences Gabriel, Centre de Recherche-Biochimie Métabolique et Nutritionnelle (LBMN), Dijon, F-21000, France

ABSTRACT

Numerous epidemiological studies show that some nutrients may protect against vascular diseases, cancers and associated inflammatory effects. Consequently, the use of phytoconstituents, namely those from the human diet, as therapeutic drugs is relevant. Various studies report the efficiency of phyto-molecules which have cellular targets similar to those of the new drugs developed by pharmaceutical companies. Indeed, more than 1600 patents are currently reported concerning flavonoids and 3000 patents concerning polyphenols. Pleiotropic pharmaceutical activities are claimed in fields such as cancer, inflammation arthritis, eye diseases and many other domains. The increase of activities after combination with other natural compounds or therapeutic drugs is also patented. In addition, the aforementioned molecules, from natural origin, generally exhibit low toxicities and often a multipotency which allow them to be able to simultaneously interfere with several signalling pathways. However, several in vivo studies revealed that polyphenols / flavonoids are efficiently absorbed by the organism, but unfortunately have a low level of bioavailability, glucuronidation and sulphation being limiting factors. Therefore, many laboratories are developing elements to increase bioavailability and consequently the biological effects of these natural molecules. For example, the modifications in the lipophilicity of molecules increase the cellular uptake and consequently involve a best absorption without loss of their activities. Moreover

* Phone : 33 3 80 39 62 37, Fax : 33 3 80 39 62 50, Email : ddelmas@u-bourgogne.fr

isomerisation and methylation of hydroxyl groups of polyphenols (e.g. resveratrol) change the cell molecular targets and are crucial to improve the molecule efficiency in blocking cell proliferation. In this review, we focus on the relevance of using flavonoid and polyphenol combinations or chemical modifications to enhance their biological effects. We discuss the innovative directions to develop a new type of drugs which may especially be used in combination with other natural components or pharmacological conventional drugs in order to obtain synergistic effects.

A) INTRODUCTION

A wide variety of plant-derived compounds, including polyphenols and flavonoids, is present in the human diet and may protect against vascular diseases, cancers and associated inflammatory effects (Figure 1).

The impetus sparking of this scientific inquiry was the result of many epidemiologic studies. For example, in France, as compared with other western countries with a fat-containing diet, the strikingly low incidences of coronary heart diseases is partly attributed to the consumption of red wine, which contains high levels of polyphenols [1]. Similarly, benefit effects may be attributed to the flavonoids of green tea.

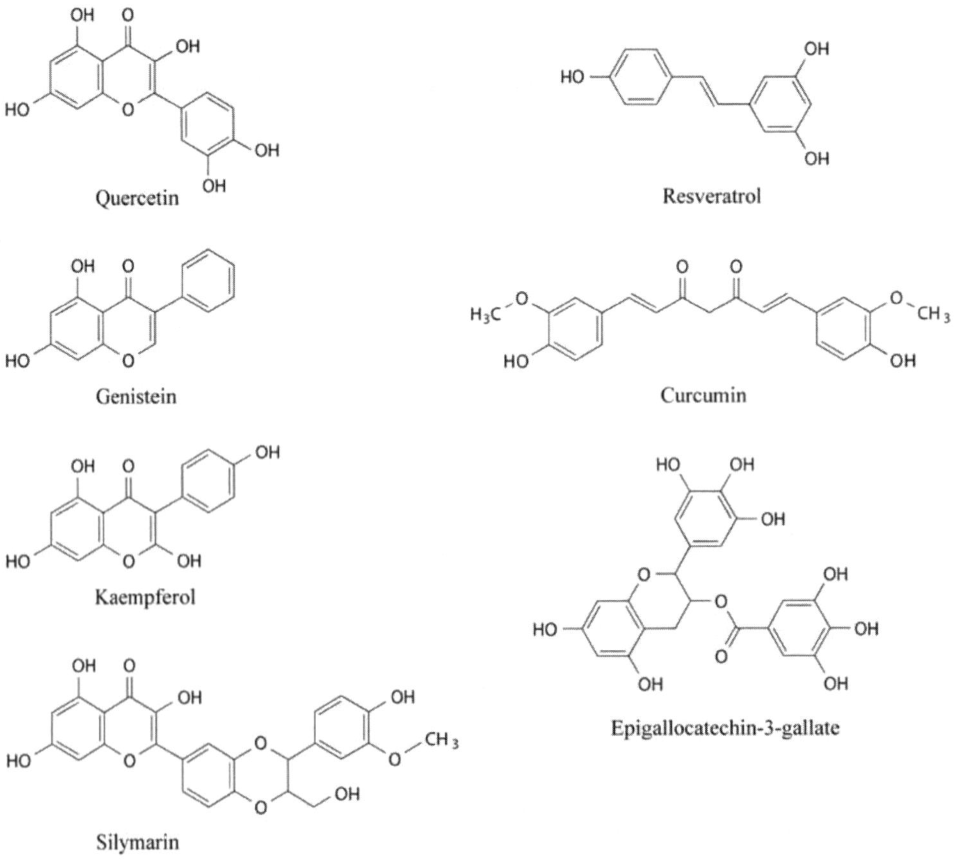

Figure 1. Examples of stilbenes / flavonoids chemical structures.

Indeed, several cohort studies demonstrate a significant inverse association between flavonoid consumption and cardiovascular risk [2]. Interestingly, other epidemiological studies reveal that phytoconstituents or micronutrients can protect against cancers [3]. Especially, Levi et al. show an inverse relation between resveratrol (a non-flavonoid polyphenol) and breast cancer risk [4]. Another cohort study in Finland [5] shows a link between flavonol consumption and reduced risk of lung cancer. These findings lead to the suggestion that polyphenols and flavonoids have beneficial health effects. Various reports from in vitro and in vivo show the pleiotropic activities of theses compounds, and interestingly, these phytoconstituents. These compounds seem to exert similar actions against general processes such as oxidation, kinases activation pathways or pro-inflammatory substances production found as well in coronary as in cancerous pathologies. In this review, we briefly summarize the pathway by which dietary microcomponents may inhibit carcinogenesis by affecting the molecular events in the initiation, promotion and progression stages. Nevertheless, there appears to be a large discrepancy between the potential effects of these compounds, as observed in vitro, and observed effects in in vivo. We show and discuss the relationship between polyphenols / flavonoids metabolism and their biological effects, and how the modifications in the lipophilicity of these molecules and the phytonaturals combinations could enhance their activities. For these practical reasons, many pharmaceutical groups develop new types of drugs that may especially be used in combination with other natural components or pharmacological conventional drugs in order to obtain synergistic effects.

B) Phytochemicals Prevent Carcinogenesis Pathways

Carcinogenesis is commonly described by three stages—initiation, promotion and progression. The initiating event can consist of a single exposure to a carcinogenic agent or, in some cases, it may be an inherited genetic defect. The initiated cell may remain dormant for months or years and unless a promoting event occurs, it may never develop into a clinical cancer case. The promotion phase is the second major step in the carcinogenesis process in which specific agents *(referred to as promoters)* trigger the further development of the initiated cells. Promoters often, but not always, interact with the cellular DNA and influence the further expression of the mutated DNA so that the initiated cell proliferates and progresses further through the carcinogenesis process. Finally, the ultimate carcinogenesis phase is the progression which is associated with the evolution of the initiated cells into a biologically malignant cell population. In this stage, a portion of the benign tumor cells may be converted into malignant forms leading to a true cancer.

1. Anti-Initiation Activities of Phytonatural Compounds

The anti-initiation activity of polyphenols and flavonoids is linked to the suppression of the metabolic activation of carcinogens and / or the detoxifying increases via a modulation of the drug-metabolizing enzymes involved either in phase I or in phase II (Figure 2).

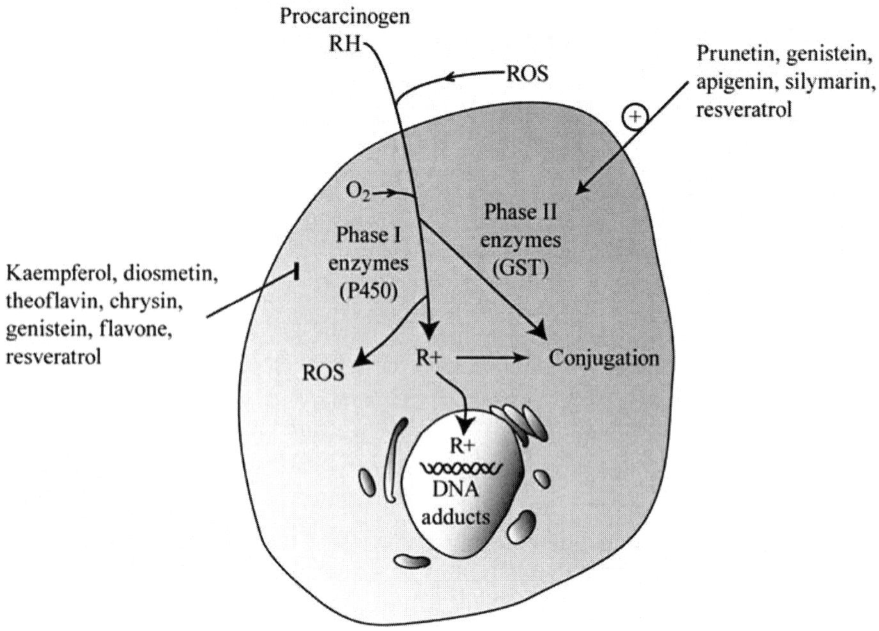

Figure 2. Polyphenols effects on tumor initiation. Polyphenols are able to prevent initiation phase by inhibition of carcinogen activation (R+) induction of carcinogen deactivation and subsequently blocking interaction between DNA and carcinogen (R+).

For example, resveratrol and genistein are able to antagonize the transactivation of genes regulated by the aryl hydrocarbon receptor (AhR) ligand, such as the 7,12-dimethylbenz[a]anthracen (DMBA) [6]. Consequently, compounds are able to reduce the number of DNA adducts induced by various chemical agents.

Moreover, polyphenolic compounds and flavonoids could induce phase II enzyme which generally protects tissues and cells from endogen and/or exogen intermediate carcinogens. Activation of phase II detoxifying enzymes by flavonoids / non flavonoids, such as UDP-glucuronyl transferase [7-9], glutathione S-transferase (GST) [10], quinone reductase [11, 12], and sulfotransferase [13] result in the detoxification of carcinogens and represent one mechanism of their anticarcinogenic effects (Figure 2).

For example, Kong et al. propose a model where an antioxidant such as butylated hydroxyanisol (BHA) and isothiocyanate sulforafane (SUL) may modulate the mitogen-activated protein kinases (MAPKs) pathway leading to transcriptional activation of the nuclear factor erythroid 2p45 related factor, Nrf2 (a basic leucine zipper transcription factor) and of the antioxidant electrophile response element (ARE), with subsequent induction of phase II detoxifying enzymes such as hemeoxygenase (HO-1), GST, NAD(P)H:quinine reductase (NQO-1) [14].

Recently, quercetin was reported to protect human hepatocytes from ethanol-induced cellular damage and this beneficial effect was mediated by a pathway involving extracellular signal-regulated protein kinase (ERK), p38, and Nrf2, with the induction of HO-1 expression [15].

In addition, the activation of Nrf2 up-regulated the induction of a phase II enzyme, NQO-1, in HepG2 cells [16]. In the same manner, resveratrol is able to up-regulate NQO-1 gene expression in human ovarian cancer PA-1 cells [17] by its activation of kinase pathways.

Furthermore, a study using a resveratrol affinity column shows that the dihydronicotinamide riboside quinone reductase 2 (NQO-2) binds resveratrol and could constitute a potential target in cancer cells [18].

2. Anti-Promotion Activities of Phytonatural Compounds

The promotion phase is the second major step in the carcinogenesis process in which specific agents *(referred to as promoters)* trigger the further development of the initiated cells. Promoters often, but not always, interact with the cellular DNA and influence the further expression of the mutated DNA so that the initiated cell proliferates and progresses further through the carcinogenesis process (Figure 3).

An intricate network of signalling pathways is involved in these control mechanisms, especially the cell cycle and the induction of apoptosis. This induction of cell death in precancerous or malignant cells is considered to be a promising strategy for chemopreventive or chemotherapeutic purpose. Natural compounds, like many cytotoxic agents, affect cell proliferation by disturbing the normal progress of the cell cycle. In fact, both stilbenes and flavonoids are able to block cell progression through the cell cycle, this blockage depends on the cell type, the natural compound concentration, and the treatment duration. Various studies report that checkpoint at both G1/S and G2/M of the cell cycle is found to be perturbed by the phyto chemicals [19-21]. Checkpoints are controlled by a family of protein kinase complexes, and each complex is composed minimally of a catalytic subunit, cyclin-dependent kinases (cdks), and its essential activating partner, cyclin.

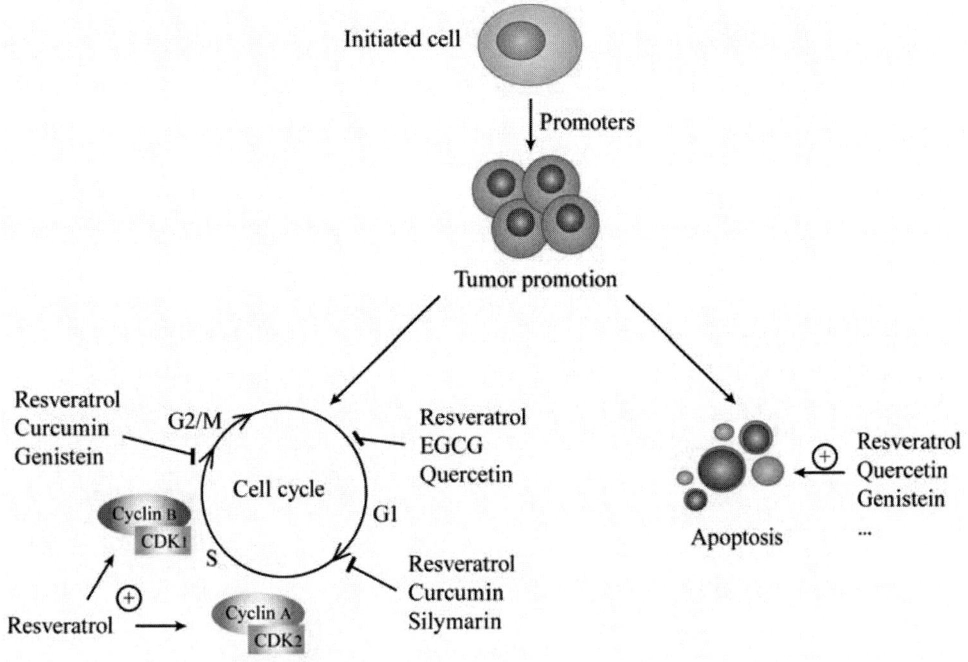

Figure 3. Polyphenols effects on tumor progression. Polyphenols are able to prevent promotion phase by inhibition of cell cycle progression and are able to induce apoptosis.

Cyclins play a key regulatory role in this process by activating their partner cdks and targeting them to the respective protein substrates [22]. Complexes-formed in this way are activated at specific intervals during the cell cycle and their inhibition blocks the cell cycle at the corresponding control point. These key regulators can be affected by these flavonoids and stilbenes leading to an arrest of the cell cycle. For example, epigallocatechin-3-gallate (EGCG), a green tea polyphenol, mediates a G1 phase arrest in various cancer cell lines such as ovarian, pancreatic through a modulation of cyclin D1 and $p21^{WAF1}$ [23, 24]. The balance between pro- and anti-apoptotic Bcl-2 family proteins favors apoptosis in prostate cancer cells also arrested in G0/G1 phase [25]. In the same manner, treatment by curcumin, resveratrol or silymarin involve an increase of $p21^{WAF1}$ and $p27^{KIP1}$ expressions and inhibit the expression of cyclin E and cyclin D1, and hyperphosphorylation of retinoblastoma (Rb) protein [26-31].

Concerning the G2/M phase, some phytochemicals can arrest the cell cycle at the transition from G2 stage to M stage such as genistein [32-35], resveratrol [36-38], curcumin and quercetin [39] in various cancer cell types (Figure 3). Biochemical analysis demonstrates that the disruption of G2 phase progression by polyphenolic compounds is accompanied by an upregulation of $p21^{WAF1}$ and an inactivation of cyclin-dependent kinase, Cdk1 [31, 35, 36, 38, 40].

In addition to cell cycle arrest, another specialized event of polyphenol compounds action involves the induction of apoptosis (Figure 3). Induction of apoptosis in precancerous or malignant cells is considered to be a promising strategy for chemopreventive or chemotherapeutic purposes. The induction of apoptosis triggered by polyphenolic compounds has been observed in various cell types with different pathways. Indeed it has been demonstrated that polyphenols are able to activate cell death by the mitochondrial pathway or by the death receptor pathway.

The mitochondrial pathway is activated in response to extracellular signals and internal disturbances such as DNA damages. We and others have shown that polyphenols such as resveratrol [41], quercetin [42, 43], genistein [44-47] induce apoptosis in various tumor cell lines by modulating pro-apoptotic Bcl-2 family proteins which are known as "BH3-only proteins" behaving as sensors of cellular damage and initiating the agents of death process. We and others have shown that polyphenols and flavonoids down-regulate Bcl-2 protein expression [41, 48-53] and gene expression [54-56], which normally stabilizes the mitochondrial potential of the membrane ($\Delta\varphi_m$), and inhibits ROS production. Cytochrome c, in the cytosol, induces oligomerization of the adapter molecule Apaf-1 to generate a complex, the apoptosome, in which caspase-9 is activated. Active caspase-9 then triggers the catalytic maturation of caspase-3 and other resultant caspases, thus leading to cell death.

Major external signals triggering apoptosis are mediated by receptor/ligand interactions (such as CD95 and tumor necrosis factor receptor). The binding of ligand to receptor induces receptor clustering and the formation of death inducing signalling complex (DISC). This complex recruits via the adaptator FADD (Fas-associated death domain protein), multiple procaspase-8 molecules resulting in caspase-8 activation. It can activate the proteolytic cascade or / and converge on the mitochondrial pathway through the activation of pro-apoptotic members of the Bcl-2 family. We and others have shown that polyphenols/flavonoids can involve this pathway in various cells lines.

The action of different polyphenols/flavonoids on the cell cycle at different stages, on the apoptosis cascade, or on the metabolizing enzymes, depends on their cellular targets, the concentrations used and the cellular type. These findings suggest a very specific mechanism of action of these phytochemical compounds. An association of these compounds or chemical modifications can modify their primary targets and amplify their biological effects.

3. Anti-Progression Activities of Phytonatural Compounds

Finally, stilbenes and flavonoids can act on the third step of carcinogenesis, the progression which is associated with the evolution of the initiated cells into a biologically malignant cell population. In this stage, a portion of the benign tumor cells may be converted into malignant forms leading to a true cancer. At this stage, tumor progression is certainly too advanced for chemopreventive intervention but not for a chemotherapeutic intervention. During tumor progression, polyphenols (resveratrol, curcumin, EGCG, silymarin, ...), as previously described, can act as antiproliferative agents by blocking cell cycle progression and inducing apoptosis of cancer cells. The phytochemical compounds can also act on events more specific of the progression / invasion step. In this final stage, invasion, can break away and start new clones of growth distant from the original site of development of the tumor. It is reported that resveratrol, quercetin, genistein show an anti-proliferative effect on highly invasive breast carcinoma cells (MDA-MB-435) [45, 49, 57]. In fact, these polyphenols can modify the key regulators of angiogenesis such as vascular endothelial growth factor (VEGF) and could inhibit matrix metalloproteinase. Indeed, resveratrol, genistein, quercetin and silymarin inhibit VEGF expression in various cancer cell lines [58-67]. One hypothesis is that polyphenols inhibition of VEGF-induced angiogenesis is mediated by disruption of ROS-dependent Src kinase activation and the subsequent VE-cadherin tyrosine phosphorylation. Efficient tumor invasion also requires partial degradation of the extracellular matrix (ECM) at the invasion front. The matrix metalloproteinases (MMPs) are the main proteases involved in remodeling the ECM contributing to invasion and metastasis, as well as tumor angiogenesis [68]. Concerning the human MMPs, the expression levels of gelatinase-A (MMP-2) and gelatinase-B (MMP-9) are associated with tumor metastasis for various human cancers [69, 70]. Resveratrol [71-73], silibin [74] and genistein [75, 76] are able to decrease the MMP-9 expression via diminished MAP kinases activation.

C) Polyphenols as Chemosensitizer Agents

An important cause of failure in cancer therapies is due to a defect of drug accumulation in cancer cells. Indeed, the action of chemopreventive or chemotherapeutic agents can be nullified by a failure of their absorption, distribution, metabolism or an increase in their excretion. Moreover, there appears to be a large discrepancy between the potential effect, as observed in vitro, and observed in vivo or in human subjects. This difference could be due to the poor bioavailability of flavonoids and polyphenols to target tissue in vivo. Metabolism of polyphenols occurs via a common pathway [77]. The chemical structure of polyphenols determines their rate and extent of intestinal absorption and the nature of the metabolites circulating in the plasma. The few bioavailability studies in humans show that the quantities of polyphenols found intact in urine vary from one phenolic compound to another [78-80]. They are particularly low for quercetin and rutin, a glycoside of quercetin (0.3–1.4%), but reach higher values for catechins from green tea, isoflavones from soy, flavanones from citrus fruits or anthocyanidins from red wine (3–26%). Interindividual variations have also been observed: 5–57% of the naringin consumed with grapefruit juice is found in urine according to the individual [81]. A major part of the polyphenols ingested (75–99%) is not found in urine. This implies they are not absorbed through the gut barrier, but excreted in the bile or metabolized by the colonic microflora or other tissues. In the same manner to chemical drugs, animal cells react to plant polyphenols exposure by recognizing these molecules as xenobiotics. As consequence, the cells transform these compounds in order to eliminate them as quick and as extended as possible. The pharmacokinetic is an essential parameter to select natural compounds based on their biological activity, especially their possible anticancer properties. For example, resveratrol is a well known promising anticancer natural molecule [82], but this molecule exhibits a low bioavailability [9, 83]. To overcome this problem, it is interesting to used: 1) phytochemicals combinations, 2) phytochemicals / therapeutics drugs association, 3) chemically modified natural polyphenols.

1. Phytochemical Combinations

The synergistic activity of phytochemical combinations can be easily tested in vitro and the combination treatment might represent a new strategy that can play a major role in the future of cancer chemoprevention [84]. Various reports show that the combination of several natural molecules or one phytochemical compound with an anticancer drug might be more effective in cancer prevention or in cancer therapy than a single molecule (Table I). By their pleiotropic actions, the use of several polyphenols can operate many cellular targets and/or decrease the phenomena of metabolisation, glucuronidation and sulfation, being limiting factors, and consequently increase the bioavailability and the biological effects of these natural molecules. It is the case for the EGCG glucuronidation [85] which is inhibited by the association with an alkaloid derived from black pepper, the piperine in the small intestine [86]. So, the bioavailability of EGCG is enhanced in mice. In a same manner, it is reported that coadministration of piperine and curcumin to humans and rats enhanced the bioavailability of curcumin by 2000% and 154%, respectively [87]. The use of flavonoids can also enhance the bioavailability of other polyphenols such as resveratrol. Indeed, many flavonoids can inhibit the hepatic glucuronidation and the hepatic/ duodenal sulphation of resveratrol and such inhibition may improve the bioavailability of this compound [88-90].

The modifications of bioavailability can enhance the toxicity of phytochemicals on cancer cells through synergistic or additive actions. For example, an antiproliferative synergy between resveratrol, quercetin and catechin is observed on human breast cancer cells [91]. No modifications is observed when compounds are used alone, but at only 0.5 μM, they significantly reduce cell proliferation and block cell cycle progression in vitro and at 5 mg/kg reduce breast tumor growth in a nude mouse model. The essential steps in tumor progression are the cell cycle and apoptosis alteration (see previously). Ellagic acid and quercetin interact synergistically with resveratrol in the induction of apoptosis and cause transient cell cycle arrest in human leukemia cells [92]. This apoptosis effect may be due to p21 overexpression and a greater p53 phosphorylation [93]. The MAP kinases, JNK1,2, and p38 are also activated in a "more than additive" manner.

Table I. Phytochemicals combination effects on cancer cell lines

Cell system	Compounds	Concentration	Action	Biological Effect	References
human platelets	quercetin	5 μM	synergy	Antagonizing the intracellular production of hydrogen peroxide	[95]
	catechin	25 μM			
B16M-F10	quercetin	20 μM	synergy	Inhibits metastatic activity	[96]
	pterostilbene	40 μM			
MOLT-4 (human leukemia cells)	quercetin	5 μM / 10 μM each	synergy	Antiproliferation, Cytotoxicity, Apoptosis	[97]
	ellagic acid				
	quercetin	20 μM each	synergy	p21, p53 and MAPK activation	[92]
	ellagic acid				
	quercetin	10 μM each	synergy	Apoptosis, cell cycle arrest	[93]
	resveratrol				
	ellagic acid	10 μM each	synergy	Apoptosis, cell cycle arrest	
	resveratrol				
	quercetin	10 μM each	synergy	Apoptosis, cell cycle arrest	
	ellagic acid				
	resveratrol				
3T3-L1 (adipocytes)	quercetin	25 μM each	synergy	Inhibition of adipogenesis, apoptosis	[98]
	resveratrol				
MDA-MB-231 (human breast cancer cells)	resveratrol	0,5 μM each	synergy	Antiproliferation, Apoptosis	[91]
	quercetin				
	catechin				

The caspase-3 activity can be synergistically induced by combinations of ellagic acid and reveratrol (combination index 0,64) or quercetin and resveratrol (combination index 0,68) [92]. A combination of EGCG and curcumin synergistically suppresses MDA-MB-231 estrogen receptor-alpha-breast cancer cells by cytotoxic effects and cell cycle arrest [94].

All those studies lead to think that polyphenols are mostly efficient against cancer when used in combinations or with other natural compounds in a plant-rich diet [95-98].

2. Polyphenols as Adjuvant for Chemosensitization

The increase in chemosensitivity is clinically relevant as it is often a limiting factor for the use of these compounds. Therefore, an increase in sensitivity should lead to a decrease of therapeutic thresholds. Taking into account the chemosensitizing agents in conventional therapy would potentially offer the possibility to improve the survival rate and decrease the toxicity of these substances for patients.

For example, the green tea polyphenol epigallocatechin-3-gallate shows synergy with 5-fluorouracil on human carcinoma cell lines [99]. Besides EGCG, various flavonoids or stilbenes can present a synergy or an additive action with anticancer drugs through a modification of anticancer drug metabolism or multiple actions on various targets. For example, various phenolic antioxidants (catechin, epicatechin, fisetin, gallic acid, morin, myricetin, naringenin, quercetin and resveratrol) can modify the paclitaxel metabolism. Indeed, Paclitaxel metabolites are virtually inactive in comparison with the parent drug. Some reports show that phenolic substances might increase paclitaxel blood concentrations during chemotherapy by inhibiting. cytochrome p450-catalyzed metabolism of paclitaxel [100]. Moreover the enhancement of paclitaxel action can be due to a complementary effect on targets [101, 102]. In resistant non-Hodgkin's lymphoma (NHL) and multiple myeloma (MM), resveratrol and paclitaxel selectively modify the expression of regulatory proteins in the apoptotic signalling pathway. Indeed, combination treatment results in apoptosis through the formation of tBid, mitochondrial membrane depolarization, cytosolic release of cytochrome c and Smac/DIABLO, activation of the caspase cascade, and cleavage of poly(adenosine diphosphate-ribose) polymerase. Combination of resveratrol with paclitaxel have minimal cytotoxicity against quiescent and mitogenically stimulated human peripheral blood mononuclear cells. Inhibition of Bcl-x(L) expression by resveratrol is critical for chemosensitization and its functional impairment mimics resveratrol-mediated sensitization to paclitaxel-induced apoptosis. Interestingly, a simultaneous exposure does not amplify the antiproliferative or pro-apoptotic effects of paclitaxel [103]. In fact, a pretreatment with resveratrol induces $p21^{WAF1}$ expression suggesting a possible arrest of cell cycle favoring the effect of paclitaxel action. This could be the case of the combination with 5-fluorouracil (5-Fu) which is a classic drug used in colorectal and hepatoma chemotherapy. Indeed, it was reported that resveratrol can exert synergic effect with this drug to inhibit hepatocarcinoma cell proliferation by the induction of apoptosis [104, 105].

Concerning cytokines, we and others have shown that polyphenols (resveratrol, quercetin, kaempferol, silibinin, genistein, apigenin) are able to sensitive to TRAIL (tumor necrosis factor-related apoptosis-inducing ligand)-induced apoptosis in cancer cells [106-114]. For example, in human colon cancer cell lines, some phytochemicals, resveratrol, quercetin, kaempferol can sensitize these cells to TRAIL-induced apoptosis [106, 108, 109, 112]. This sensitization by quercetin and resveratrol involves an increase of formation of a functional DISC at plasma membrane level [108, 112] and activates a caspase-dependent pathway that escapes Bcl-2-mediated expression [112]. The cholesterol sequestering agent nystatin prevents resveratrol or quercetin-induced death receptor redistribution and cell sensitization to death receptor stimulation, suggesting that polyphenols-induced redistribution of death receptors in lipid rafts is an essential step in their sensitizing effects expression [108, 112]. The sensitization by resveratrol involves also a cell cycle arrest-mediated survivin depletion and an upregulation of p21 [106].

3. Chemical Modifications of Natural Polyphenols to Improve Their Efficacy

Previous studies have documented that stilbenes and flavonoids, despite an efficient absorption by the organism, have unfortunately a low level bioavailability, glucuronidation and sulfation being limiting factors [78-80].

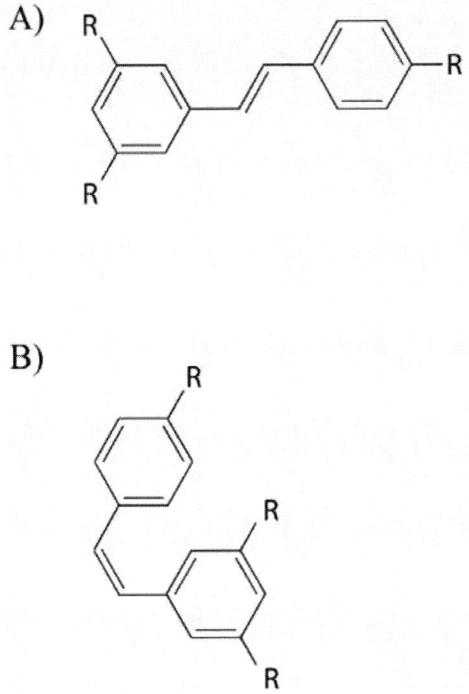

Figure 4. Chemical structures of resveratrol and derivatives. Chemical structures of *Trans* (A) or *Cis* (B) resveratrol (R=OH); resveratrol triacetate (R=CH_3COO); trimethoxyresveratrol (R=CH_3O).

Nevertheless, some elements may increase phytochemicals bioavailability such as the acetylation of polyphenol molecules (Figure 4). Indeed, recent studies show that acetylation can enhance biological activities and increase bioavailability of natural compounds such as epigallocatechin-3-gallate [115, 116]. Besides these compounds, we have recently developed acetylated forms of resveratrol and oligomers, showing that acetylation of *trans*-resveratrol inhibits colon cancer cell proliferation in the same manner as resveratrol [117]. It seems that the acetylation of the molecules does not change the targets compared to the parent molecule such as the cyclin in the cell cycle progression or the caspase activation in the apoptosis induction. These results attract major interest since an esterification of the three phenol groups leads to important modifications in the lipophilicity of the molecule and could therefore improve their intestinal absorption and cell permeability [118]. Consequently, the enhancement of cellular uptake of these molecules without loss of their activities is of great interest such as is observed with the anticancer drug, declopramide [119].

On the contrary, the isomerization of molecules and the methylation of hydroxyl groups change the cell molecular targets and are crucial to strengthened efficiency of the molecule such as resveratrol for blocking the cell cycle. Indeed, Cardile *et al.* prepared a series of acylated, methylated and hydrogenated resveratrol analogs and subjected them to bioassay towards human prostate tumor cell cultures DU-145 [120]. The results shows that the most active compound is the *cis* (Z)-3,5,4′-trimethoxystilbene, which is considerably more efficient than *trans* (E) resveratrol. Other literature data [121] reports that polymethoxystilbenes and related compounds as resveratrol analogs show interesting antitumor properties such as potent antiproliferative, pro-apoptotic activity or strong inhibition of TNFα-induced activation of NF-*k*B [122]. Further studies indicate that polymethoxystilbenes undergo different metabolic conversion and have a higher bioavailability with respect to resveratrol. Recently, Saiko et al., reported the influence of several *trans*-resveratrol analogs on HT 29 human colon cancer cell proliferation inhibition and apoptosis [123]. Indeed, a poor effect with 3,5, 4',5' tetramethoxy-*trans*-resveratrol is observed while a strong effect of 3,5 4' trimethoxy-*trans*-resveratrol and of 3,3',4,5'-tetramethoxy-*trans*-stilbene lead to remarkable changes of the cell cycle distribution on HT29 cells. Interestingly, after treatment with 3,5 4' trimethoxy-*trans*-resveratrol, growth arrest occurrs mainly in the G2-M phase, whereas incubation with 3,3',4,5'-tetramethoxy-*trans*-stilbene resulted in arrest in the G0-G1 phase of the cell cycle. The presence of hydroxylated group does not significantly change the antiproliferative effect. This is in agreement with results of Ovesna *et al.*, reporting that hydroxylation mainly protect against DNA damage [124]. However experiments are done on established cell lines which are already initiated. The only visible effect can be seen on promotion step.

Moreover, the isomerisation could modulate the activity of these compounds. Indeed, methoxylated *Z*-stilbenoids have a structural analogy with combretastatin A4, a potent antimitotic which interacts with tubulin like colchicines [125]. In the majority of cases where pairs of *E*- and *Z*-isomers were evaluated for antitumor activity, the *cis* (*Z*)-isomers proved significantly more active effects than their *trans* (*E*) analogs; nevertheless, the antiproliferative / apoptotic activity ratio between the *E*/Z isomers reported show wide variations and in some cases both either have comparable activities or the *E*-isomer may be even more active, as for *E* and *Z*-resveratrol. The strong effect of *cis* (Z) 3,5,4'-trimethylresveratrol is due to its inhibition of the microtubule polymerisation [126, 127], leading to a blockade of the cell division. This blockade provokes an increase of cell death, probably by mitotic catastrophe [128]. Other compounds exhibit a similar antiproliferative activity to *trans* (E) resveratrol, but their action mechanism is very different: resveratrol accumulates cells in S phase, while most of the other synthetic derivatives stop mitosis (M phase). The stronger effect of *cis* (*Z*) methoxy derivatives than the *trans* (*E*) counterparts is not linked to the lack of anti-oxidative effect (diseappearence of hydroxyl groups) but would be due to a steric mechanism leading to interference with different pathways as compared to the *trans* derivatives.

When the analogs of phenolics compounds is used, it is important to choose the methods to estimate the biological effects such as antiproliferative activity. Indeed, we and others have shown that methods commonly used to measure cytotoxic and/or antiproliferative effects could lead to a pitfall resulting from a differential sensitivity to natural compounds [117, 129]. For example, in the human colorectal cancer cell, SW480, we observed that resveratrol triacetate and a preparation containing resveratrol (16 %) and ε-viniferin (20 %) can induce an increase in the MTT-reducing activity [117]. These observations are very important since the MTT test can mask antiproliferative activities and could be a possible pitfall in cell sensitization determination. In genistein-treated cells, it was suggest that this increase of MTT-reducing activity could be due to an increase of the cell volume and of the number of mitochondria [130]. Similarly, resveratrol and its acetylated form induce an increase in cell volume and also induce an accumulation of SW480 cells in S phase [117]. Bernhard et al. [129] suggest that this phenomenon is associated with the differentiation process. This hypothesis is supported by the ability of resveratrol to induce differentiation of colon carcinoma cells via nuclear receptor [131]. However, it was not the case with ε-viniferin and its acetylated form which have no effect on the cell volume and differentiation, probably because these polyphenols may interact with the redox activities of mitochondria and consequently contribute to the reduction of MTT.

Consequently, it is necessary to evaluate methods used for cytotoxic determinations and to evaluate the absence of toxicities in normal cells. Several studies have shown that polyphenols compounds such as resveratrol and viniferin have no cytotoxic effect on normal hematopoietic progenitor cells, in contrast to leukemic cells. In addition, resveratrol shows specific cytotoxic effects toward tumor cells when compared with normal lung [132] and blood cells [133]. Furthermore, at the concentrations inducing growth inhibition and cell cycle arrest in colon carcinoma cells, polyphenols compounds and vineatrol did not impair the viability of human normal peripheral blood mononuclear cells (PBMC) and much higher concentrations were required to induce a cytotoxic effect in these cells [52], but what are the effects of derivatives compounds on the normal cells ? This point is very critical for a potential use of these compounds in therapeutics and more studies should be carried out to determine the absence of toxicity on normal cell and in animal models.

E) Pattern of Various Combinations of Chemical Modifications

Increase of activities after combination with natural compounds or therapeutic drugs or chemical modifications is also protected. In addition, these molecules, from natural origin, generally exhibit a lower toxicity and often a multipotency which allow them to be able to simultaneously interfere with several signalling pathways.

Although a large number of patents are available in data bases (more than 3000 results using the text word "polyphenol" on November 6th, 2008 in Esp@cenet.com worldwide) patent filing remains at a very high level.

Diversity of technical and scientific approaches as well as patent arguments is still a subject of surprise for people not familiar with the words polyphenol and flavonoid. Pharmacology activity profile of flavonoid is focused on cancer, control of inflammation, hair loss skin disorders and color.

Apart the "classical" anticancer and cardiovascular activity profile of polyphenol such as resveratrol new applications are claimed especially in cosmetic field, central nervous system, food complements and preparations etc... As described in figure 5, four approaches can be identified to develop innovation in polyphenol and flavonoid use:

1) modification of the production methods leads to increase of production or identification of new compounds;
2) in a second way new chemical structures are obtained by total synthesis or hemi synthesis from raw materials;
3) the third approach is related to formulation leading to increase of compliance and activity;
4) and finally combination therapy with various other components leads to increase or even synergy of activity. Due to the large of amount patents and projects this review will focus only on the more recent information.

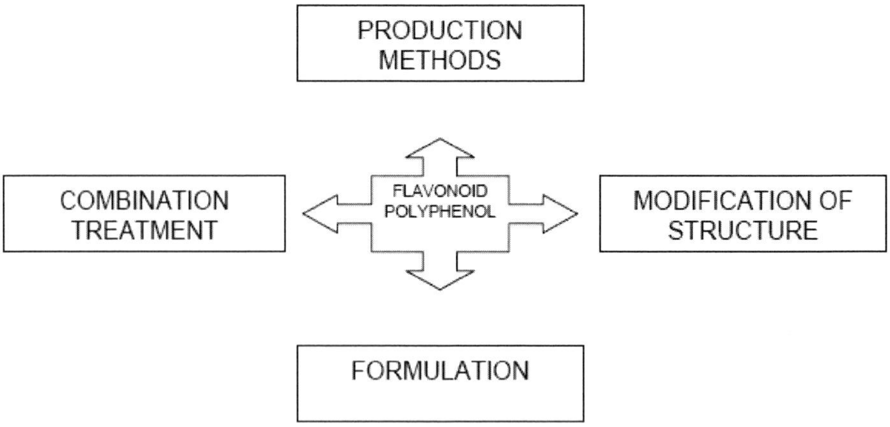

Figure 5. The four approaches for innovation in polyphenol use.

1. Production Methods

New plants are reported to be powerful producers of polyphenols with strong activity in traditional pharmaceutical domains (inflammation, cancer, cardiovascular…) including algae (EP1977756) and a new plant species from *Fallopia* named *igniscum* (DE102007011676) (Table II).

Table II. Optimization of production methods for polyphenols

Patent Number and date of filling	Inventor , company	Claims and commentaries
EP1977756, 2008-10-08	M Besnard, Diana Naturals	High quantity of polyphenols in the phylum of brown algae (Phaeophyceae) is reported with activity in inflammation domain
DE102007011676 2008-09-18	J H Wilhelm	Active substances from the leafage and/or the rhizome of the new plant species from Fallopia named igniscum is claimed
JP2008037839 2008-02-21	K Masao Cosmo Oil Ltd	The agent for increasing the polyphenol content in a plant contains 5-aminolevulinic acid derivatives
CA2621922 2007-03-15	J Page Nat. Res. Council	DNA Sequences involved in prenylflavonoid synthesis in hops are use for modification of prenylflavonoid plants production
CN101199355 2008-06-18	W Liu High Tech Res Cter of Shangai	Improvement of the resveratrol production by a genetically modified peanut kernel with a full-long resveratrol synthase gene and a specific promoter Arah1P.
JP2007089430 2007-04-12	Y Tsurunaga Matsushita Ltd	Irradiation of leaves by a white lamp 2 emitting visible light, and a fluorescent light 3 emitting UV-B light. To increase polyphenol production.
CN101160393 2008-04-09	M Katz Fluxome Sciences	Metabolically engineered cells for the production of resveratrol or an oligomeric or glycosidically-bound

Table III. Optimization of production methods for flavonoids

Patent Number and date of filling	Inventor , company	Claims and commentaries
CN101229328 2008-07-30	Central South Univ of FO	*Method of extracting eucalyptus and bamboo wood flavonoid*
WO2008125433 2008-10-23	Poole Mervin C UNILEVER	The invention relates to a method for producing a plant tissue, preferably a fruit with an increased content of a flavonoid component and to a plant tissue obtained by transfection of transcripts of TDR4.
WO2008096354 2008-08-14	Levin I Israel State	*Means and methods for providing an AFT gene encoding a protein characterized by at least 80% identity with the amino acid sequence from LA1996 Seq is reported. The AFT gene confers higher concentrations of flavonoids to the plants compared with prior art cultivated plants. Transgenic plants expressing metabolites of the flavonoid pathway, especially anthocyanin or flavonols, in plants, plant parts or seeds thereof, carrying particular DNA sequences recombinable into a plurality of one or more transformation and/or expression vectors, useful for transformation and/or expression in plants are disclosed. Methods of obtaining same are disclosed.*
US2008200537 2008-08-21	Cleveland T	Increased biosynthesis of the isoflavonoid phytoalexin compounds, Glyceollins I, II and III, in soy plants is obtained after grown under stressed conditions (elicited soy). Compounds exhibit marked anti-estrogenic effects on ER function with inhibition of proliferation of ER-positive estrogen dependent breast cancer cells and inhibiting ER-dependent gene expression of progesterone receptor (PgR) and stromal derived factor-1 (SDF1/CXCL12).
JP2008161184 2008-07-17	Chin-Wen H Tatung Univ	The in vitro flavonoid-rich rhizome tissue of N. gracilis, which is obtained from a tissue culture-prepared product variable in the flavonoid content of Neomarica gracilis, contains tectorigenin which is not the case from the original plant
US2008134356 2008-06-05	Rommens C	The present invention relates to increasing at least one antioxidant level in a plant or plant product by expressing a polynucleotide that encodes a transcription factor, which is active in a flavonoid pathway. Overexpression of, for instance, a novel and newly-identified gene, the mCai gene, in a plant, results in increased accumulation of chlorogenic acid and other related phenolics, which, in turn, increases the levels of beneficial antioxidant in the plant
NZ543387 (A) 2008-04-30	Spangenberg G Agres Ltd	The present invention relates to nucleic acids and nucleic acid fragments encoding amino acid sequences for flavonoid biosynthetic enzymes in plants, and the use thereof for the modification of flavonoid biosynthesis in plants. (chalcone isomerase (CHI), chalcone synthase (CHS), chalcone reductase (CHR), dihydroflavonol 4-reductase (DFR), leucoanthocyanidin reductase (LCR), flavonoid 3', 5' hydrolase (F3'5'H), flavanone 3-hydroxylase (F3H), flavonoid 3'-hydroxylase (F3'H), phenylalanine ammonia-olyase (PAL) and vestitone reductase (VR)) (originating from WO03031622 2003-04-17)

Optimization of polyphenol production is obtained by stimulation of production by compounds (JP2008037839), genetic manipulations (CA2621922 and CN101199355) as well as treatment of plants before final extraction (JP2007089430 using lamp illumination of plants). Modification of bacteria for production of polyphenols is also feasible (CN101160393). Concerning more specifically flavonoids, new plants are reported to be powerful producer of flavonoids with strong activity in traditional pharmaceutical domains (inflammation, cancer cardiovascular…). Development of new extraction method to obtain significant quantity of compounds is claimed especially from China unfortunately without direct translation of patents (See bamboo origin in CN101229328) (Table III). Genetic transformation of plants is also used to increase flavonoid production by the use of genes involved in the synthesis pathway or transcription factors (WO2008125433, WO2008096354 US2008134356).

In a more simple approach, stress induction of production is also described in soybeans for example (US2008200537). In vitro culture is also reported to induce original production of flavonoid (JP2008161184).

2. Modification of Structures

Syntheses of new analogs of polyphenol remain a good approach for innovation (Table IV). In CA2617213 inhibition of inflammation, recruitment and cell proliferation is claimed according to chemical modifications. Rather complex compounds are also reported (example in EP1901735 or CN101115763) with questionable possibility for final pharmaceutical production (Figure 6A). Chemical modification of resveratrol remains hardly explored especially in anticancer and cardiovascular fields (see US2005240062 as an example). Association of polyphenols with fatty acids is again reported for increased activity (US2008176956 and WO2007099162).

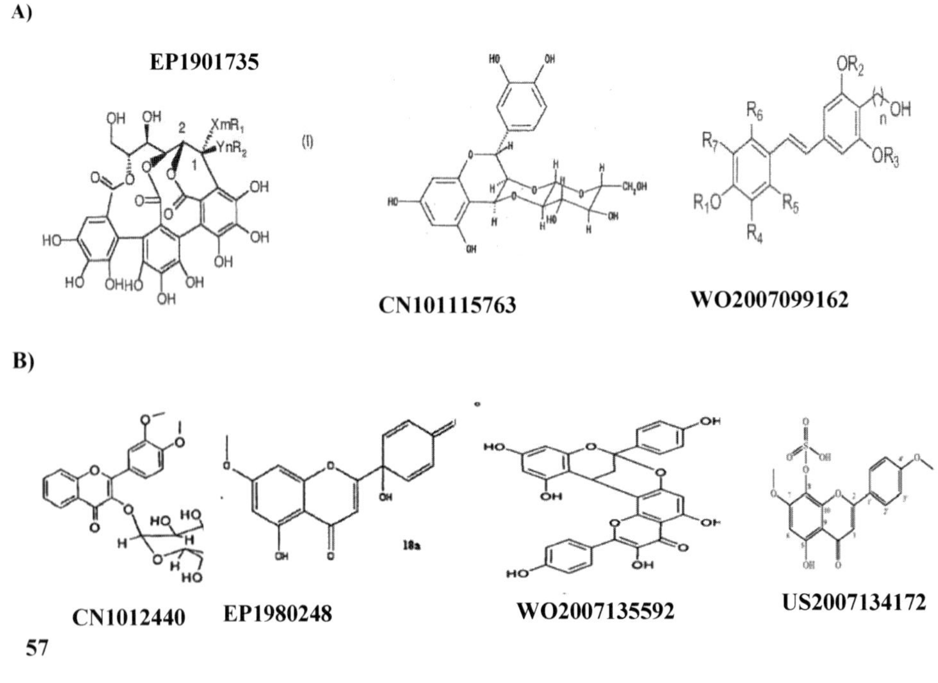

Figure 6. Some examples of structures with a patent.

Table IV. Chemical modifications by synthesis or hemi synthesis of polyphenol drugs

Patent Number and date of filling	1rst Inventor , company	Claims and commentaries
CA2617213 2007-02-08	F Chiacchia Resverlogix Corp	Polyphenol-like compounds that are useful f or inhibiting VCAM-1 expression, MCP-1 expression and/or SMC proliferation for inflammation and cardiovascular problems
EP1901735 2008-03-26	G Depierre Bordeaux Univ	Polyphenols active on cell proliferation especially on cancer cells
CN101115763 2008-01-30	K Nagamine Nichirei Biosciences Inc	Polyphenol glycoside from acerola associated with an antioxidant, a glucosidase inhibitor, a food, a cosmetic, and a skin preparation for external use, each of which comprises such compound
US2005240062 2005-10-27	G Pettit	Structural modifications of resveratrol and combretastatin A-4 for the production of novel compounds having antineoplastic and antimicrobial activity
US2008176956 2008-07-24	S Hsu Georgia Res Inst	Production of green tea polyphenols with one on more ester-linked fatty acids.
WO2007099162 2007-09-07	L Bang CNRS	Hydroxylated long chain resveratrol derivatives useful as neurotrophic agents.
CN101072815 2007-11-14	T Numata Univ Tsukuba	Therapeutic agent for mitochondrial disease for preventive/therapeutic agent for diabetes mellitus with polymeric polphenol extracted for fermented tea

Table V. Chemical modifications by synthesis or hemi synthesis of flavonoid drugs

Patent Number and date of filling	1rst Inventor , company	Claims and commentaries
US2008287374 2008-11-20	Yamazaki R	Flavonoid and glycosides, esters, or salts mixed with an anticancer agent are claimed to be anticancer agent (no structure available) with inhibition of BCRP (an ABC transporter)
CN101244057 2008-08-20	Yongsheng J Second Military Med Univ	"3-substituted oxygen group-3',4'-dimethoxy flavonoid compound with blood fat reducing function" (Patent in Chinese language)
EP1980248 2008-10-15	A-Shen Lin Kaohsiung Med Univ.	Flavonoid compound with modification of rings with increased anticancer activity.
US2007134172 2007-06-14	Buchholz H	Novel flavonoid derivative, to an extract comprising the flavonoid derivative, to the cosmetic and pharmaceutical use thereof, to preparations comprising the flavonoid derivative or extract, and to a process for the preparation of the flavonoid derivative or extract.
WO2008076767 2008-06-26	Cushman M Purdue Res Found.	Substituted flavonoid compounds, and pharmaceutical formulations of flavonoid compounds are described. Optimization of structure on cell proliferation and apoptosis induction is reported
CN101205233 2008-06-25	Yonghong L South Chiba Sea Inst Ocean.	Novel dimeric flavonoid compound for the treatment of cancers, especially the cervical cancer, gastric cancer and liver cancer, from the roots of the Ephedra sinica. Activity is reported on HeLa cervical carcinoma cells, SGC-7901 gastric cancer cells and HepG2 hepatocellular carcinoma cells.
WO2007135592 2007-11-29	Chan T Univ Hong Kong Polytech.	A series of flavonoid dimers are found to be efficient P-gp modulators that increase cytotoxicity of anticancer drugs in vitro and dramatically enhance their intracellular drug accumulation.

Surprisingly, polymerization of natural polyphenols is claimed to increase pharmacologic activity in metabolic disease (CN101072815) (Table IV). Concerning syntheses of new analogs of flavonoids remain as well as polyphenols a good approach for innovation (Table V). In US2008287374 and EP1980248 flavonoids and esters are demonstated as anticancer agents. WO2008076767 reports substituted flavonoid compounds, and more specifically, racemic abyssinone II, zapotin, and analogs useful for treating cancer. Substituted flavonoids in CN101244057 are described to be hypolipidemic agents (Figure 6B).

3. Formulation

Polyphenol administration is complex due to high level of astringency and bitterness and low absorption associated with questionable gut stability. Therefore new ways for increasing compliance and oral availability are under study in many companies. Microencapsulation (US2008213441) or association with new vehicle (WO2008072155) as well as nanoencapsulation (CN101214225) and nanocrystallization (CN101195559) are good ways to increase stability and facilitate absorption (Table VI).

Table VI. New formulation approaches for polyphenols use

Patent Number and date of filling	1rst Inventor , company	Claims and commentaries
US2008213441 2008-09-04	C J Ludwig	Reduction of astringency in polyphenol and protection from oxidation, enzymatic degradation, while maintaining gastrointestinal bioavailability within the digestive system by microencapsulation
WO2008072155 2008-06-19	E Amal Firmenich and Cie	The ingredient delivery system comprises polyphenol in combination with porous apatite grains and an amorphous metal salt in order to increase stability and availability
CN101214225 2008-07-09	Ouyangwuqing Northwest univ	Production of a resveratrol nano-emulsion anticancer drug which is characterized in that the particle size of the nano-emulsion anticancer drug is between 1nm and 100nm
CN101195559 2008-06-11	Y Wang	Resveratrol nano-crystallization relates to skin-care cosmetic technical field, relates to a method for preparing white chenopodium album alcohol nanometer crystal and application
S2008095866 2008-04-24	L Declercq Ajinomoto Monichem	Phosphorylated polyphenols combination with a carrier provide a means for delayed delivery to keratinous tissues, such as skin, hair and nails, with enzymes of the keratinous tissue dephosphorylating the polyphenol, and returning it to its native active form.
EP1893555 2008-03-05	S Delaire Rhone Poulenc Chimie	Bioprecursor of formula [A]n -PP - [B]m wherein: PP represents a polyphenol radical where each hydroxyl function is protected by a group a saturated or unsaturated alkyl chain, comprising 1 to 20 carbon atoms able to form the initial polyphenol after enzymatic digestion.
US2008213456 2008-09-04	M Chimel Mars Inc	Bars and Confectioneries with a high cocoa polyphenol content and sterol/stanol esters are produced with processes able to maintain high level of active compounds.

If required optimization of topical use of polyphenol is also hardly worked for the treatment of skin disorders. S2008095866 claims increase of topical availability of polyphenols with phosphorylated polyphenols. An original approach with the synthesis of bioprecursors of polyphenol is also reported in EP1893555 especially for topic targets. In that case bioprocessing of these molecules will lead to in situ production of active polyphenols. Food industry is also concerned by polyphenol use as demonstrated by US2008213456 showing incorporation of extracts into bars (Table VI).

Flavonoid usage is also complex due to instability of the compounds. Topical use is limited due to interaction with UV light, therefore stabilization of the drug with antioxidant compounds is necessary (WO2008140440) (Table VII).

Table VII. New formulation approaches for flavonoid use

Patent Number and date of filling	1rst Inventor , company	Claims and commentaries
WO2008140440 2008-11-20	Mercier M F	Stable flavonoid solutions including antioxidant drugs in combination with other compounds and the use of these solutions in treating dermatologic conditions are reported.
JP2008174553 2008-07-31	Glico Daily Products Co	Promoting the absorption of flavonoid with pectin derived from an apple or a citrus as an effective ingredient.
JP2008174507 2008-07-31	Suntory Ltd	Production of a flavonoid (catechin or its methylated form) glycoside (from maltotriose residue-containing carbohydrate (preferably, maltotriose, maltotetraose, maltopentaose, maltohexaose, maltoheptaose, a dextrin, [gamma]-cyclodextrin, a soluble starch) highly soluble in water, better in taste and increased in stability.
DE102007005507 2008-08-07	Wellness and Health Care GMBH	Mixture of Piperin (black pepper), flavonoids (grapefruit), and a third component containing amino acids (lysine) and niacin.
CN101180319 (A) 2008-05-14	Lang Zhuo Agency Sciencde Techn and Res.	Polymer carrier with C6 or C8 position of the flavonoid A ring is used to form delivery vehicles to deliver high doses of flavonoids, and may also be used as delivery vehicles to deliver an additional bioactive agent.
GB2443576 2008-05-07	Managoli N B Sahajanand Biotech Ltd.	Implantable medical devices, such as stents, that comprise a composition for controlled delivery of flavonoids or a derivative thereof.
JP2007223914 2007-09-06	Takayanagi K Unitika Ltd	Oral administration formulation with, a carotenoid such as cryptoxanthin or its fatty acid ester, a flavonoid such as hesperidin, its derivative or hesperitin and/or its derivative and has anti-diabetes action and/or an ameliorative action for impaired glucose tolerance.

In order to increase oral availability mixture with pectin from citrus and other origin is also reported (JP2008174553). Modification of taste and increase of water solubility is obtained after glycosylation of compounds (JP2008174507). Complex mixtures are also claimed to increase oral absorption (DE102007005507). In CN101180319 chemical linkage with polymer is shown to increase local availability of flavonoid even after in vivo injection. Local effect of flavonoid is also found after inclusion of compound into medical devices for example in implantable stents for the prevention of restenosis (GB2443576) (Table VII).

4. Combination Treatment

A mixture of natural compounds is an old pharmaceutical approach in polyphenol use. However a clear synergy of activity is rarely demonstrated. Some recent patents describe this type of result (combination of fatty acids and polyphenol in US2008234361 and US2008004342 and combination of natural extracts in CN101156839, WO2008120220, EP1782802, US2007219146 and US2007054868) (Table VIII). Example of synergy of activity on cancer cell proliferation in vitro is shown in figure 7. Sophisticated in vitro demonstration of activity is under development (see SNARE target in WO2008111796 for the demonstration of compound activity on central nervous system diseases or inhibition of proteasome in US2008015248 for inhibition of cancer cell proliferation). AMPK target is also reported for control of cancer cells (US2007244202) and sirtuins for the control of aging (US2008255382).

Use of polyphenols as a nutrient is claimed in UA80692 or US2008262081 leading to improvements of cancer and inflammation. In rather the same domain WO2007009187 reports a combination with probiotics in order to increase cardiovascular health. In another approach (N101138569) polyphenols are claimed to increase antineoplastic activity of drugs such as indol-3-methanol. It is also remarkable to notice that biological activity is not necessary while ORAC value appears to be acceptable for patent filling. (US2008254135) (*ORAC Value* Is the *Value* Given to a Fruit's Oxygen Radical Absorbance Capacity). Activity on metabolic disease such as diabetes and obesity is increasing especially in patent from Asia (example in CN101199647).

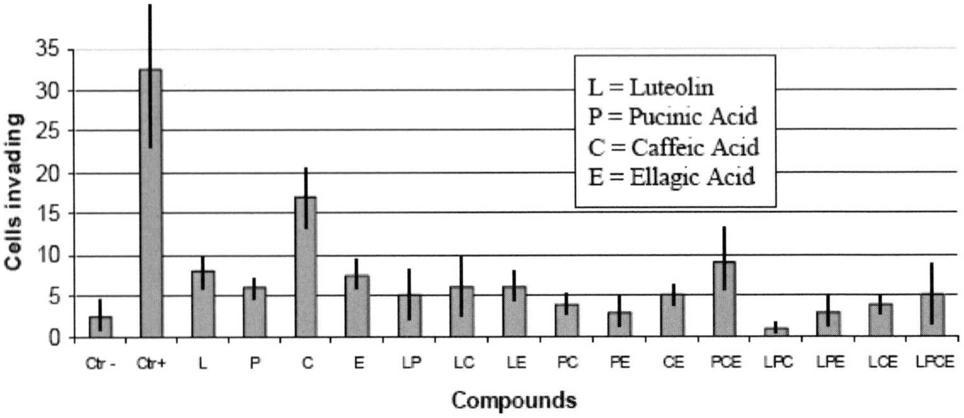

Figure 7. Synergy of activity after mixing polyphenol and conjugated fatty acids on prostate cancer cells. (US2008234361) (according to patent number US2008234361).

Table VIII. Combination treatment

Patent Number and date of filling	1[rst] Inventor , company	Claims and commentaries
US2008234361 2008-09-25	E Lansky Rimonest Ltd	Mixture of conjugated fatty acid(s) and polyphenol(s) for the treatment of obesity, diabetes, cancer and heart disease.
US2008004342 2008-01-03	G P Zaloga	The biologically active formulation of a fatty acid and a complex phenol is used to inhibit mammalian cell growth and/or metastasis of malignant cells.
CN101156839 2008-04-09	S Zhang Beijing Xinghao Med St	Resveratrol in combination with other drugs demonstrates synergism and enhancement function on prevention and treatment of ischemia-refilling cardiac muscle cell.
WO2008120220 2008-10-09	G Ganra Raju	Enriched 3- O-acetyl-11-keto-ss-boswellic acid and enriched demethylated curcuminoids, demonstrate synergistic effect on specific inhibition of- COX-2 and 5-LOX with anti-inflammatory, antiulcerogenic and antioxidant activities.
EP17828022007-05-09	J M Estrela Ariquel Univ Valencia	Combined use of pterostilbene and quercetin for the production of cancer treatment medicaments with decrease of cell proliferation inv tro and in in vivo experiments.
US200721914620 07-09-20	B Sunil	Diabetes Mellitus is treated by synergistic mixture of polyphenol of concentration ranging between 85 to 95% (w/w) GAE, theobromine of concentration ranging between 1 to 5% (w/w), and moisture content ranging between 0.5 to 10% (v/w).
US2007054868 2007-03-08	I B Weinstein	Treating or preventing cancer in a subject with a Synergistic Polyphenol Compound or composition thereof (no results available)
WO2008111796 2008-09-18	W Dae-Hyuk Sungkyunkwan Univ	Naturally extracted polyphenols suppresses the formation of a SNARE complex with claimed about the control of central nervous system dysfunction.
US2008015248 2008-01-17	Q P Dou	Synthetic green tea derived polyphenolic compounds are produced and used for inhibition of proteasomal activity for treating cancers
US2007244202 2007-10-18	M Takatoshi Kao Corp	AMPK activator containing resveratrol as an active ingredient was described
US2008255382 2008-10-16	A Merritt Univ Brigham	Novel sirtuin activating compounds and methods for making the same with methods for preparing resveratrol, resveratrol esters and substituted and unsubstituted stilbenes
UA80692 2007-10-25	M Rat	Nutrient pharmaceutical formulation with ascorbic acid, L-lysine, L-proline and polyphenol compound are used for the treatment if cancer
US2008262081 2008-10-23	D Raerdersorff	Nutraceutical compositions with Resveratrol for delaying aging and/or for the treatment or prevention of age-related diseases in animals, in particular in mammals including humans
WO2007009187 2007-01-25	S Keith Tarac Tech	Polyphenol from grape seed, apple, pear, green tea or cocoa extracts, in combination with lactobacilli and bifidobacteria species improves cardiovascular health
N101138569 2008-03-12	J Zhou Beijing Weimingbao Bio	Increase of the curative effect of anti-cancer Indole-3-methanol (I3C) and derivatives with resveratrol
US2008254135 2008-10-16	M Heuer	Components having high ORAC values and supplying polyphenols and antioxidants in amounts equal to or greater than the recommended daily requirements found in fruits and vegetables are able to enhance cardioprotective and immune system functions.
CN101199647 2008-06-18	B Zhao Chinese Acad Sci	Mixture of epigallocatechin-3-gallate, any kind of tea polyphenol and cyclocarya paliurus (Batal.) iljinsk water extracts are active on type II diabetes mellitus and reverse insulin resistance

The patent approach remains especially active in the polyphenol field. New formulations and mixtures seem to be especially appreciated. New mechanisms of action in relation with published scientific results can be observed (sirtuin phenomenon). The number of patents is relatively stable according to a year of filing, indicating that the situation will remain relatively stable for the future.

Conclusion

We have established that one of the goals is to increase bioavailability and consequently the biological effects of natural molecules. Increase in the lipophilicity of molecules should improve the cellular uptake and consequently lead to better absorption without loss of their activities. We presented the idea that isomerisation and methylation of hydroxyl groups of some polyphenols especially resveratrol are crucial to improve the molecule efficiency in blocking cell proliferation by changing the cell molecular targets. We focused on the relevance of using flavonoid and polyphenol combinations or chemical modifications to enhance their biological effects. We suggested innovative directions to develop new types of drugs which may especially be used in combination with other natural components or pharmacological conventional drugs in order to obtain a synergistic effect.

Acknowledgments

This project was supported by the "Conseil Régional de Bourgogne", BIVB and Ligue contre le Cancer, comités Côte d'Or et Jura.

References

[1] Frankel, E.N., Waterhouse, A.L. and Kinsella, J.E., Inhibition of human LDL oxidation by resveratrol, *Lancet*. 1993, *341*, 1103-1104.

[2] Maron, D.J., Flavonoids for reduction of atherosclerotic risk, *Curr Atheroscler Rep*. 2004, *6*, 73-78.

[3] Renaud, S.C., Gueguen, R., Schenker, J. and d'Houtaud, A., Alcohol and mortality in middle-aged men from eastern France, *Epidemiology*. 1998, *9*, 184-188.

[4] Levi, F., Pasche, C., Lucchini, F., Ghidoni, R., Ferraroni, M. and La Vecchia, C., Resveratrol and breast cancer risk, *Eur J Cancer Prev*. 2005, *14*, 139-142.

[5] Knekt, P., Jarvinen, R., Seppanen, R., Hellovaara, M., Teppo, L., Pukkala, E. and Aromaa, A., Dietary flavonoids and the risk of lung cancer and other malignant neoplasms, *Am J Epidemiol*. 1997, *146*, 223-230.

[6] Chan, H.Y. and Leung, L.K., A potential protective mechanism of soya isoflavones against 7,12-dimethylbenz[a]anthracene tumour initiation, *Br J Nutr*. 2003, *90*, 457-465.

[7] Walle, T., Otake, Y., Galijatovic, A., Ritter, J.K. and Walle, U.K., Induction of UDP-glucuronosyltransferase UGT1A1 by the flavonoid chrysin in the human hepatoma cell line hep G2, *Drug Metab Dispos*. 2000, *28*, 1077-1082.

[8] Galijatovic, A., Walle, U.K. and Walle, T., Induction of UDP-glucuronosyltransferase by the flavonoids chrysin and quercetin in Caco-2 cells, *Pharm Res*. 2000, *17*, 21-26.

[9] Lancon, A., Hanet, N., Jannin, B., Delmas, D., Heydel, J.M., Lizard, G., Chagnon, M.C., Artur, Y. and Latruffe, N., Resveratrol in human hepatoma HepG2 cells: metabolism and inducibility of detoxifying enzymes, *Drug Metab Dispos*. 2007, *35*, 699-703.

[10] Nijhoff, W.A., Bosboom, M.A., Smidt, M.H. and Peters, W.H., Enhancement of rat hepatic and gastrointestinal glutathione and glutathione S-transferases by alpha-angelicalactone and flavone, *Carcinogenesis*. 1995, *16*, 607-612.

[11] Miranda, C.L., Aponso, G.L., Stevens, J.F., Deinzer, M.L. and Buhler, D.R., Prenylated chalcones and flavanones as inducers of quinone reductase in mouse Hepa 1c1c7 cells, *Cancer Lett*. 2000, *149*, 21-29.

[12] Yannai, S., Day, A.J., Williamson, G. and Rhodes, M.J., Characterization of flavonoids as monofunctional or bifunctional inducers of quinone reductase in murine hepatoma cell lines, *Food Chem Toxicol*. 1998, *36*, 623-630.

[13] Eaton, E.A., Walle, U.K., Lewis, A.J., Hudson, T., Wilson, A.A. and Walle, T., Flavonoids, potent inhibitors of the human P-form phenolsulfotransferase. Potential role in drug metabolism and chemoprevention, *Drug Metab Dispos*. 1996, *24*, 232-237.

[14] Kong, A.N., Yu, R., Hebbar, V., Chen, C., Owuor, E., Hu, R., Ee, R. and Mandlekar, S., Signal transduction events elicited by cancer prevention compounds, *Mutat Res*. 2001, *480-481*, 231-241.

[15] Murakami, A., Ashida, H. and Terao, J., Multitargeted cancer prevention by quercetin, *Cancer Lett*. 2008, *269*, 315-325.

[16] Tanigawa, S., Fujii, M. and Hou, D.X., Action of Nrf2 and Keap1 in ARE-mediated NQO1 expression by quercetin, *Free Radic Biol Med*. 2007, *42*, 1690-1703.

[17] Yang, S.H., Kim, J.S., Oh, T.J., Kim, M.S., Lee, S.W., Woo, S.K., Cho, H.S., Choi, Y.H., Kim, Y.H., Rha, S.Y., Chung, H.C. and An, S.W., Genome-scale analysis of resveratrol-induced gene expression profile in human ovarian cancer cells using a cDNA microarray, *Int J Oncol*. 2003, *22*, 741-750.

[18] Wang, Z., Hsieh, T.C., Zhang, Z., Ma, Y. and Wu, J.M., Identification and purification of resveratrol targeting proteins using immobilized resveratrol affinity chromatography, *Biochem Biophys Res Commun*. 2004, *323*, 743-749.

[19] Traganos, F., Ardelt, B., Halko, N., Bruno, S. and Darzynkiewicz, Z., Effects of genistein on the growth and cell cycle progression of normal human lymphocytes and human leukemic MOLT-4 and HL-60 cells, *Cancer Res*. 1992, *52*, 6200-6208.

[20] Hosokawa, N., Hosokawa, Y., Sakai, T., Yoshida, M., Marui, N., Nishino, H., Kawai, K. and Aoike, A., Inhibitory effect of quercetin on the synthesis of a possibly cell-cycle-related 17-kDa protein, in human colon cancer cells, *Int J Cancer*. 1990, *45*, 1119-1124.

[21] Zi, X., Grasso, A.W., Kung, H.J. and Agarwal, R., A flavonoid antioxidant, silymarin, inhibits activation of erbB1 signaling and induces cyclin-dependent kinase inhibitors, G1 arrest, and anticarcinogenic effects in human prostate carcinoma DU145 cells, *Cancer Res*. 1998, *58*, 1920-1929.

[22] Morgan, D.O., Principles of CDK regulation, *Nature*. 1995, *374*, 131-134.

[23] Huh, S.W., Bae, S.M., Kim, Y.W., Lee, J.M., Namkoong, S.E., Lee, I.P., Kim, S.H., Kim, C.K. and Ahn, W.S., Anticancer effects of (-)-epigallocatechin-3-gallate on ovarian carcinoma cell lines, *Gynecol Oncol*. 2004, *94*, 760-768.

[24] Hsieh, T.C. and Wu, J.M., Suppression of cell proliferation and gene expression by combinatorial synergy of EGCG, resveratrol and gamma-tocotrienol in estrogen receptor-positive MCF-7 breast cancer cells, *Int J Oncol.* 2008, *33*, 851-859.

[25] Hastak, K., Gupta, S., Ahmad, N., Agarwal, M.K., Agarwal, M.L. and Mukhtar, H., Role of p53 and NF-kappaB in epigallocatechin-3-gallate-induced apoptosis of LNCaP cells, *Oncogene.* 2003, *22*, 4851-4859.

[26] Lah, J.J., Cui, W. and Hu, K.Q., Effects and mechanisms of silibinin on human hepatoma cell lines, *World J Gastroenterol.* 2007, *13*, 5299-5305.

[27] Srivastava, R.K., Chen, Q., Siddiqui, I., Sarva, K. and Shankar, S., Linkage of curcumin-induced cell cycle arrest and apoptosis by cyclin-dependent kinase inhibitor p21(/WAF1/CIP1), *Cell Cycle.* 2007, *6*, 2953-2961.

[28] Ahmad, N., Adhami, V.M., Afaq, F., Feyes, D.K. and Mukhtar, H., Resveratrol causes WAF-1/p21-mediated G(1)-phase arrest of cell cycle and induction of apoptosis in human epidermoid carcinoma A431 cells, *Clin Cancer Res.* 2001, *7*, 1466-1473.

[29] Adhami, V.M., Afaq, F. and Ahmad, N., Involvement of the retinoblastoma (pRb)-E2F/DP pathway during antiproliferative effects of resveratrol in human epidermoid carcinoma (A431) cells, *Biochem Biophys Res Commun.* 2001, *288*, 579-585.

[30] Kim, Y.A., Lee, W.H., Choi, T.H., Rhee, S.H., Park, K.Y. and Choi, Y.H., Involvement of p21WAF1/CIP1, pRB, Bax and NF-kappaB in induction of growth arrest and apoptosis by resveratrol in human lung carcinoma A549 cells, *Int J Oncol.* 2003, *23*, 1143-1149.

[31] Deep, G. and Agarwal, R., Chemopreventive efficacy of silymarin in skin and prostate cancer, *Integr Cancer Ther.* 2007, *6*, 130-145.

[32] Lian, F., Bhuiyan, M., Li, Y.W., Wall, N., Kraut, M. and Sarkar, F.H., Genistein-induced G2-M arrest, p21WAF1 upregulation, and apoptosis in a non-small-cell lung cancer cell line, *Nutr Cancer.* 1998, *31*, 184-191.

[33] Pagliacci, M.C., Smacchia, M., Migliorati, G., Grignani, F., Riccardi, C. and Nicoletti, I., Growth-inhibitory effects of the natural phyto-oestrogen genistein in MCF-7 human breast cancer cells, *Eur J Cancer.* 1994, *30A*, 1675-1682.

[34] Casagrande, F. and Darbon, J.M., p21CIP1 is dispensable for the G2 arrest caused by genistein in human melanoma cells, *Exp Cell Res.* 2000, *258*, 101-108.

[35] Davis, J.N., Singh, B., Bhuiyan, M. and Sarkar, F.H., Genistein-induced upregulation of p21WAF1, downregulation of cyclin B, and induction of apoptosis in prostate cancer cells, *Nutr Cancer.* 1998, *32*, 123-131.

[36] Wolter, F., Akoglu, B., Clausnitzer, A. and Stein, J., Downregulation of the cyclin D1/Cdk4 complex occurs during resveratrol-induced cell cycle arrest in colon cancer cell lines, *J Nutr.* 2001, *131*, 2197-2203.

[37] Schneider, Y., Vincent, F., Duranton, B., Badolo, L., Gosse, F., Bergmann, C., Seiler, N. and Raul, F., Anti-proliferative effect of resveratrol, a natural component of grapes and wine, on human colonic cancer cells, *Cancer Lett.* 2000, *158*, 85-91.

[38] Delmas, D., Passilly-Degrace, P., Jannin, B., Malki, M.C. and Latruffe, N., Resveratrol, a chemopreventive agent, disrupts the cell cycle control of human SW480 colorectal tumor cells, *Int J Mol Med.* 2002, *10*, 193-199.

[39] Choi, J.A., Kim, J.Y., Lee, J.Y., Kang, C.M., Kwon, H.J., Yoo, Y.D., Kim, T.W., Lee, Y.S. and Lee, S.J., Induction of cell cycle arrest and apoptosis in human breast cancer cells by quercetin, *Int J Oncol.* 2001, *19*, 837-844.

[40] Liang, Y.C., Tsai, S.H., Chen, L., Lin-Shiau, S.Y. and Lin, J.K., Resveratrol-induced G2 arrest through the inhibition of CDK7 and p34CDC2 kinases in colon carcinoma HT29 cells, *Biochem Pharmacol.* 2003, *65*, 1053-1060.

[41] Delmas, D., Rebe, C., Lacour, S., Filomenko, R., Athias, A., Gambert, P., Cherkaoui-Malki, M., Jannin, B., Dubrez-Daloz, L., Latruffe, N. and Solary, E., Resveratrol-induced apoptosis is associated with Fas redistribution in the rafts and the formation of a death-inducing signaling complex in colon cancer cells, *J Biol Chem.* 2003, *278*, 41482-41490.

[42] Mouria, M., Gukovskaya, A.S., Jung, Y., Buechler, P., Hines, O.J., Reber, H.A. and Pandol, S.J., Food-derived polyphenols inhibit pancreatic cancer growth through mitochondrial cytochrome C release and apoptosis, *Int J Cancer.* 2002, *98*, 761-769.

[43] Granado-Serrano, A.B., Martin, M.A., Bravo, L., Goya, L. and Ramos, S., Quercetin induces apoptosis via caspase activation, regulation of Bcl-2, and inhibition of PI-3-kinase/Akt and ERK pathways in a human hepatoma cell line (HepG2), *J Nutr.* 2006, *136*, 2715-2721.

[44] Li, Y., Upadhyay, S., Bhuiyan, M. and Sarkar, F.H., Induction of apoptosis in breast cancer cells MDA-MB-231 by genistein, *Oncogene.* 1999, *18*, 3166-3172.

[45] Li, Y., Bhuiyan, M. and Sarkar, F.H., Induction of apoptosis and inhibition of c-erbB-2 in MDA-MB-435 cells by genistein, *Int J Oncol.* 1999, *15*, 525-533.

[46] Alhasan, S.A., Pietrasczkiwicz, H., Alonso, M.D., Ensley, J. and Sarkar, F.H., Genistein-induced cell cycle arrest and apoptosis in a head and neck squamous cell carcinoma cell line, *Nutr Cancer.* 1999, *34*, 12-19.

[47] Katdare, M., Osborne, M. and Telang, N.T., Soy isoflavone genistein modulates cell cycle progression and induces apoptosis in HER-2/neu oncogene expressing human breast epithelial cells, *Int J Oncol.* 2002, *21*, 809-815.

[48] Kim, Y.A., Choi, B.T., Lee, Y.T., Park, D.I., Rhee, S.H., Park, K.Y. and Choi, Y.H., Resveratrol inhibits cell proliferation and induces apoptosis of human breast carcinoma MCF-7 cells, *Oncol Rep.* 2004, *11*, 441-446.

[49] Hsieh, T.C., Burfeind, P., Laud, K., Backer, J.M., Traganos, F., Darzynkiewicz, Z. and Wu, J.M., Cell cycle effects and control of gene expression by resveratrol in human breast carcinoma cell lines with different metastatic potentials, *Int J Oncol.* 1999, *15*, 245-252.

[50] Surh, Y.J., Hurh, Y.J., Kang, J.Y., Lee, E., Kong, G. and Lee, S.J., Resveratrol, an antioxidant present in red wine, induces apoptosis in human promyelocytic leukemia (HL-60) cells, *Cancer Lett.* 1999, *140*, 1-10.

[51] Roman, V., Billard, C., Kern, C., Ferry-Dumazet, H., Izard, J.C., Mohammad, R., Mossalayi, D.M. and Kolb, J.P., Analysis of resveratrol-induced apoptosis in human B-cell chronic leukaemia, *Br J Haematol.* 2002, *117*, 842-851.

[52] Billard, C., Izard, J.C., Roman, V., Kern, C., Mathiot, C., Mentz, F. and Kolb, J.P., Comparative antiproliferative and apoptotic effects of resveratrol, epsilon-viniferin and vine-shots derived polyphenols (vineatrols) on chronic B lymphocytic leukemia cells and normal human lymphocytes, *Leuk Lymphoma.* 2002, *43*, 1991-2002.

[53] Lee, D.H., Szczepanski, M. and Lee, Y.J., Role of Bax in quercetin-induced apoptosis in human prostate cancer cells, *Biochem Pharmacol.* 2008, *75*, 2345-2355.

[54] Zhou, H.B., Yan, Y., Sun, Y.N. and Zhu, J.R., Resveratrol induces apoptosis in human esophageal carcinoma cells, *World J Gastroenterol.* 2003, *9*, 408-411.

[55] Kaneuchi, M., Sasaki, M., Tanaka, Y., Yamamoto, R., Sakuragi, N. and Dahiya, R., Resveratrol suppresses growth of Ishikawa cells through down-regulation of EGF, *Int J Oncol.* 2003, *23*, 1167-1172.
[56] Zhou, H.B., Chen, J.J., Wang, W.X., Cai, J.T. and Du, Q., Anticancer activity of resveratrol on implanted human primary gastric carcinoma cells in nude mice, *World J Gastroenterol.* 2005, *11*, 280-284.
[57] Dechsupa, S., Kothan, S., Vergote, J., Leger, G., Martineau, A., Berangeo, S., Kosanlavit, R., Moretti, J.L. and Mankhetkorn, S., Quercetin, Siamois 1 and Siamois 2 induce apoptosis in human breast cancer MDA-mB-435 cells xenograft in vivo, *Cancer Biol Ther.* 2007, *6*, 56-61.
[58] Aggarwal, B.B., Bhardwaj, A., Aggarwal, R.S., Seeram, N.P., Shishodia, S. and Takada, Y., Role of resveratrol in prevention and therapy of cancer: preclinical and clinical studies, *Anticancer Res.* 2004, *24*, 2783-2840.
[59] Brakenhielm, E., Cao, R. and Cao, Y., Suppression of angiogenesis, tumor growth, and wound healing by resveratrol, a natural compound in red wine and grapes, *Faseb J.* 2001, *15*, 1798-1800.
[60] Kim, J.D., Liu, L., Guo, W. and Meydani, M., Chemical structure of flavonols in relation to modulation of angiogenesis and immune-endothelial cell adhesion, *J Nutr Biochem.* 2006, *17*, 165-176.
[61] Luo, H., Jiang, B.H., King, S.M. and Chen, Y.C., Inhibition of cell growth and VEGF expression in ovarian cancer cells by flavonoids, *Nutr Cancer.* 2008, *60*, 800-809.
[62] Guo, Y., Wang, S., Hoot, D.R. and Clinton, S.K., Suppression of VEGF-mediated autocrine and paracrine interactions between prostate cancer cells and vascular endothelial cells by soy isoflavones, *J Nutr Biochem.* 2007, *18*, 408-417.
[63] Kim, M.H., Flavonoids inhibit VEGF/bFGF-induced angiogenesis in vitro by inhibiting the matrix-degrading proteases, *J Cell Biochem.* 2003, *89*, 529-538.
[64] Jiang, C., Agarwal, R. and Lu, J., Anti-angiogenic potential of a cancer chemopreventive flavonoid antioxidant, silymarin: inhibition of key attributes of vascular endothelial cells and angiogenic cytokine secretion by cancer epithelial cells, *Biochem Biophys Res Commun.* 2000, *276*, 371-378.
[65] Yang, S.H., Lin, J.K., Chen, W.S. and Chiu, J.H., Anti-angiogenic effect of silymarin on colon cancer LoVo cell line, *J Surg Res.* 2003, *113*, 133-138.
[66] Garvin, S., Ollinger, K. and Dabrosin, C., Resveratrol induces apoptosis and inhibits angiogenesis in human breast cancer xenografts in vivo, *Cancer Lett.* 2006, *231*, 113-122.
[67] Cao, Z., Fang, J., Xia, C., Shi, X. and Jiang, B.H., trans-3,4,5'-Trihydroxystibene inhibits hypoxia-inducible factor 1alpha and vascular endothelial growth factor expression in human ovarian cancer cells, *Clin Cancer Res.* 2004, *10*, 5253-5263.
[68] Sternlicht, M.D. and Werb, Z., How matrix metalloproteinases regulate cell behavior, *Annu Rev Cell Dev Biol.* 2001, *17*, 463-516.
[69] Sato, H., Takino, T., Okada, Y., Cao, J., Shinagawa, A., Yamamoto, E. and Seiki, M., A matrix metalloproteinase expressed on the surface of invasive tumour cells, *Nature.* 1994, *370*, 61-65.
[70] Sato, H. and Seiki, M., Regulatory mechanism of 92 kDa type IV collagenase gene expression which is associated with invasiveness of tumor cells, *Oncogene.* 1993, *8*, 395-405.

[71] Li, Y.T., Shen, F., Liu, B.H. and Cheng, G.F., Resveratrol inhibits matrix metalloproteinase-9 transcription in U937 cells, *Acta Pharmacol Sin*. 2003, *24*, 1167-1171.

[72] Woo, J.H., Lim, J.H., Kim, Y.H., Suh, S.I., Min do, S., Chang, J.S., Lee, Y.H., Park, J.W. and Kwon, T.K., Resveratrol inhibits phorbol myristate acetate-induced matrix metalloproteinase-9 expression by inhibiting JNK and PKC delta signal transduction, *Oncogene*. 2004, *23*, 1845-1853.

[73] Gunther, S., Ruhe, C., Derikito, M.G., Bose, G., Sauer, H. and Wartenberg, M., Polyphenols prevent cell shedding from mouse mammary cancer spheroids and inhibit cancer cell invasion in confrontation cultures derived from embryonic stem cells, *Cancer Lett*. 2006.

[74] Lee, S.O., Jeong, Y.J., Im, H.G., Kim, C.H., Chang, Y.C. and Lee, I.S., Silibinin suppresses PMA-induced MMP-9 expression by blocking the AP-1 activation via MAPK signaling pathways in MCF-7 human breast carcinoma cells, *Biochem Biophys Res Commun*. 2007, *354*, 165-171.

[75] Owen, J.L., Torroella-Kouri, M. and Iragavarapu-Charyulu, V., Molecular events involved in the increased expression of matrix metalloproteinase-9 by T lymphocytes of mammary tumor-bearing mice, *Int J Mol Med*. 2008, *21*, 125-134.

[76] Li, Y. and Sarkar, F.H., Down-regulation of invasion and angiogenesis-related genes identified by cDNA microarray analysis of PC3 prostate cancer cells treated with genistein, *Cancer Lett*. 2002, *186*, 157-164.

[77] Scalbert, A. and Williamson, G., Dietary intake and bioavailability of polyphenols, *J Nutr*. 2000, *130*, 2073S-2085S.

[78] Xu, X., Wang, H.J., Murphy, P.A., Cook, L. and Hendrich, S., Daidzein is a more bioavailable soymilk isoflavone than is genistein in adult women, *J Nutr*. 1994, *124*, 825-832.

[79] Hollman, P.C., van Trijp, J.M., Buysman, M.N., van der Gaag, M.S., Mengelers, M.J., de Vries, J.H. and Katan, M.B., Relative bioavailability of the antioxidant flavonoid quercetin from various foods in man, *FEBS Lett*. 1997, *418*, 152-156.

[80] Lee, M.J., Wang, Z.Y., Li, H., Chen, L., Sun, Y., Gobbo, S., Balentine, D.A. and Yang, C.S., Analysis of plasma and urinary tea polyphenols in human subjects, *Cancer Epidemiol Biomarkers Prev*. 1995, *4*, 393-399.

[81] Fuhr, U. and Kummert, A.L., The fate of naringin in humans: a key to grapefruit juice-drug interactions? *Clin Pharmacol Ther*. 1995, *58*, 365-373.

[82] Delmas, D., Lancon, A., Colin, D., Jannin, B. and Latruffe, N., Resveratrol as a chemopreventive agent: a promising molecule for fighting cancer, *Curr Drug Targets*. 2006, *7*, 423-442.

[83] [83] Niles, R.M., Cook, C.P., Meadows, G.G., Fu, Y.M., McLaughlin, J.L. and Rankin, G.O., Resveratrol is rapidly metabolized in athymic (nu/nu) mice and does not inhibit human melanoma xenograft tumor growth, *J Nutr*. 2006, *136*, 2542-2546.

[84] Sporn, M.B. and Suh, N., Chemoprevention: an essential approach to controlling cancer, *Nat Rev Cancer*. 2002, *2*, 537-543.

[85] Lambert, J.D., Lee, M.J., Lu, H., Meng, X., Hong, J.J., Seril, D.N., Sturgill, M.G. and Yang, C.S., Epigallocatechin-3-gallate is absorbed but extensively glucuronidated following oral administration to mice, *J Nutr*. 2003, *133*, 4172-4177.

[86] Lambert, J.D., Hong, J., Kim, D.H., Mishin, V.M. and Yang, C.S., Piperine enhances the bioavailability of the tea polyphenol (-)-epigallocatechin-3-gallate in mice, *J Nutr.* 2004, *134*, 1948-1952.

[87] Shoba, G., Joy, D., Joseph, T., Majeed, M., Rajendran, R. and Srinivas, P.S., Influence of piperine on the pharmacokinetics of curcumin in animals and human volunteers, *Planta Med.* 1998, *64*, 353-356.

[88] de Santi, C., Pietrabissa, A., Mosca, F. and Pacifici, G.M., Glucuronidation of resveratrol, a natural product present in grape and wine, in the human liver, *Xenobiotica.* 2000, *30*, 1047-1054.

[89] De Santi, C., Pietrabissa, A., Spisni, R., Mosca, F. and Pacifici, G.M., Sulphation of resveratrol, a natural compound present in wine, and its inhibition by natural flavonoids, *Xenobiotica.* 2000, *30*, 857-866.

[90] De Santi, C., Pietrabissa, A., Spisni, R., Mosca, F. and Pacifici, G.M., Sulphation of resveratrol, a natural product present in grapes and wine, in the human liver and duodenum, *Xenobiotica.* 2000, *30*, 609-617.

[91] Schlachterman, A., Valle, F., Wall, K.M., Azios, N.G., Castillo, L., Morell, L., Washington, A.V., Cubano, L.A. and Dharmawardhane, S.F., Combined resveratrol, quercetin, and catechin treatment reduces breast tumor growth in a nude mouse model, *Transl Oncol.* 2008, *1*, 19-27.

[92] Mertens-Talcott, S.U. and Percival, S.S., Ellagic acid and quercetin interact synergistically with resveratrol in the induction of apoptosis and cause transient cell cycle arrest in human leukemia cells, *Cancer Lett.* 2005, *218*, 141-151.

[93] Mertens-Talcott, S.U., Bomser, J.A., Romero, C., Talcott, S.T. and Percival, S.S., Ellagic acid potentiates the effect of quercetin on p21waf1/cip1, p53, and MAP-kinases without affecting intracellular generation of reactive oxygen species in vitro, *J Nutr.* 2005, *135*, 609-614.

[94] Somers-Edgar, T.J., Scandlyn, M.J., Stuart, E.C., Le Nedelec, M.J., Valentine, S.P. and Rosengren, R.J., The combination of epigallocatechin gallate and curcumin suppresses ER alpha-breast cancer cell growth in vitro and in vivo, *Int J Cancer.* 2008, *122*, 1966-1971.

[95] Pignatelli, P., Pulcinelli, F.M., Celestini, A., Lenti, L., Ghiselli, A., Gazzaniga, P.P. and Violi, F., The flavonoids quercetin and catechin synergistically inhibit platelet function by antagonizing the intracellular production of hydrogen peroxide, *Am J Clin Nutr.* 2000, *72*, 1150-1155.

[96] Ferrer, P., Asensi, M., Segarra, R., Ortega, A., Benlloch, M., Obrador, E., Varea, M.T., Asensio, G., Jorda, L. and Estrela, J.M., Association between pterostilbene and quercetin inhibits metastatic activity of B16 melanoma, *Neoplasia.* 2005, *7*, 37-47.

[97] Mertens-Talcott, S.U., Talcott, S.T. and Percival, S.S., Low concentrations of quercetin and ellagic acid synergistically influence proliferation, cytotoxicity and apoptosis in MOLT-4 human leukemia cells, *J Nutr.* 2003, *133*, 2669-2674.

[98] Yang, J.Y., Della-Fera, M.A., Rayalam, S., Ambati, S., Hartzell, D.L., Park, H.J. and Baile, C.A., Enhanced inhibition of adipogenesis and induction of apoptosis in 3T3-L1 adipocytes with combinations of resveratrol and quercetin, *Life Sci.* 2008, *82*, 1032-1039.

[99] Navarro-Peran, E., Cabezas-Herrera, J., Campo, L.S. and Rodriguez-Lopez, J.N., Effects of folate cycle disruption by the green tea polyphenol epigallocatechin-3-gallate, *Int J Biochem Cell Biol.* 2007, *39*, 2215-2225.

[100] Vaclavikova, R., Horsky, S., Simek, P. and Gut, I., Paclitaxel metabolism in rat and human liver microsomes is inhibited by phenolic antioxidants, *Naunyn Schmiedebergs Arch Pharmacol.* 2003, *368*, 200-209.

[101] Jazirehi, A.R. and Bonavida, B., Resveratrol modifies the expression of apoptotic regulatory proteins and sensitizes non-Hodgkin's lymphoma and multiple myeloma cell lines to paclitaxel-induced apoptosis, *Mol Cancer Ther.* 2004, *3*, 71-84.

[102] Duraj, J., Bodo, J., Sulikova, M., Rauko, P. and Sedlak, J., Diverse resveratrol sensitization to apoptosis induced by anticancer drugs in sensitive and resistant leukemia cells, *Neoplasma.* 2006, *53*, 384-392.

[103] Kubota, T., Uemura, Y., Kobayashi, M. and Taguchi, H., Combined effects of resveratrol and paclitaxel on lung cancer cells, *Anticancer Res.* 2003, *23*, 4039-4046.

[104] Sun, Z.J., Pan, C.E., Liu, H.S. and Wang, G.J., Anti-hepatoma activity of resveratrol in vitro, *World J Gastroenterol.* 2002, *8*, 79-81.

[105] Fuggetta, M.P., D'Atri, S., Lanzilli, G., Tricarico, M., Cannavo, E., Zambruno, G., Falchetti, R. and Ravagnan, G., In vitro antitumour activity of resveratrol in human melanoma cells sensitive or resistant to temozolomide, *Melanoma Res.* 2004, *14*, 189-196.

[106] Fulda, S. and Debatin, K.M., Sensitization for tumor necrosis factor-related apoptosis-inducing ligand-induced apoptosis by the chemopreventive agent resveratrol, *Cancer Res.* 2004, *64*, 337-346.

[107] Russo, M., Nigro, P., Rosiello, R., D'Arienzo, R. and Russo, G.L., Quercetin enhances CD95- and TRAIL-induced apoptosis in leukemia cell lines, *Leukemia.* 2007, *21*, 1130-1133.

[108] Psahoulia, F.H., Drosopoulos, K.G., Doubravska, L., Andera, L. and Pintzas, A., Quercetin enhances TRAIL-mediated apoptosis in colon cancer cells by inducing the accumulation of death receptors in lipid rafts, *Mol Cancer Ther.* 2007, *6*, 2591-2599.

[109] Yoshida, T., Konishi, M., Horinaka, M., Yasuda, T., Goda, A.E., Taniguchi, H., Yano, K., Wakada, M. and Sakai, T., Kaempferol sensitizes colon cancer cells to TRAIL-induced apoptosis, *Biochem Biophys Res Commun.* 2008, *375*, 129-133.

[110] Son, Y.G., Kim, E.H., Kim, J.Y., Kim, S.U., Kwon, T.K., Yoon, A.R., Yun, C.O. and Choi, K.S., Silibinin sensitizes human glioma cells to TRAIL-mediated apoptosis via DR5 up-regulation and down-regulation of c-FLIP and survivin, *Cancer Res.* 2007, *67*, 8274-8284.

[111] Jin, C.Y., Park, C., Cheong, J., Choi, B.T., Lee, T.H., Lee, J.D., Lee, W.H., Kim, G.Y., Ryu, C.H. and Choi, Y.H., Genistein sensitizes TRAIL-resistant human gastric adenocarcinoma AGS cells through activation of caspase-3, *Cancer Lett.* 2007, *257*, 56-64.

[112] Delmas, D., Rebe, C., Micheau, O., Athias, A., Gambert, P., Grazide, S., Laurent, G., Latruffe, N. and Solary, E., Redistribution of CD95, DR4 and DR5 in rafts accounts for the synergistic toxicity of resveratrol and death receptor ligands in colon carcinoma cells, *Oncogene.* 2004, *23*, 8979-8986.

[113] Gill, C., Walsh, S.E., Morrissey, C., Fitzpatrick, J.M. and Watson, R.W., Resveratrol sensitizes androgen independent prostate cancer cells to death-receptor mediated apoptosis through multiple mechanisms, *Prostate*. 2007, *67*, 1641-1653.
[114] Horinaka, M., Yoshida, T., Shiraishi, T., Nakata, S., Wakada, M. and Sakai, T., The dietary flavonoid apigenin sensitizes malignant tumor cells to tumor necrosis factor-related apoptosis-inducing ligand, *Mol Cancer Ther*. 2006, *5*, 945-951.
[115] Lambert, J.D., Sang, S., Hong, J., Kwon, S.J., Lee, M.J., Ho, C.T. and Yang, C.S., Peracetylation as a means of enhancing in vitro bioactivity and bioavailability of epigallocatechin-3-gallate, *Drug Metab Dispos*. 2006, *34*, 2111-2116.
[116] Fragopoulou, E., Nomikos, T., Karantonis, H.C., Apostolakis, C., Pliakis, E., Samiotaki, M., Panayotou, G. and Antonopoulou, S., Biological activity of acetylated phenolic compounds, *J Agric Food Chem*. 2007, *55*, 80-89.
[117] Marel, A.K., Lizard, G., Izard, J.C., Latruffe, N. and Delmas, D., Inhibitory effects of trans-resveratrol analogs molecules on the proliferation and the cell cycle progression of human colon tumoral cells, *Mol Nutr Food Res*. 2008, *52*, 538-548.
[118] Riva, S., Monti, D., Luisetti, M. and Danieli, B., Enzymatic modification of natural compounds with pharmacological properties, *Ann N Y Acad Sci*. 1998, *864*, 70-80.
[119] Hua, J., Sheng, Y., Bryngelsson, C., Kane, R. and Pero, R.W., Comparison of antitumor activity of declopramide (3-chloroprocainamide) and N-acetyl-declopramide, *Anticancer Res*. 1999, *19*, 285-290.
[120] Cardile, V., Lombardo, L., Spatafora, C. and Tringali, C., Chemo-enzymatic synthesis and cell-growth inhibition activity of resveratrol analogues, *Bioorg Chem*. 2005, *33*, 22-33.
[121] Pettit, G.R., Grealish, M.P., Jung, M.K., Hamel, E., Pettit, R.K., Chapuis, J.C. and Schmidt, J.M., Antineoplastic agents. 465. Structural modification of resveratrol: sodium resverastatin phosphate, *J Med Chem*. 2002, *45*, 2534-2542.
[122] Heynekamp, J.J., Weber, W.M., Hunsaker, L.A., Gonzales, A.M., Orlando, R.A., Deck, L.M. and Jagt, D.L., Substituted trans-stilbenes, including analogues of the natural product resveratrol, inhibit the human tumor necrosis factor alpha-induced activation of transcription factor nuclear factor KappaB, *J Med Chem*. 2006, *49*, 7182-7189.
[123] Saiko, P., Pemberger, M., Horvath, Z., Savinc, I., Grusch, M., Handler, N., Erker, T., Jaeger, W., Fritzer-Szekeres, M. and Szekeres, T., Novel resveratrol analogs induce apoptosis and cause cell cycle arrest in HT29 human colon cancer cells: inhibition of ribonucleotide reductase activity, *Oncol Rep*. 2008, *19*, 1621-1626.
[124] Ovesna, Z., Kozics, K., Bader, Y., Saiko, P., Handler, N., Erker, T. and Szekeres, T., Antioxidant activity of resveratrol, piceatannol and 3,3',4,4',5,5'-hexahydroxy-trans-stilbene in three leukemia cell lines, *Oncol Rep*. 2006, *16*, 617-624.
[125] de Lima, D.P., Rotta, R., Beatriz, A., Marques, M.R., Montenegro, R.C., Vasconcellos, M.C., Pessoa, C., de Moraes, M.O., Costa-Lotufo, L.V., Frankland Sawaya, A.C. and Eberlin, M.N., Synthesis and biological evaluation of cytotoxic properties of stilbene-based resveratrol analogs, *Eur J Med Chem*. 2008.
[126] Schneider, Y., Fischer, B., Coelho, D., Roussi, S., Gosse, F., Bischoff, P. and Raul, F., (Z)-3,5,4'-Tri-O-methyl-resveratrol, induces apoptosis in human lymphoblastoid cells independently of their p53 status, *Cancer Lett*. 2004, *211*, 155-161.

[127] Seiler, N., Schneider, Y., Gosse, F., Schleiffer, R. and Raul, F., Polyploidisation of metastatic colon carcinoma cells by microtubule and tubulin interacting drugs: effect on proteolytic activity and invasiveness, *Int J Oncol.* 2004, *25*, 1039-1048.
[128] Mansilla, S., Bataller, M. and Portugal, J., Mitotic catastrophe as a consequence of chemotherapy, *Anticancer Agents Med Chem.* 2006, *6*, 589-602.
[129] Bernhard, D., Schwaiger, W., Crazzolara, R., Tinhofer, I., Kofler, R. and Csordas, A., Enhanced MTT-reducing activity under growth inhibition by resveratrol in CEM-C7H2 lymphocytic leukemia cells, *Cancer Lett.* 2003, *195*, 193-199.
[130] Pagliacci, M.C., Spinozzi, F., Migliorati, G., Fumi, G., Smacchia, M., Grignani, F., Riccardi, C. and Nicoletti, I., Genistein inhibits tumour cell growth in vitro but enhances mitochondrial reduction of tetrazolium salts: a further pitfall in the use of the MTT assay for evaluating cell growth and survival, *Eur J Cancer.* 1993, *29A*, 1573-1577.
[131] Ulrich, S., Loitsch, S.M., Rau, O., von Knethen, A., Brune, B., Schubert-Zsilavecz, M. and Stein, J.M., Peroxisome Proliferator-Activated Receptor {gamma} as a Molecular Target of Resveratrol-Induced Modulation of Polyamine Metabolism, *Cancer Res.* 2006, *66*, 7348-7354.
[132] Lu, J., Ho, C.H., Ghai, G. and Chen, K.Y., Resveratrol analog, 3,4,5,4'-tetrahydroxystilbene, differentially induces pro-apoptotic p53/Bax gene expression and inhibits the growth of transformed cells but not their normal counterparts, *Carcinogenesis.* 2001, *22*, 321-328.
[133] Clement, M.V., Hirpara, J.L., Chawdhury, S.H. and Pervaiz, S., Chemopreventive agent resveratrol, a natural product derived from grapes, triggers CD95 signaling-dependent apoptosis in human tumor cells, *Blood.* 1998, 92, 996-1002.

In: Flavonoids: Biosynthesis, Biological Effects…
Editor: Raymond B. Keller
ISBN: 978-1-60741-622-7

Chapter 6

EFFECT OF A DIET RICH IN COCOA FLAVONOIDS ON EXPERIMENTAL ACUTE INFLAMMATION

***M. Castell*[*,1,4]*, A. Franch*[1,2,4]*, S. Ramos-Romero*[1]*, E. Ramiro-Puig*[3]*, F. J. Pérez-Cano*[1,4] *and C. Castellote*[1,2,4]**

[1]Department of Physiology, Faculty of Pharmacy, University of Barcelona, Barcelona, Spain

[2]CIBER *Epidemiología y Salud Pública*, Barcelona, Spain

[3]INSERM U793, Faculté Necker-Enfants Malades, Paris, France

[4]Members of *Institut de Recerca en Nutrició i Seguretat Alimentària* (INSA, University of Barcelona)

ABSTRACT

Cocoa has recently become an object of interest due to its high content of flavonoids, mainly the monomers epicatechin and catechin and various polymers derived from these monomers called procyanidins. Previous *in vitro* studies have shown the ability of cocoa flavonoids to down-regulate inflammatory mediators produced by stimulated macrophages, but there are no studies that consider the effects of *in vivo* cocoa intake on inflammatory response. In the present article, we report the *in vivo* cocoa inhibitory effect on the acute inflammatory response. Female Wistar rats received Natural Forastero cocoa containing 21.2 mg flavonoids/g for 7 days (2.4 or 4.8 g per rat kg, p.o.). Then, acute inflammation was induced by means of carrageenin, histamine, serotonin, bradykinin or PGE_2 hind-paw injection. Rats fed 4.8 g/kg/day cocoa showed a significant reduction in the hind-paw edema induced by carrageenin from the first hour after induction ($P<0.05$). However, cocoa intake did not modify the edema induced by histamine, serotonin or PGE_2. Only a certain protective effect was observed at the lowest dose of cocoa in the bradykinin model. Moreover, peritoneal macrophages from rats that received 4.8 g/kg/day cocoa for 7 days showed a reduced ability to produce radical oxygen species (ROS), nitric oxide (NO), tumor necrosis factor α (TNFα) and interleukin 6 (IL-6). This fact could justify, at least partially, the beneficial effect of cocoa on carrageenin-induced inflammation. In summary, a diet rich in cocoa flavonoids was able to down-regulate the acute inflammatory response by decreasing the inflammatory potential of macrophages.

---

* E-mail: margaridacastell@ub.edu

1. INTRODUCTION

One of the foods with a relatively high content of flavonoids is cocoa, which is obtained from the beans of the *Theobroma cacao* tree (Lee, 2003). The beneficial effects of cocoa were known as early as 600 BC: the Mayans and Aztecs roasted and ground cocoa beans to prepare a divine beverage called *xocolatl*, which was mainly used to cure fatigue, fever, infections, and heart pain (Hurst et al., 2002). Although most people presently see cocoa and its derivatives only as snacks, scientific evidence of the health benefits of cocoa known by the ancients is emerging now.

In addition to being a rich source of fiber (26–40%), proteins (15–20%), carbohydrates (~15%), and lipids (10–24%), cocoa powder contains minerals, vitamins (A, E, B and folic acid) and a high amount of flavonoids. However, cocoa flavonoid content is difficult to establish because it depends on geographic origin, climate, storage methods and manufacturing processes (Manach et al., 2004; McShea et al., 2008). Cocoa powder mainly contains the flavanols (-)-epicatechin, (+)-catechin and polymers derived from these monomers called procyanidins; it is reported to contain up to 70 mg/g of polyphenols (Vinson et al., 1999). Epicatechin and catechin are biologically active, but epicatechin is more efficiently absorbed than catechin (Baba et al., 2001). Procyanidins are the major flavonoids in cocoa and chocolate products ranging from 2.16 to 48.70 mg/g (Gu et al., 2006). Short procyanidins (dimers and trimers) are absorbed in the small intestine and rapidly detected in plasma (Baba et al., 2000). However, large procyanidins are less efficiently absorbed in its polymeric form, but can be metabolized by colon microflora to phenolic acids and then absorbed (Manach et al., 2004). Quercetin and its derivatives, naringenin, luteolin and apigenin, are also present in smaller quantities (Sanchez-Rabaneda et al., 2003).

Experimental and clinical data suggest that the consumption of cocoa flavonoids can produce positive clinical benefits in the cardiovascular system (review by Buijsse et al., 2006 and Cooper et al., 2008) and also in brain function (reviewed by McShea et al., 2008). Cocoa intake reduces the risk of cardiovascular disease by modulating blood pressure (Grassi et al., 2005; Taubert et al., 2007) as well as decreasing blood cholesterol (Baba et al., 2007), moreover it produces vasodilatation and inhibits platelet activation and aggregation (Hermann et al., 2006). *In vitro* assays and studies in animal models suggest that cocoa has beneficial effects on neurodegenerative disorders such as Alzheimer's disease and Parkinson's disease (Datla et al., 2007; Ramiro-Puig et al., 2009a). However, it remains to establish doses and length of treatment because a recent trial in healthy adults does not find neuropsychological effects after a short-term dark chocolate intake (Crews et al., 2008). Biological effects of cocoa are mainly attributed to the high content of antioxidant polyphenols (reviewed in Ramiro-Puig et al., 2009b). Cocoa has a potent antioxidant capacity compared to products traditionally considered high in antioxidants (Lee et al., 2003; Vinson et al., 2006). Flavonoids act as antioxidants by directly neutralizing free radicals, chelating Fe^{2+} and Cu^{+} which enhance highly aggressive ROS, inhibiting xanthine oxidase that is responsible for ROS production, and up-regulating or protecting antioxidant defense (Cotelle, 2001). Epicatechin and catechin are very effective in neutralizing several types of free radicals (Hatano et al., 2002; Yilmaz et al., 2004). Procyanidins account for the highest percentage of antioxidants in cocoa products (Gu et al., 2006) and they also scavenge radicals with an activity that is proportional to the number of monomeric units they contain (Counet et al.,

2003). In addition, quercetin and other compounds such as methylxanthines contribute to cocoa's antioxidant activity (Lamuela-Raventos at al., 2001; Azam et al., 2003). The antioxidant properties of flavonoids in cocoa lead us to consider it as a potential beneficial ingredient able to down-regulate the inflammatory response. *In vitro* studies showed that cocoa flavonoids modulate cytokines and eicosanoids produced during inflammation (Mao et al., 2000; Schramm et al., 2001). In response to inflammatory stimulus, macrophages produce nitric oxide (NO) and cytokines, mainly tumor necrosis factor-α (TNFα) and interleukin (IL-) 1, IL-6, and IL-12, and chemokines, such as monocyte chemoattractant protein 1 (MCP-1) (reviewed by Medzhitov, 2008). *In vitro* studies have demonstrated the regulatory effects of cocoa on secretion of inflammatory mediators (reviewed by Ramiro-Puig et al., 2009b). Flavonoid-rich cocoa extract added to LPS-stimulated macrophages decreases secretion of TNFα, MCP-1, and NO (Ono et al., 2003; Ramiro et al., 2005). However, other studies with purified cocoa flavonoid fractions show an enhanced secretion of TNFα, IL-1, IL-6 and IL-10 from stimulated human peripheral blood mononuclear cells (Kenny et al., 2007). Although these *in vitro* studies concerning the anti-inflammatory ability of cocoa flavonoids, alone or in the whole product, few studies focus on the *in vivo* effect. It has been described that supplementation with cocoa products in humans did not affect markers of inflammation (Mathur et al., 2002); however, a recent cross-sectional analysis shows that the regular intake of dark chocolate by a healthy population from southern Italy is inversely related to serum C-reactive protein concentration (di Giuseppe et al., 2008).

The aim of this study was, firstly, to ascertain the potential anti-inflammatory activity induced by cocoa intake and, secondly, to test this potential on several rat models of acute inflammation. The first goal was developed in peritoneal macrophages obtained from rats that had received daily cocoa for a week, and was focused on the production of oxidants (ROS and NO) and cytokines (TNFα and IL-6). Secondly, in rats with the same cocoa diet, the development of acute inflammation was determined after induction with carrageenin, histamine, serotonin, bradykinin and prostaglandin E_2 (PGE_2).

2. Material and Methods

2.1. Animals

Eight-week-old female Wistar rats were obtained from Harlan (Barcelona, Spain). Rats were housed 3 per cage in controlled conditions of temperature and humidity in a 12:12 light:dark cycle. Rats had free access to food (chow ref. 2014, Harlan Teklad, Madison, WI, USA) and water. Animals were randomly distributed in 3-4 experimental groups in each experimental design (n = 8-10/group). Two of them were daily administered, by oral gavage, with cocoa in mineral water at doses of 2.4 g/kg/day and 4.8 g/kg/day for 7 days. We used Natural Forastero cocoa (Nutrexpa, Barcelona, Spain) containing 21.2 mg of total phenols/g according to the Folin-Ciocalteu method (Singleton et al., 1999). The remaining animals received the same volume of vehicle (mineral water). Handling was done in the same time range to avoid the influence of biological rhythms. At the end of the study rats were sacrificed by CO_2 inhalation. Studies were performed in accordance with the institutional guidelines for the care and use of laboratory animals established by the Ethical Committee for Animal Experimentation at the University of Barcelona and approved by the Catalonian Government.

2.2. Isolation of Peritoneal Macrophages

After 7 days of cocoa or vehicle administration p.o., rats were anaesthetized with ketamine/xylacine (i.m., 90 mg/kg and 10 mg/kg, respectively) to obtain peritoneal macrophages. 40 mL ice-cold sterile phosphate buffer solution (PBS) pH 7.2 was injected to peritoneal cavity. Abdominal massages were immediately performed to induce cell migration. Cell suspension was aspirated, centrifuged (170 *g*, 5 min, 4 °C) and resuspended in cold DMEM+GlutaMAX media (Invitrogen, Paisley, UK) containing 10% fetal bovine serum (PAA, Pashing, Austria), 100 IU/mL streptomycin-penicillin (Sigma-Aldrich, St Louis, MO, USA) (DMEM-FBS). Cell count and viability was determined by double staining with acridine orange and ethidium bromide (Sigma) followed by fluorescence light microscopical analysis. Cells were plated and cultured in different conditions according to the assay.

2.3. ROS Production by DCF Assay

To determine the effects of cocoa on ROS production, peritoneal macrophages (25×10^3 cells/100 µL in DMEM-FBS) were plated in 96 well black plates (Corning Inc, NY, USA) and allowed to attach overnight (37 °C, 5% CO_2). Macrophages were washed once with warm RPMI-1640 medium without phenol red (Sigma) containing 100 IU/mL streptomycin-penicillin and incubated with 20 µmol/L of reduced 2',7'-dichlorofluorescein diacetate (H_2DCF-DA, Invitrogen) probe for 30 min at 37 °C. H_2DCF-DA diffuses through the cell membrane and is enzymatically hydrolyzed by intracellular esterases to form non-fluorescent 2',7'-dichlorofluorescein (H_2DCF) which is oxidized by ROS to a fluorescent compound (DCF). Thus, DCF fluorescence intensity is proportional to intracellular ROS production. Fluorescence was measured every 30 min by fluorometry (excitation 538 nm, emission 485 nm) up to 3.5 h. For each animal, background from corresponding wells without fluorescent probe was subtracted.

2.4. Cytokine and NO Production

Immediately after isolation, macrophages were plated in 12-well flat-bottom plate (TPP, Trasadingen, Switzerland) at 1.2×10^6/mL in DMEM-FBS (37 °C, 5% CO_2) overnight to allow macrophage adhesion. Non-adherent cells were removed by washing three times with warm sterile PBS. The attached macrophages were stimulated by addition of 1 µg/mL lypopolysaccharide (LPS) from *E.coli* O55:B5 (Sigma). Supernatants were collected for quantification of TNFα after 6 h and IL-6 and NO after 24 h. Supernatants were stored at -80 °C until evaluation. Cells were harvested to determine cell viability. The concentration of TNFα and IL-6 in supernatants was quantified using rat ELISA sets from BD Pharmingen (Erembodegen, Belgium), following the manufacturer's instructions.

Stable end product of NO, NO_2^-, was quantified by a modification of Griess reaction. Briefly, macrophage supernatants (100 µL) were mixed with 60 µL sulphanilamide 1% (in 1.2 N HCl) and 60 µL N-(1-naphthyl)ethylene-diamine dihydrochloride 0.3% (in distilled water) for 10 min at room temperature. Absorbance was read spectrophotometrically at 540 nm. The concentration of NO_2^- was calculated using known concentration of $NaNO_2$.

2.5. Induction of Acute Inflammation in Rat Hind Paws

Five rat models of acute inflammation were induced by subplantar injection of carrageenin λ, histamine, serotonin, bradykinin or PGE_2, all from Sigma-Aldrich. After 7 days of cocoa or vehicle administration p.o., animals were injected with 0.1 mL carrageenin λ (10 mg/mL), histamine (5 mg/mL), serotonin (5 mg/mL), bradykinin (0.08 mg/mL) or PGE_2 (0.01 mg/mL), in saline solution. The left hind paw was injected with the same volume of saline solution. A reference treatment group was constituted by animals administered with vehicle during 7 days that received one dose of indomethacin (p.o., 10 mg/kg, Sigma in 0.1% CMC-Tween 20) 1 h prior to the induction of inflammation.

2.6. Inflammation Assessment

Paw volume was measured by using a water plethysmometer (UGO Basile, Comerlo, VA, Italy). Left and right hind paws were measured just before the induction (time 0). After carrageenin injection, paw volumes were quantified at 30 min and every hour until 6 h. In the other 4 experimental models, the measurements were performed each 15 min during the first hour, and each 30 min up to 2 h. All determinations were performed in a blinded manner. Paw volumes were expressed as percentage of increase with respect to time 0. Area under curve (AUC) was calculated between time 0 and the end of the inflammatory period evaluation.

2.7. Statistics

The software package SPSS 16.0 (SPSS Inc., Chicago, IL, USA) was used for statistical analysis. Conventional one-way ANOVA was performed, considering the experimental group as independent variable. When treatment had a significant effect on dependent variable, Scheffe's test was applied. Significant differences were accepted when $P<0.05$.

3. RESULTS

3.1. Peritoneal Macrophages Viability

Peritoneal macrophages were obtained from rats after cocoa intake (2.4 or 4.8 g/kg/day) or vehicle for 7 days. Cells were 98% viable when isolated. After overnight culture and washing, some cells were LPS-stimulated and 6 h later, they showed a viability of about 40%

whereas non-stimulated cultures were ~50% viable. However, 24 h after LPS stimulation, macrophage viability reached ~70% and 75% in LPS-stimulated and non-stimulated macrophages, respectively. There were no differences among cells obtained from both cocoa-administered rats and those from reference animals.

3.2. ROS and NO Production by Peritoneal Macrophages

ROS production from peritoneal macrophages increased progressively along the 3.5 h assay (Figure 1A). Cells obtained from 2.4 g/kg cocoa animals produced the same ROS levels as reference macrophages. Macrophages isolated from animals that received 4.8 g/kg/day of cocoa synthesized lower ROS than reference cells already at 0.5 h and all along the studied period. Differences between both groups were higher as later measurements were made but they did not reach statistically significant results because of the high variability.

NO production was detected in macrophage culture medium after 24 h of LPS-stimulation or in resting conditions (Figure 1B).

Macrophages obtained from rats that received 2.4 g/kg/day of cocoa showed NO levels similar to those from reference group, both in LPS-stimulation and in resting conditions. Nevertheless, NO secretion by macrophages isolated from animals with an intake of 4.8 g/kg/day of cocoa was lower than that quantified in the reference group in any culture condition (P<0.05, Figure 1B).

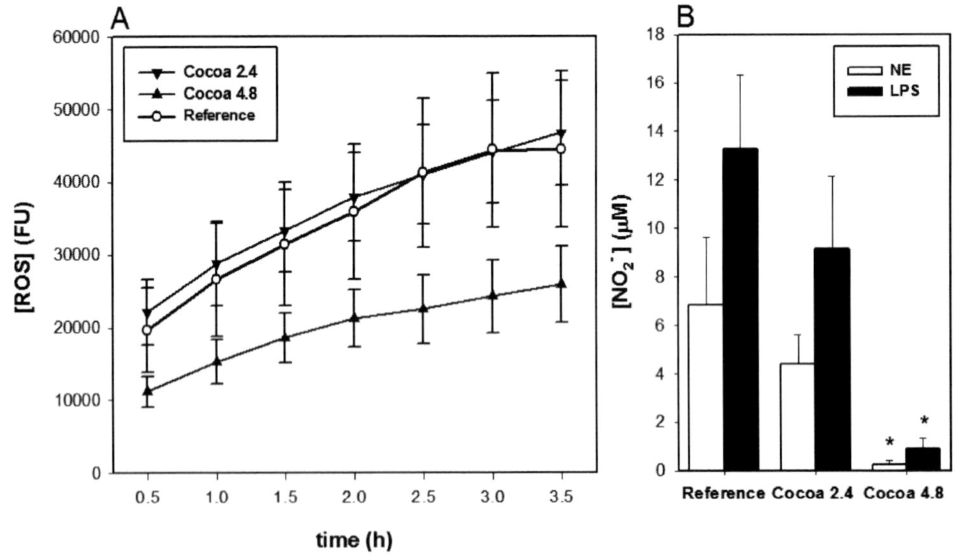

Figure 1. ROS and NO production by peritoneal macrophages. Time-course of ROS production from peritoneal macrophages (A) was determined by means of DCF assay. NO cell production, quantified as NO_2^- concentration (B), was measured by modified Griess assay in LPS-stimulated and resting macrophages. Values are summarized as mean ± SEM (n = 8-9). * P<0.05 compared with reference group.

3.3. TNFα and IL-6 Secretion from Peritoneal Macrophages

TNFα secretion was quantified in LPS-stimulated and resting macrophages. Macrophages from animals administered with 4.8 g/kg/day of cocoa produced lower TNFα levels than those of reference cells (P<0.05, Figure 2A). The reduction of TNFα levels was about 75% and 82% in both non-stimulated and LPS-stimulated conditions, respectively. Conversely, macrophages from animals that received 2.4 g/kg/day of cocoa did not modify the secretion of this cytokine.

In addition, 4.8 g/kg/day of cocoa intake diminished the IL-6 secretion by non-stimulated and LPS-stimulated macrophages (P<0.01, Figure 2B). In this case, the IL-6 inhibition got up to 94% in non-stimulated macrophages and to 88% in LPS-stimulated ones with respect to reference cells. No significant differences in IL-6 levels were found in macrophage cultures from animals administered with 2.4 g/kg cocoa.

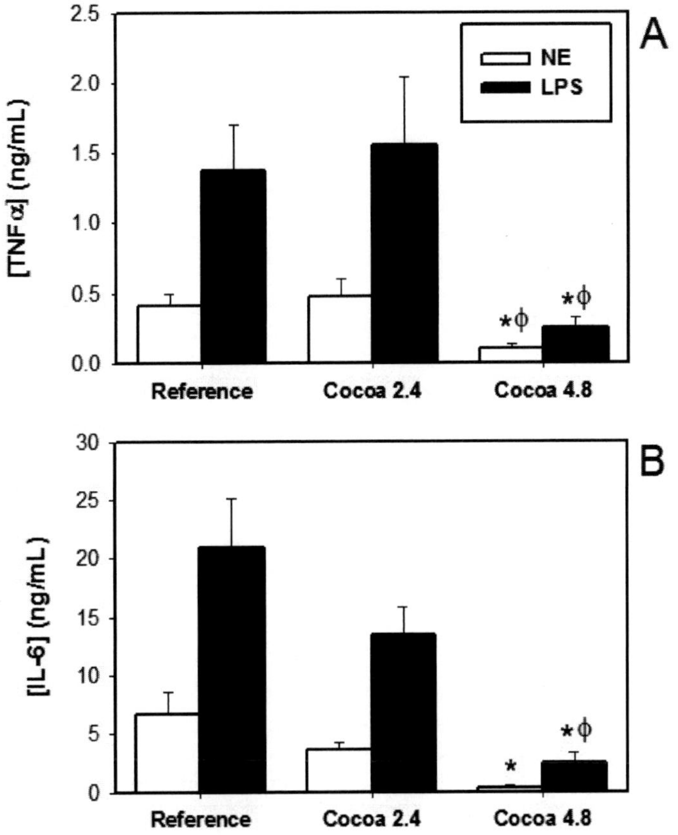

Figure 2. TNFα and IL-6 secretion from peritoneal macrophages. TNFα (A) and IL-6 (B) concentration (ng/mL) in cell culture supernatants was determined by means of ELISA assay. Values are summarized as mean ± SEM (n = 8-9). * P<0.05 compared with reference group. ϕ P<0.05 compared with 2.4 g/kg cocoa group.

3.4. Paw Edema Induced by Carrageenin

The time-course of hind-paw volume increase after carrageenin injection is summarized in Figure 3A. Paw edema was detected in the reference group from 30 min after carrageenin injection. Thereafter, it rose reaching a maximum increase of ~80% with respect to time 0 at 5-6 h post-injection. Indomethacin showed its anti-inflammatory effect from 1 h post-induction ($P<0.05$) and during all the study ($P<0.01$). Animals from 2.4 g/kg cocoa group displayed a lower paw volume increase than reference group during the first hour ($P<0.05$); thereafter, however, their paw edema fit the reference pattern. Animals that had taken 4.8 g/kg/day of cocoa showed a significant paw edema improvement which was already detected 2 h after carrageenin injection ($P<0.05$), and remained until the end of the study ($P<0.05$). At this time, the inflammation developed in the 4.8 g/kg cocoa group was the 68% of that of the reference group.

AUC from paw edema time-course was calculated between 0 and 6 h post-induction (Figure 3B). AUC from 4.8 g/kg cocoa animals was 30% lower than that in reference group ($P<0.001$), whereas, indomethacin inhibition was of about 44% ($P<0.001$).

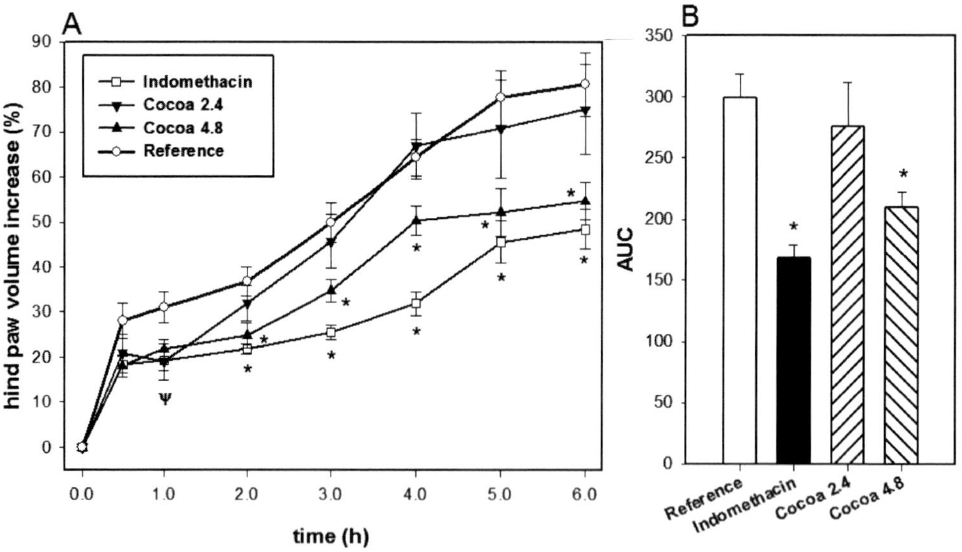

Figure 3. Time-course of carrageenin-induced paw edema. Percentage of hind-paw volume increase respect to time 0 (A) along 6 h from carrageenin-injection. Area under the curve (B) determined between time 0 and 6 h post-induction. Values are summarized as mean ± SEM (n = 8-10). * $P<0.05$ compared with reference group. ψ $P<0.05$ all treated groups compared with reference group.

3.5. Acute Paw Edema Induced by Inflammatory Mediators

Time-course of acute inflammation induced by histamine, serotonin, bradykinin and PGE_2 are showed in Figure 4. Paw edema induced by histamine (Figure 4A) or bradykinin (Figure 4C) was maximum at 0.5 h after injection, rising up to 40%. Paw edema induced by serotonin (Figure 4B) reached increase of 55% at 2 h of induction and hind-paw volumes increased until 30% for animals injected with PGE_2 solution (Figure 4D).

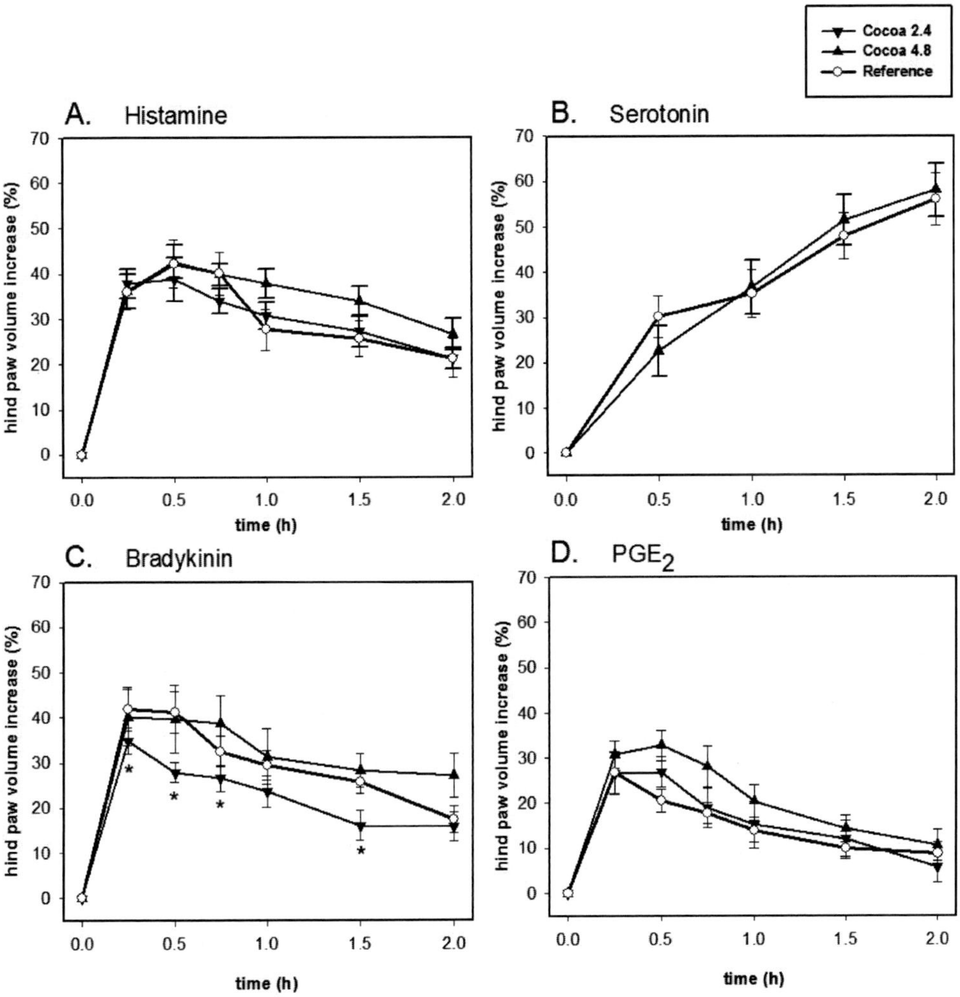

Figure 4. Time-course of paw edema in acute inflammatory models. Time-course of histamine- (A), serotonin- (B), bradykinin- (C), and PGE_2-induced acute inflammation (D) in the studied groups. Values are summarized as mean ± SEM (n = 8-10). * $P<0.05$ compared with reference group.

Cocoa-enriched diet did not protect from the development of histamine-, serotonin- and PGE_2-induced paw edema. Nevertheless, a significant reduction of paw volume increase was detected in 2.4 g/kg cocoa group in the bradykinin model. These animals showed lower inflammation at 15 min post-injection ($P<0.05$) and during all studied period ($P<0.01$). Daily intake of 2.4 g/kg cocoa reduced up to 28% the AUC of hind paw volume evolution ($P<0.05$, data not shown). Indomethacin did not show anti-inflammatory effects in these models of acute inflammation (data not shown).

Discussion

This study shows the *in vivo* anti-inflammatory power of a high cocoa intake for a week. Although several studies demonstrate the regulatory effect of cocoa flavonoids *in vitro* on cells under inflammatory stimulus (Mao et al., 2000; Ono et al., 2003; Ramiro et al., 2005), there are few evidences of the effect of cocoa on inflammatory response in physiological conditions. Here we show two *in vivo* evidences that allow suggesting the inflammation inhibition by a cocoa diet.

The first part of this study shows that a high cocoa intake for a week reduces the inflammatory potential of macrophages. During an inflammatory response, macrophages are crucial cells participating in the secretion of mediators that eventually induce vasodilatation, vascular permeability increase and leukocyte migration (Medzhitov, 2008). Moreover, macrophages produce a battery of reactive oxygen, nitrogen and halogen species which are proposed to cause damage to surrounding tissues (Son et al., 2008). In the present study, macrophages from animals that had taken a high dose of cocoa produced lower levels of reactive nitrogen species and also had a tendency to synthesize lower reactive oxygen species. These results agree with *in vitro* studies showing that cells from different origins treated with cocoa fractions or flavonoids alone decrease the production of ROS in a dose-dependent manner (Sanbongi et al., 1997, Erlejman et al., 2006; Granado-Serrano et al., 2007; Ramiro-Puig et al., 2009a). Moreover, cocoa fractions are reported to reduce the levels of NO when produced in inflammatory conditions (Ono et al., 2003; Lyu et al., 2005; Ramiro et al., 2005). These results seem to be contradictory with the effects of cocoa flavonoids in vascular tissue where they are reported to promote NO bioactivity and then to cause vasodilatation and decrease blood pressure (Sies et al., 2005; Taubert et al., 2007). These opposite effects seem to be related to the enzyme isoform involved in NO synthesis: eNOS in the endothelial region, or iNOS after an aggressive stimulus (Karim et al., 2000; Ono et al., 2003). Therefore, cocoa compounds would have contrary effects depending on these enzyme isoforms.

In a similar way, macrophages isolated from animals that had taken a high dose of cocoa for a week showed a lower ability to secrete two essential cytokines in the inflammatory process, TNFα and IL-6. These results agree with those previously obtained after adding a cocoa extract on a macrophage cell line (Ramiro et al., 2005), although there are controversial results when cocoa flavonoid fractions were used on blood mononuclear cells (Mao et al., 2000; Kenny et al., 2007). In any case, an important difference between these *in vitro* studies and those showed here consists in the compounds that achieve cells. In a more physiological approach, the present study suggests that metabolites derived from cocoa absorbed fractions have anti-inflammatory properties. How macrophages down-regulate their inflammatory response in the presence of cocoa metabolites remains to be established. However, some *in vitro* studies show that flavonoids such as epicatechin, catechin, dimeric procyanidins and quercetin can modify the NF-κB pathway (Mackenzie et al., 2004; Comalada et al., 2005) involved in the production of inflammatory products. Therefore, it can be suggested that the cocoa absorbed fraction, flavonoids or even other compounds, can also interact with this transduction pathway.

After demonstrating the effect of cocoa in reducing some inflammatory mediators *ex vivo*, the second part of this study was focused on ascertaining whether a cocoa enriched diet was able to directly modulate a local inflammation *in vivo*. Specifically, we examined the effect of cocoa on the local inflammatory response induced by carrageenin in the rat hind paw (Winter et al., 1962). This model is widely applied for the screening of anti-inflammatory drugs which provokes a progressive local edema during 4–6 h, that remains even up to 24 h. Carrageenin-induced edema is accompanied with prostanoids and pro-inflammatory cytokines increase in paw tissues, mainly consisting in an early increase of TNFα followed by elevations in IL-1β and IL-6 (Guay et al., 2004; Rocha et al., 2006; Loram et al., 2007). As shown here, rats that received cocoa for a week developed a lower carrageenin-induced paw edema than reference animals. This regulatory effect was seen at the first hour of induction by both cocoa doses (2.4 and 4.8 g/kg/day) and, in those animals with the high cocoa dose, remained until the end of the study. These results confirm preliminary studies using a higher dose (Ramos-Romero et al., 2008). Although the cocoa compounds responsible for this effect remain to be established, flavonoids are good candidates because two s.c. or i.v. injections of catechin and epicatechin produced a significant reduction of paw edema in the carrageenin model (Matsuoka et al., 1995). Moreover, quercetin, also present in small quantities in cocoa, inhibited the carrageenin-induced paw edema when administered i.p. to mice (Rotelli et al., 2003), and also diminished the carrageenin-induced air pouch when administered locally to rats (Morikawa et al., 2003). In addition, other isolated flavonoids (Ferrándiz et al., 1991) or plant extracts (Autore et al., 2001; Chakradhar et al., 2005; Ghule et al., 2006) have shown an inhibitory effect on carrageenin-induced edema.

The anti-inflammatory effect of cocoa on carrageenin-induced edema may be due to its action on different events during the inflammatory response. In the carrageenin model, it has been described that histamine and serotonin released from local mast cells are responsible for the inflammation in the first phase, followed by kinins and therefore by the local production of prostaglandins (Morris, 2003). To analyze which mechanism/s could be influenced by cocoa, we have tested the effect of cocoa intake on acute inflammatory models induced by several single mediators. Cocoa intake had no protective effect in edema induced by histamine or serotonin. These results allow us to suggest that cocoa compounds did not counteract the actions of vasoactive amine. This fact could be explained by the vasodilator effect of cocoa (Hermann et al., 2006) that would add to the vasoactive inflammatory mediators. In contrast, other flavonoid-enriched plant extracts or isolated flavonoids have shown anti-inflammatory effect in histamine- and serotonin-induced acute inflammation. In these cases, however, there are different routes of administration and a short period between administration and inflammation induction (Sala et al., 2003; Gupta et al., 2005; Zhou et al., 2006; Paulino et al., 2006). On the other hand, cocoa intake could modulate the release of these inflammatory mediators because the down-regulatory role of some flavonoids on mast cell activation and histamine release has been recently described (Park et al., 2008; Shimoda et al., 2008).

In the present study, cocoa intake also produced no inhibition on PGE_2-induced inflammation. Despite these results, it has been described that some flavonoids may inhibit cyclooxigenase pathways and PGE_2 synthesis (de Pascual-Teresa et al., 2004; Delporte et al., 2005). Therefore, although cocoa could not counteract PGE_2 effects when it was injected, it remains to know if it could regulate its synthesis.

Interestingly, rats receiving the lowest dose of cocoa (2.4 g/kg/day) developed a significant reduction of paw edema induced by bradykinin. This effect may be partially attributed to the fact that flavonoids are able to bind bradykinin (Richard et al., 2006) and then antagonize its effects (Yun-Choi et al., 1993). Moreover, it has been suggested that bradykinin stimulate TNFα release from macrophages (Loram et al., 2007), a process that can be down-modulated by cocoa intake as shown here. On the other hand, bradykinin acts on endothelial cells causing vasodilatation, and on non-myelinated afferent neurons, mediating pain (Marceau et al., 2004). These actions would not be affected by a cocoa diet and then would explain the mild effect of cocoa on the bradykinin model. In addition, the beneficial properties of cocoa on this model were not observed at the highest dose. This lack of effect could be explained by the vasodilator consequences of cocoa intake, which at high concentration would predominate over the antagonistic action of flavonoids on bradykinin.

Therefore, from the experimental models induced by single inflammatory mediators, it could be suggested that the anti-inflammatory effect of 2.4 g/kg/day cocoa was due at least partially by regulating bradykinin actions. This effect could explain the inhibition observed with this dose during the first hour in the carrageenin model. Later, the same dose would not be able to counteract the macrophage activation phase, which agrees with results from peritoneal macrophages. On the contrary, higher doses of cocoa inhibit carrageenin-induced edema longer, which could be the result of the down-regulation of mediators produced by macrophages as reactive oxygen and nitrogen species and cytokines.

In summary, a high intake of cocoa could produce anti-inflammatory effects *in vivo*, as shown *in vitro*. Although it remains to be ascertained the precise mechanism of action of cocoa and its effectiveness in other inflammatory processes, cocoa seems a good candidate to be considered as a functional food.

Acknowledgments

S.R. is the recipient of fellowships from the Ministerio de Educación y Ciencia (BES-2006-13640). The present study was supported by the Ministerio de Educación y Ciencia, Spain (AGL2005-002823) and from SGR 2005-0083 of the Generalitat de Catalunya.

References

Autore, G., Rastrelli, L., Lauro, M.R., Marzocco, S., Sorrentino, R., Sorrentino, U., Pinto, A., and Aquino, R. (2001). Inhibition of nitric oxide synthase expression by a methanolic extract of *Crescentia alata* and its derived flavonols. *Life Sci., 70,* 523-534.

Azam, S., Hadi, N., Khan, U. N., and Hadi, S. M. (2003). Antioxidant and prooxidant properties of caffeine, theobromine and xanthine. *Med. Sci. Monit., 9,* 325-330.

Baba, S., Natsume, M., Yasuda, A., Nakamura, Y., Tamura, T., Osakabe, N., Kanegae, M., and Kondo K. (2007). Plasma LDL and HDL cholesterol and oxidized LDL concentrations are altered in normo- and hypercholesterolemic humans after intake of different levels of cocoa powder. *J. Nutr., 137,* 1436-1441.

Baba, S., Osakabe, N., Natsume, M., Muto, Y., Takizawa, T., and Terao, J. (2001). Absorption and urinary excretion of (-)-epicatechin after administration of different levels of cocoa powder or (-)-epicatechin in rats. *J. Agric. Food Chem., 49,* 6050-6056.

Baba, S., Osakabe, N., Natsume, M., Yasuda, A., Takizawa, T., Nakamura, T., and Terao, J. (2000). Cocoa powder enhances the level of antioxidative activity in rat plasma. *Br. J. Nutr., 84,* 673-680.

Buijsse, B., Feskens, E. J. M., Kok, F. J., and Kromhout, D. (2006). Cocoa intake, blood pressure, and cardiovascular mortality. *Arch. Intern. Med., 166,* 411-417.

Chakradhar, V., Babu, Y. H., Ganapaty, S., Prasad, Y. R., Rao, N. K. (2005) Anti-inflammatory activity of a flavonol glycoside from *Tephrosia spinosa. Nat. Prod. Sci., 11,* 63-66.

Comalada, M., Camuesco, D., Sierra, S., Ballester, I., Xaus, J., Gálvez, J., and Zarzuelo, A. (2005). In vivo quercitrin anti-inflammatory effect involves release of quercetin, which inhibits inflammation through down-regulation of the NF-κB pathway. *Eur. J. Immunol., 35,* 584-592.

Cooper, K. A., Donovan, J. L., Waterhouse, A. L., and Williamson, G. (2008). Cocoa and health: a decade of research. *Br. J. Nutr., 99,* 1-11.

Cotelle, N. (2001). Role of flavonoids in oxidative stress. *Curr. Top Med. Chem., 1,* 569-590.

Counet, C., and Collin, S. (2003). Effect of the number of flavanol units on the antioxidant activity of procyanidin fractions isolated from chocolate. *J. Agric. Food Chem., 51,* 6816-6822.

Crews, W. D. Jr., Harrison, D. W., and Wright, J. W. (2008). A double-blind, placebo-controlled, randomized trial of the effects of dark chocolate and cocoa on variables associated with neuropsychological functioning and cardiovascular health: clinical findings from a sample of healthy, cognitively intact older adults. *Am. J. Clin. Nutr., 87,* 872-880.

Datla KP, Zbarsky V, Rai D, Parkar, S., Osakabe, N., Aruoma, O. I., and Dexter, D. T. (2007). Short-term supplementation with plant extracts rich in flavonoids protect nigrostriatal dopaminergic neurons in a rat model of Parkinson's disease. *J. Am. Coll. Nutr., 26,* 341-349.

de Pascual-Teresa, S., Johnston, K. L., DuPont, M. S., O'Leary, K. A., Needs, P. W., Morgan, L. M., Clifford, M. N., Bao, Y., and Williamson, G. (2004). Quercetin metabolites downregulate cyclooxygenase-2 transcription in human lymphocytes ex vivo but not in vivo. *J. Nutr., 134,* 552-557.

Delporte, C., Backhouse, N., Erazo, S., Negrete, R., Vidal, P., Silva, X., López-Pérez J. L., Feliciano, A. S., and Muñoz, O. (2005). Analgesic-antiinflammatory properties of *Proustia pyrifolia. J. Ethnopharmacol., 99,* 119-124.

di Giuseppe, R., di Castelnuovo, A., Centritto, F., Zito, F., de Curtis, A., Costanzo, S., Vohnout, B., Sieri, S., Krogh, V., Donati, M. B., de Gaetano, G., and Iacoviello, L. (2008). Regular consumption of dark chocolate is associated with low serum concentrations of C-reactive protein in a healthy Italian population. *J. Nutr., 138,* 1939-1945.

Erlejman, A. G., Fraga, C. G., and Oteiza, P. I. (2006). Procyanidins protect Caco-2 cells from bile acid- and oxidant-induced damage. *Free Radic. Biol. Med., 41,* 1247-1256.

Ferrándiz, M. L. and Alcaraz, M. J. (1991). Anti-inflammatory activity and inhibition of arachidonic acid metabolism by flavonoids. *Agents Actions, 32,* 283-288.

Ghule, B. V., Ghante, M. H., Saoji, A. N. and Yeole, P. G. (2006). Hypolipidemic and antihyperlipidemic effects of *Lagenaria siceraria* (Mol.) fruit extracts. *Indian J. Exp. Biol., 44,* 905-909.

Granado-Serrano, A. B., Martín, M. A., Izquierdo-Pulido, M., Goya, L., Bravo, L., and Ramos, S. (2007). Molecular mechanisms of (-)-epicatechin and chlorogenic acid on the regulation of the apoptotic and survival/proliferation pathways in a human hepatoma cell line. *J. Agric. Food Chem., 55,* 2020-2027.

Grassi, D., Necozione, S., Lippi, C., Croce, G., Valeri, L., Pasqualetti, P., Desideri, G., Blumberg, J. B., and Ferri, C. (2005) Cocoa reduces blood pressure and insulin resistance and improves endothelium-dependent vasodilation in hypertensives. *Hypertension, 46,* 398–405.

Gu, L., House, S. E., Wu, X., Ou, B., and Prior, R. L. (2006) Procyanidin and catechin contents and antioxidant capacity of cocoa and chocolate products. *J. Agric. Food Chem., 54,* 4057-4061.

Guay, J., Bateman, K., Gordon, R., Manzini, J., and Riendeau, D. (2004). Carrageenan-induced paw edema in rat elicits a predominant prostaglandin E_2 (PGE_2) response in the central nervous system associated with the induction of microsomal PGE_2 synthase-1. *J. Biol. Chem., 279,* 24866-24872.

Gupta, M., Mazumder, U. K., Kumar, R. S., Gomathi, P., Rajeshwar, Y., Kakoti, B. B., and Selven, V. T. (2005). Anti-inflammatory, analgesic and antipyretic effects of methanol extract from *Bauhinia racemosa* stem bark in animal models. *J. Ethnopharmacol., 98,* 267-273.

Hatano, T., Miyatake, H., Natsume, M., Osakabe, N., Takizawa, T., Ito, H., and Yoshida, T. (2002). Proanthocyanidin glycosides and related polyphenols from cacao liquor and their antioxidant effects. *Phytochemistry, 59,* 749-758.

Hermann, F., Spieker, L. E., Ruschitzka, F., Sudano, I., Hermann, M., Binggeli, C., Lüscher, T. F., Riesen, W., Noll, G., and Corti, R. (2006). Dark chocolate improves endothelial and platelet function. *Heart, 92*, 119-120.

Hurst, W. J., Tarka, S. M. Jr., Powis, T. G., Valdez, F. Jr. and Hester, T. R. (2002). Cacao usage by the earliest Maya civilization. *Nature, 418,* 289-290.

Karim, M., McCormick, K., and Kappagoda, C. T. (2000). Effects of cocoa extracts on endothelium-dependent relaxation. *J. Nutr., 130,* S2105–S2108.

Kenny, T. P., Keen, C. L., Schmitz, H. H., and Gershwin, M. E. (2007). Immune effects of cocoa procyanidin oligomers on peripheral blood mononuclear cells. *Exp. Biol. Med. (Maywood), 232,* 293-300.

Lamuela-Raventos R. M., Andres-Lacueva, C., Permanyer, J., and Izquierdo-Pulido, M. (2001). More antioxidants in cocoa. *J. Nutr., 131,* 834-835.

Lee, K. W., Kim, Y. J., Lee, H. J. and Lee, C. Y. (2003). Cocoa has more phenolic phytochemicals and a higher antioxidant capacity than teas and red wine. *J. Agric. Food Chem., 51,* 7292-7295.

Loram, L. C., Fuller, A., Fick, L. G., Cartmell, T., Poole, S., and Mitchell, D. (2007). Cytokine profiles during carrageenan-induced inflammatory hyperalgesia in rat muscle and hind paw. *J. Pain, 8,* 127-136.

Lyu, S., Rhim, J., and Park, W. (2005) Antiherpetic activities of flavonoids against herpes simplex virus type 1 (HSV-1) and type 2 (HSV-2) in vitro. *Arch. Pharm. Res., 28,* 1293-1301.

Mackenzie, G. G., Carrasquedo, F., Delfino, J. M., Keen, C. L., Fraga, C. G., and Oteiza, P. I. (2004) Epicatechin, catechin, and dimeric procyanidins inhibit PMA-induced NF-κB activation at multiple steps in Jurkat T cells. *FASEB J., 18,* 167-169.

Manach, C., Scalbert, A., Morand, C., Remesy, C. and Jimenez, L. (2004). Polyphenols: food sources and bioavailability. *Am. J. Clin. Nutr., 79,* 727-747.

Mao, T., Van De Water, J., Keen, C. L., Schmitz, H. H., and Gershwin, M. E. (2000). Cocoa procyanidins and human cytokine transcription and secretion. *J. Nutr., 130,* S2093–S2099.

Marceau, F., and Regoli, D. (2004). Bradykinin receptor ligands: therapeutic perspectives. *Nat. Rev. Drug Discov., 3,* 845-852.

Mathur, S., Devaraj, S., Grundy, S. M., and Jialal, I. (2002). Cocoa products decrease low density lipoprotein oxidative susceptibility but do not affect biomarkers of inflammation in humans. *J. Nutr., 132,* 3663–3667.

Matsuoka, Y., Hasegawa, H., Okuda, S., Muraki, T., Uruno, T., and Kubota, K. (1995). Ameliorative effects of tea catechins on active oxygen-related nerve cell injuries. *J. Pharmacol. Exp. Ther.*, 274, 602-608.

McShea, A., Ramiro-Puig, E., Munro, S. B., Casadesus, G., Castell, M., and Smith, M. A. (2008). Clinical benefit and preservation of flavonols in dark chocolate manufacturing. *Nutr. Rev., 66,* 630-641.

Medzhitov, R. (2008). Origin and physiological roles of inflammation. *Nature, 454,* 428-435.

Morikawa, K., Nonaka, M., Narahara, M., Torii, I., Kawaguchi, K., Yoshikawa, T., Kumazawa, Y., and Morikawa, S. (2003). Inhibitory effect of quercetin on carrageenan-induced inflammation in rats. *Life Sci., 74,* 709-721.

Morris, C. J. (2003). Carrageenan-induced paw edema in the rat and mouse. *Method. Mol. Biol., 225,* 115-121.

Ono, K., Takahashi, T., Kamei, M., Mato, T., Hashizume, S., Kamiya, S., and Tsutsumi, H. (2003). Effects of an aqueous extract of cocoa on nitric oxide production of macrophages activated by lipopolysaccharide and interferon-gamma. *Nutrition, 19,* 681-685.

Park, H. H., Lee, S., Son, H. Y., Park, S. B., Kim, M. S., Choi, E. J., Singh, T. S., Ha, J. H., Lee, M. G., Kim, J. E., Hyun, M. C., Kwon, T. K., Kim, Y. H., and Kim, S. H. (2008) Flavonoids inhibit histamine release and expression of proinflammatory cytokines in mast cells. *Arch. Pharm. Res., 31,* 1303-1311.

Paulino, N., Teixeira, C., Martins, R., Scremin, A., Dirsch, V. M., Vollmar, A. M., Abreu, S. R., de Castro, S. L., and Marcucci, M. C. (2006). Evaluation of the analgesic and anti-inflammatory effects of a Brazilian green propolis. *Planta Med., 72,* 899-906.

Ramiro, E., Franch, A., Castellote, C., Perez-Cano, F., Permanyer, J., Izquierdo-Pulido, M., and Castell, M. (2005). Flavonoids from *Theobroma cacao* down-regulate inflammatory mediators. *J. Agric. Food Chem., 53,* 8506-8511.

Ramiro-Puig, E., Casadesús, G., Lee, H. G., Zhu, X., McShea, A., Perry, G., Pérez-Cano, F. J., Smith, M. A., and Castell, M. (2009a) Neuroprotective effect of cocoa flavonoids on *in vitro* oxidative stress. *Eur. J. Nutr., 48*, 54-61.

Ramiro-Puig, E., and Castell, M. (2009b) Cocoa: antioxidant and immunomodulator. *Br. J. Nutr., 101*, 931-40.

Ramos-Romero, S., Ramiro-Puig, E., Pérez-Cano, F. J., Castellote, C., Franch, A. and Castell, M. (2008). Anti-inflammatory effects of cocoa in rat carrageenin-induced paw oedema. *Proc. Nutr. Soc., 67,* E65.

Richard, T., Lefeuvre, D., Descendit, A., Quideau, S., and Monti, J. P. (2006). Recognition characters in peptide-polyphenol complex formation. *Biochim. Biophys. Acta, 1760,* 951-958.

Rocha, A. C., Fernandes, E. S., Quintao, N. L., Campos, M. M., and Calixto, J. B. (2006). Relevance of tumour necrosis factor-alpha for the inflammatory and nociceptive responses evoked by carrageenan in the mouse paw. *Br. J. Pharmacol., 5,* 688-695.

Rotelli, A. E., Guardia, T., Juarez, A. O., de la Rocha, N. E., and Pelzer, L. E. (2003). Comparative study of flavonoids in experimental models of inflammation. *Pharmacol. Res., 48,* 601-606.

Sala, A., Recio, M. C., Schinella, G. R., Máñez, S., Giner, R. M., Cerdá-Nicolás, M., and Rosí, J. L. (2003). Assessment of the anti-inflammatory activity and free radical scavenger activity of tiliroside. *Eur. J. Pharmacol. 461,* 53-61.

Sanbongi, C., Suzuki, N., and Sakane, T. (1997). Polyphenols in chocolate, which have antioxidant activity, modulate immune functions in humans in vitro. *Cell Immunol., 177,* 129-136.

Sanchez-Rabaneda, F., Jáuregui, O., Casals, I., Andres-Lacueva, C., Izquierdo-Pulido, M., and Lamuela-Raventos, R. M. (2003). Liquid chromatographic/ electrospray ionization tandem mass spectrometric study of the phenolic composition of cocoa (*Theobroma cacao*). *J. Mass Spectrom., 38,* 35-42.

Schramm, D. D., Wang, J. F., Holt, R. R., Ensunsa, J. L., Gonsalves, J. L., Lazarus, S. A., Schmitz, H. H., German, J. B., and Keen, C. L. (2001) Chocolate procyanidins decrease the leukotriene-prostacyclin ratio in humans and human aortic endothelial cells. *Am. J. Clin. Nutr., 73,* 36–40.

Shimoda, K., Kobayashi, T., Akagi, M., Hamada, H., and Hamada H. (2008) Synthesis of Oligosaccharides of Genistein and Quercetin as Potential Anti-inflammatory Agents. *Chem. Let., 37,* 876-877.

Sies, H., Schewe, T., Heiss, C., and Kelm, M. (2005). Cocoa polyphenols and inflammatory mediators. *Am. J. Clin. Nutr., 81,* S304-12.

Singleton, V. L., Orthofer R., and Lamuela-Raventós, R. M (1999). Analysis of total phenols and other oxidation substrates and antioxidants by means of Folin-Ciocalteu reagent. *Method. Enzymol., 299,* 152-178.

Son, J., Pang, B., McFaline, J. L., Taghizadeh, K., and Dedon, P. C. (2008). Surveying the damage: the challenges of developing nucleic acid biomarkers of inflammation. *Mol. Biosyst., 4,* 902-908.

Taubert, D., Roesen, R., Lehmann, C., Jung, N., and Schomig, E. (2007) Effects of low habitual cocoa intake on blood pressure and bioactive nitric oxide: a randomized controlled trial. *JAMA., 298,* 49-60.

Vinson, J. A., Proch, J., and Zubik, L. (1999). Phenol antioxidant quantity and quality in foods: cocoa, dark chocolate, and milk chocolate. *J. Agric. Food Chem., 47,* 4821-4824.

Vinson, J. A., Proch, J., Bose, P., Muchler, S., Taffera, P., Shuta, D., Samman, N., and Agbor, G. A. (2006). Chocolate is a powerful ex vivo and in vivo antioxidant, an antiatherosclerotic agent in an animal model, and a significant contributor to antioxidants in the European and American Diets. *J. Agric. Food Chem., 54,* 8071-8076.

Winter, C. A., Risley, E. A., and Nuss, G. W. (1962). Carrageenan-induced edema in hind paw of the rat as an assay for anti-inflammatory drugs. *Proc. Soc. Exp. Biol., 111,* 544-547.

Yilmaz, Y., and Toledo, R. T. (2004). Major flavonoids in grape seeds and skins: antioxidant capacity of catechin, epicatechin, and gallic acid. *J. Agric. Food Chem., 52,* 255-260.

Yun-Choi H. S., Chung, H. S., and Kim, Y. J. (1993) Evaluation of some flavonoids as potential bradykinin antagonist. *Arch. Pharm. Res., 16,* 283-288.

Zhou, H., Wong, Y. F., Cai, X., Liu, Z. Q., Jiang, Z. H., Bian, Z. X., Xu, H. X., and Liu, L. (2006). Suppressive effects of JCICM-6, the extract of an anti-arthritic herbal formula, on the experimental inflammatory and nociceptive models in rodents. *Biol. Pharm. Bull., 29,* 253-260.

In: Flavonoids: Biosynthesis, Biological Effects... ISBN: 978-1-60741-622-7
Editor: Raymond B. Keller

Chapter 7

MECHANISMS AT THE ROOT OF FLAVONOID ACTION IN CANCER: A STEP TOWARD SOLVING THE RUBIK'S CUBE

Maria Marino* and Pamela Bulzomi
Department of Biology, University Roma Tre, Viale G. Marconi, 446, I-00146 Roma, Italy

ABSTRACT

The biological activity of flavonoids was first recognized when the antiestrogenic principle present in red clover that caused infertility in sheep in Western Australia was discovered. These adverse effects of flavonoids placed these substances in the class of endocrine-disrupting chemicals. On the other hand, flavonoids are recently claimed to prevent several cancer types and to reduce incidence of cardiovascular diseases, osteoporosis, neurodegenerative diseases, as well as chronic and acute inflammation. Despite these controversial effects, a huge number of plant extracts or mixtures, containing varying amounts of isolated flavonoids, are commercially available on the market as dietary supplements and healthy products. The commercial success of these supplements is evident, even though the activity and mechanisms of flavonoid action are still unclear.

Owing to their chemical structure, the most obvious feature of flavonoids is their ability to quench free radicals. However, in the last few years many exciting new indication in elucidating the mechanisms of flavonoid actions have been published. Flavonoids inhibit several signal transduction-involved kinases and affect protein functions via competitive or allosteric interactions. Among others, flavonoids interact with and affect the cellular responses mediated by estrogen receptors (ERα and ERβ). In particular, our recent data indicate that some flavonoids (i.e., naringenin and quercetin) decouple specific ERα action mechanisms, important for cell proliferation, driving cells to the apoptosis. Therefore, distinct complex mechanisms of actions, possibly interacting one another, for nutritional molecules on cell signalling and response can be hypothesized.

---

* Tel. 0039-06-57336345; fax 0039-06-57336321. e-mail address: m.marino@uniroma3.it (M. Marino)

Aim of this review is to provide an updating picture about mechanisms by which flavonoids play a role in cellular response and in preventing human pathologies such as cancer. In particular, their direct interaction with nuclear receptors and/or by their ability to modulate the activity of key enzymes involved in cell signaling and antioxidant responses will be presented and discussed.

1. Introduction

Flavonoids, phenylbenzo-pyrones (phenylchromones), are a large group of non nutrient compounds naturally produced from plants as part of their defence mechanisms against stresses of different origins. They are present in all terrestrial vascular plants; whereas, in mammals, flavonoids occur only through dietary intake (Birt et al., 2001). Flavonoids, have an assortment of structures based on a common three-ring nucleus (Middleton et al., 2000) in which primary substituents (eg, hydroxyl, methoxyl, or glycosyl groups) can be further substituted (e.g., additionally glycosylated or acylated) sometimes yielding highly complex structures (Cheynier, 2005) (Figure 1). More than 4,000 different flavonoids, have been described and categorized into 6 subclasses as a function of the type of heterocycle involved: flavonols, flavones, flavanols, flavanonols, flavanones, and isoflavones (Figure 1) (Birt et al., 2001; Manach et al., 2004).

First recognized in '40 as the antiestrogenic principle present in red clover that caused infertility in sheep in Western Australia (Bennetts et al., 1946; Galluzzo and Marino, 2006), more recently, the use of flavonoids to curb menopausal symptoms and provide a "natural" and presumably cancer risk-free estrogenic replacement (Ling et al., 2004) has become popular in Western countries.

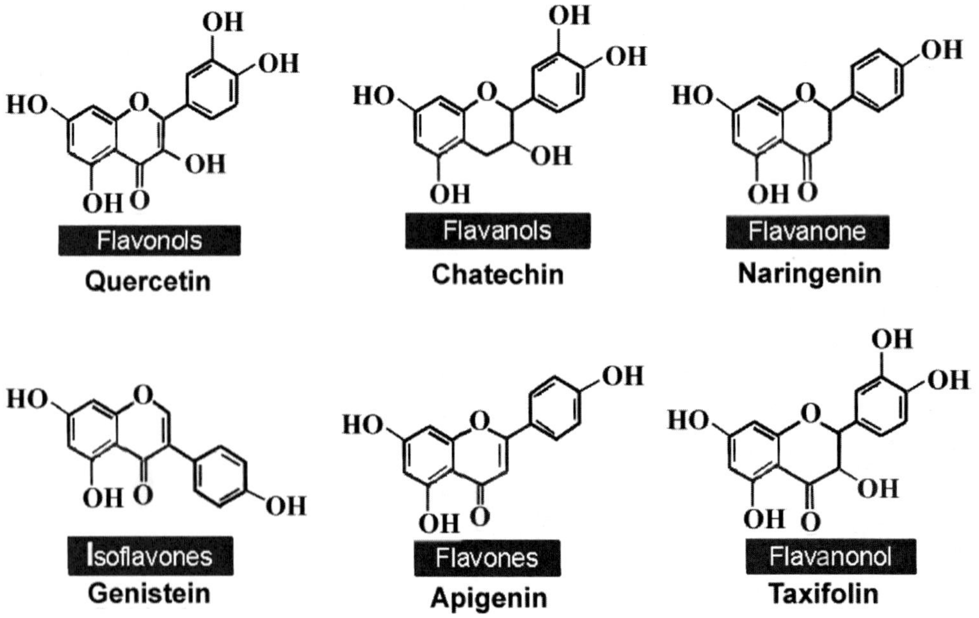

Figure 1. Chemical structures of commonly occurring plant flavonoids.

Thus, a huge number of preparations are now commercially available on the market as health food products. As dietary supplements they are obtainable as plant extracts or mixtures, containing varying amounts of isolated or concentrate flavonoids in bakery, dairy, infant formulas (Tomar and Shiao, 2008). The commercial success of these supplements is evident and the consumption of these compounds in Western countries is increasing even if different and opposite flavonoid effects have been reported.

In particular, epidemiological data show that in pre-menopausal women, assuming daily soy, follicle stimulating and luteinizing hormone levels significantly decreased, increasing menstrual cycle length (Jacobs and Lewis, 2002). Hyperplasia of mammary glands in both sexes, aberrant or delayed spermatogenesis, histological changes in the vagina and ovary, mineralization of renal tubules in males, modulation of natural killer cell activity, and myelotoxicity had been observed in rats exposed to isoflavone genistein through placental transfer or lactational exposure, or ingestion (Flynn et al., 2000; Delclos et al., 2001; Guo et al., 2005; Doerge et al., 2006). On the other hand, a positive association between the increased intake of phytoestrogen and reduced amount of neurodegenerative diseases, improvement of cognition and learning (Kirk et al., 1998), and fewer tendency to osteoporosis (Zhang et al., 2003; Adlercreutz et al., 2004) have also been reported. In addition, diets rich in flavonoids also lead to lower serum cholesterol levels, low-density lipoproteins, and triglycerides (Delclos et al., 2001), thus reducing the incidence of cardiovascular diseases (Doerge et al., 2006). Finally, the close relationship between flavonoids and cancer is suggested by the large variation in rates of specific cancers in different countries and by the spectacular changes observed in the incidence of cancer in migrating populations (Guo et al., 2005; Béliveau and Gingras, 2007; Benavente-García and Castillo, 2008). These observations are strengthened by many experimental data obtained from studies using cellular and animal models (Caltagirone et al., 2000; Fenton and Hord, 2004; Albini et al., 2005; Béliveau and Gingras, 2007; Espìn et al., 2007; Benavente-García and Castillo, 2008).

Flavonoids have been considered able to modulate this wide spectrum of responses due to their chemical structure compatible with putative antioxidant properties which can interact with reactive oxygen-nitrogen species (RONS)-mediated intracellular signaling (Virgili and Marino, 2008). However, different cellular effects not directly related to flavonoid antioxidant capacity have been recently reported. Flavonoids could modulate the activity of several kinases and could affect protein functions (e.g. receptors) via competitive or allosteric interactions. Thus, flavonoids should be considered pleiotropic substances which possess distinct mechanisms of action possibly interacting each other.

Aim of this review is to provide an update about mechanisms by which flavonoids play a role in cellular response and in preventing cancer.

2. Prooxidant/Antioxidant Activity of Flavonoids

RONS, including nitric oxide (NO) and hydrogen peroxide (H_2O_2), are endogenously synthesized in several cells were participate, as second messengers, in cytokine and/or growth factor signals (Stone and Jang, 2006). On the other hand, RONS are the principal responsible of oxidative stress initiation when their production exceeds cellular antioxidant defenses. The consequence of RONS action is the damage of membrane lipids, proteins, and DNA with the subsequent onset of various diseases (Moskaug et al., 2005).

RONS, either directly or indirectly, regulates the activity of some of the most well-known signaling enzymes including guanylyl cyclase, phospholipase C, phospholipase A2, phospholipase D, activating protein-1 (AP-1), nuclear factor κB (NF-κB), insulin receptor, c-Src, Jun N-terminal kinase, and p38 kinase (MAPK) (Hehner et al., 2000). Moreover, a significant inhibition of phosphatase activity, paralleled by the net increase of phosphorylation level, has been reported (O'Loghlen et al., 2003, Hao et al., 2006).

Due to their chemical structure, flavonoids are able to quench free radicals by forming resonance-stabilized phenoxyl radicals *in vitro*, in cell cultures, and in cell free systems (Hanasaki et al., 1994, Ursini et al., 1994, Birt et al., 2001). In addition, these compounds have been considered able to impair the RONS-mediated intracellular signaling by directly inhibiting the involved enzymes or by chelating trace elements involved in free radical production or up-regulating the antioxidant cellular response (Surh, 2003, Lee et al., 2005, Chiang et al., 2006, Kweon et al., 2006). Thus, an high intake of flavonoids should be associated with a reduced risk of degenerative diseases such as cardiovascular disease and cancer. Experimental data have shown that flavonoids block the progression of latent microtumors (Béliveau and Gingras, 2007) and this effect could be elicited via the modulation of the enzymatic systems responsible for neutralizing free radicals (Conney, 2003; Ioannides and Lewis 2004) and/or by directly inducing cancer cell death by apoptosis. For example, phenethyl isothiocyanate from cruciferous vegetables, curcumin from turmeric, resveratrol from grapes, and naringenin from oranges have all been shown to possess strong pro-apoptotic activity against cells isolated from a variety of tumors (Totta et al., 2004; Karunagaran et al., 2005; Totta et al., 2005). Thus, the antioxidant activity of flavonoids could represent the close relationship between flavonoids and cancer chemoprevention.

However, flavonoids also possess pro-oxidant properties which could contribute to their anti-cancer activity (Galati et al., 2000). Flavonoid pro-oxidant activity seems to be involved in the inhibition of mitochondrial respiration and is related to their *in vitro* ability to undergo to auto-oxidation to produce superoxide anions. On the other hand, transition metals, which catalyze auto-oxidation, result linked to proteins *in vivo* and it is unlikely they could significantly participate in the auto-oxidation of polyphenols. As alternative mechanism flavonoids pro-oxidant activity could be dependent from the activity of peroxidases (O'Brien, 2000). As an example, the apigenin in the presence of myeloperoxidase forms a peroxyl radical *in vitro* (Galati et al., 2001) which leads to the intracellular production of ROS and contributes to the apoptotic and necrotic cell death (Wang et al., 1999; Morrissey et al., 2005; Vargo et al., 2006; Miyoshi et al., 2007). Baicalin-apoptosis induction is also accompanied with the generation of intracellular ROS and the increase of the cytochrome c release (Ueda et al., 2002). Cytochrome c release and mitochondrial transmembrane potential disruption precedes the apoptosoma activation in MCF-7 cell treated with 200μM of the stilbene trans-resveratrol (Filomeni et al., 2007). Contrasting results have been obtained treating cells with quercetin. This flavonoid possess an high antioxidant activity preventing the H_2O_2-induced ROS production in a dose-dependent manner not related with its pro-apoptotic effect. In addition, the cell treatment with 50 μM quercetin induces an increase of ROS production in a cell context dependent way (Galluzzo et al., 2008 and literature cited therein). Thus, other action mechanism(s) independent from antioxidant/pro-oxidant effects of flavonoids should be evoked to explain the potential chemopreventive and chemoprotective effect of these substances.

3. Flavonoids as Kinase Inhibitors

Cancer progression arrest and tumor cell growth inhibition have been associated with the strong affinity of flavonoid for proteins involved in a variety of cellular processes.

The flavonoid-induced inhibition of the epidermal growth factor receptor (EGF-R), protein kinase C (PKC), phosphatydil inositol 3 kinase (PI3K) and extracellular regulated kinase (ERK) have been described (Hagiwara et al., 1988; Spencer et al., 2003; Kim et al., 2008). As a possible mechanism their competition with ATP for the binding to the protein catalytic site has been evoked (Chao, 2000; Manthey, 2000). However, in most reports, direct demonstration of such inhibition was not shown. Indeed, although EGF stimulation of EGF-R tyrosine auto-phosphorylation in prostate and breast cancer cells was blocked by tyrphostins (synthetic tyrosine kinase inhibitors), genistein had no effect (Peterson and Barnes, 1996). In rats treated with genistein, the reduced reactivity of EGF-R with anti-phosphotyrosine antibodies was shown instead to result from a reduction in the amount of EGF-R protein (Dalu et al., 1998). These data suggest that genistein elicits its effects through transcriptional processes rather than directly on tyrosine kinase activity.

Moreover, flavonoids can block enzyme activity modulating redox-sensitive transcription factors. Curcumin (diferuloylmethane) and epigallocatechin-3-gallate (EGCG) induce hemeoxygenase-1 (HO-1), an enzyme with antioxidant properties which influences the apoptosis, promoting nuclear translocation of the nuclear factor (erythroid-derived 2)-related factor (Nrf2) (Andreadi et al., 2006).

There is growing evidence that phytoestrogens could have a protective effect on the initiation or progression of breast cancer by inhibiting the local production of estrogens from circulating precursors in breast tissue. Indeed *in vitro* experiments have shown that phytoestrogens, mainly flavones and flavonones, inhibit the activity of key steroidogenic enzymes (i.e., aromatase and 17β-hydroxysteroid dehydrogenase) involved in the synthesis of estradiol from circulating androgens and estrogen sulphate (Rice and Whitehead, 2006).

Flavonoid ability to prevent cell invasion and matrix degradation, as well as alterations of cellular metabolism, has been associated to their effect on cancer progression reduction (Manna et al., 2000; Pellegatta et al., 2003; El Bedoui et al., 2005; Wung et al., 2005). In particular, the alteration of glucose homeostasis by the inhibition of glycogen phosphorylase activity has been reported (Jakobs et al., 2006). The glucose uptake could be also inhibited directly by flavonoid binding to the glucose transporter 4, or indirectly by inhibiting PI3K/AKT pathway-induced by insulin receptor (IR) phosphorylation (Nomura et al., 2008).

However, flavonoids-dependent kinases inhibition is present at high flavonoid concentration (>50 μM). At present the relative importance of each of these pathways and their putative cross-talk remains to be established as well as the clinical significance in nutritionally relevant flavonoid concentration (i.e., 0.1-10 μM) remain unsolved.

4. Flavonoids as Nuclear Receptor Ligands

Nuclear receptors (NR) are ligand-activated transcription factors sharing a common evolutionary history (Gronemeyer et al., 2004), having similar sequence features at the protein level (Figure 2). A specific corresponding endogenous ligand for some of the NRs is not known, and therefore these receptors have been named "orphan receptors." This group includes the lipid-regulating peroxisome proliferator-activated receptors (PPARs), the liver X receptor, the farnesoid X receptor, and the pregnane nuclear receptor (PXR). Fibrates or glitazones, oxysterols, bile acids, and xenobiotics could activate the orphan receptors of the NR1 subfamily and produce effects that resemble some of the actions caused by flavonoid intake (Virgili ad Marino, 2008).

Resveratrol, has been found to selectively activate PPARα and PPARγ transcriptional activity by 15- to 30-fold above control levels. This activation was dose dependent at quite high concentrations (10, 50, and 100 μM) in endothelial cells (Shay and Banz, 2005). Experimental data demonstrate that genistein could act as a ligand for PPARγ with a K_i comparable to that of some known PPARγ ligands (Iqbal et al., 2002; Dang et al., 2003). In particular genistein seems to be an PPARα agonists. In fact female obese Zucker rats consuming a high isoflavone diet improved their glucose tolerance and displayed liver triglyceride and cholesterol and plasma cholesterol levels significantly lower than controls (Mezei et al., 2003).

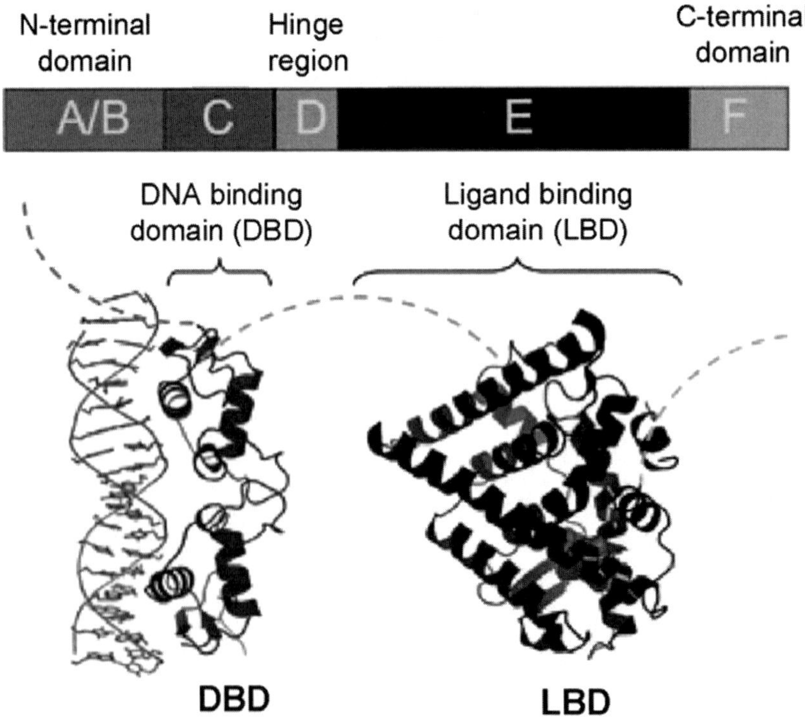

Figure 2. NRs share an evolutionarily conserved structure consisting of the high variable *N*-amino-terminal region involved in transactivation (A and B domains), the conserved DNA binding region (DBD, C domain), the hinge region, the ligand binding domain (LBD; E domain), and the *C*-terminal region (F domain). For details, see text.

This data is consistent with the hypothesis that soy isoflavones improve lipid metabolism and have an antidiabetic effect by activating PPAR receptors and is in agreement with observations in humans treated with antidiabetic PPARα agonists (e.g. GW501516) used to treat hyperlipidemia and type 2 diabetes (Elisaf et al., 2002).

Mixtures of isoflavones and isolated isoflavones have been reported to induce PXR transcriptional activity (Ricketts et al., 2005) which has been shown to be activated by a chemically and structurally diverse set of xenobiotic and endogenous compounds and to regulate gene expression pathways involved in metabolism and transport of these same classes of compounds (Moore and Kliewer, 2000; Wang et al., 2007). Notably, PXR has been shown to directly regulate the cytochrome P450 3A gene, a phase I drug metabolism gene, whose product is responsible for the metabolism of drugs (Moore and Kliewer, 2000; Wang et al., 2007). Other authors reported that genistein, formononetin, kaempferol, and apigenin did not exhibit PXR ligand activity (Mnif et al., 2007). Thus, at present the contribution of PXR signaling to the flavonoid effects on human health remains elusive. Contrasting data have also been reported about flavonoids effects on AhR. Quercetin, galangin, diosmin, and diosmetin increase the expression of phase I enzymes, important for the prevention of cancer, by binding to AhR receptor (Kang et al., 1999).

Computer docking analyses and mammalian two-hybrid experiments indicate that isoflavones (i.e., genistein, daidzein, and biochanin A) and one flavone (trihydroxyflavone) are relatively poor ligands of estrogen related receptor γ (ERRγ, NR3) but they can act as agonists of ERRα and ERRβ activity (Suetsugi et al., 2003).

4.1. Flavonoids as Estrogen Receptor Ligands

At concentrations more physiologically achievable in the plasma (from 0.1 μM to 10 μM) after the consumption of meals rich in flavonoids (Manach et al., 2004), flavonoids can bind to and, consequently, modulate ER activity (Birt et al., 2001; Totta et al., 2004) leading to estrogenic or antiestrogenic effects. Because of their ability to interfere with E2 action, flavonoids are actually defined as dietary phytoestrogen (Saarinen et al., 2006).

Flavonoids interfere with organ and tissue responses to 17β-estradiol (E2) by binding to estrogen receptors ERα and ERβ. ERα and ERβ are encoded by two different genes and belong to the nuclear receptor superfamily (NR3A1 and NR3A2, respectively) (Figure 2) (Nilsson et al., 2001). E2 binding to its receptors causes ER dissociation from heat shock proteins, ER dimerization (omo/eterodimerization) and binding to specific DNA sequences [estrogen response element (ERE)] thus triggering to the transcription of responsive genes (Ascenzi et al., 2006). Moreover, ERα, but not ERβ, can regulate gene transcription through its indirect interaction with the transcription factors stimulating protein 1 (Sp-1) and AP-1 (Ascenzi et al., 2006). Both in the direct and indirect action modes, ERs need to interact with coregulatory proteins (coactivators or corepressors) which provide a platform upon which additional proteins are assembled (Ascenzi et al., 2006).

A growing number of reports indicate E2 effects in living cells are mediated by various pathways rather than by a single uniform mechanism. E2 rapid effects have been attributed in most cells to a population of ERs present on the plasma membranes (Levin 2005). We recently demonstrated that ERα undergoes *S*-palmitoylation on a cysteine residue (Cys447) present in the ligand binding domain (LBD) which allows receptor anchoring to plasma membrane, association to caveolin-1, and which accounts for the ability of E2 to activate different signaling pathways (Acconcia et al., 2005a). The Cys399 residue present in the LBD of ERβ is also subjected to *S*-palmitoylation (Galluzzo et al., 2007) indicating that a similar mechanism also works for ERβ localization to the plasma membrane and association to caveolin-1. Thus, ERα and ERβ have to be considered as a population of protein(s) which localization in the cell can dynamically change, shuttling from membrane to cytosol and to the nucleus on the dependence of E2 binding (Acconcia et al., 2005a; Levin, 2005). As a consequence, rapid and more prolonged E2 actions could be more finely coordinated. The physiological significance of ERs-dependent rapid pathways is quite clarified, at least for some E2 target tissues. The mechanism by which E2 exerts proliferative properties has been assumed to be exclusively mediated by ERα-induced rapid membrane-starting actions (Marino et al., 2005; Ascenzi et al., 2006), whereas E2 induces cell death through ERβ non-genomic signaling (Acconcia et al., 2005b). In the nervous system, E2 influences neural functions (e.g., cognition, behavior, stress responses, and reproduction) in part inducing such rapid responses (Farach-Carson and Davis, 2003). In the liver, rapid E2-induced signals are deeply linked to the expression of LDL-receptor and to the decreased cholesterol-LDL levels in the plasma (Distefano et al., 2002). An important mode of E2-mediated atheroprotection is linked to E2 capability to rapidly activate endothelial NOS and NO production (Chambliss et al., 2002).

These rapid effects (E2 extranuclear signals) include the activation of mitogen-activated protein kinase (MAPK) (i.e., p38, extranuclear regulated kinases [ERK]), PI3K, signal transducer and activator of transcription, epidermal growth factor receptor, Src kinase, Shc kinase, protein kinase C, adenylate cyclase, GTP-binding proteins, and NOS (Dang and Lowik, 2005). Microarray analysis of gene expression in vascular endothelial cells treated with E2 for 40 min showed that 250 genes were up-regulated; this could be prevented by Ly294002, a PI3K inhibitor. Interestingly, the transcriptional activity of the E2-ERα complex could be inhibited by pre-treating cells with PD98059 and U0126, two ERK inhibitors (Ascenzi et al., 2006). These findings support the idea that E2-induced rapid signals synergize with genomic events to maintain the pleiotropic hormone effects in the body (Galluzzo and Marino, 2006).

A plethora of papers indicates the ability of flavonoids to bind both ER isoforms maintaining the ERs gene transcriptional ability, nevertheless several epidemiological and experimental data show that flavonoid effects can be both estrogen mimetic and antiestrogenic. Several groups have demonstrated that flavonoid affinity to ERs is lower than E2 (Kuiper et al., 1997). Competition binding studies confirm that nutritional molecules (e.g., genistein, coumestrol, daidzein, and equol) show a distinct preference for ERβ (Kuiper et al., 1997; Mueller et al., 2004; Escande et al., 2006), although the prenylated chalcone occurring in hops, 8-prenylnaringenin, has been found to be a potent ERα agonist, but a weak agonist of ERβ in E2 competition assays (Stevens and Page, 2004). Phytochemicals as the isoflavonoids daidzein and genistein, the flavanone naringenin, and the flavonol quercetin increase the activity of ERE-luciferase reporter gene construct in cells expressing ERα or ERβ (Mueller, 2002; Totta et al., 2004; Virgili et al., 2004; Totta et al., 2005), but impair ERα interaction with Sp-1 and AP-1 (Peach et al., 1997; Liu et al., 2002; Virgili et al., 2004). Cluster analysis of DNA microarray in MCF-7 cells show a very similar profiles between estrogen responding genes and 10 μM genistein (Terasaka et al., 2004) while the expression of only five genes is affected by daidzein with respect to E2 in TM4 Sertoli cells. These five genes were related to cell signaling, cell proliferation, and apoptosis, suggesting a possible correlation with the inhibition of cell viability reported after treatment with daidzein (Adachi et al., 2005).

The capability of flavonoids to influence E2 rapid actions in both reproductive and non-reproductive E2-target tissues and how such effects may impact the normal development and physiological properties of cells largely have not been tackled until very recently (Somjen, 2005; Watson, 2005). In fact, scarce information is available on the non genomic signal transduction pathways activated after the formation of flavonoids:ERα and flavonoids:ERβ complexes. Recent evidence favors the idea that besides coactivator association, the ER-LBD is essential and sufficient also for activation of rapid E2-induced signals (Marino et al., 2005). Thus, it is possible that flavonoids could induce different conformational changes of ER, also precluding the activation of rapid signaling cascades (Galluzzo et al., 2008). As support of this hypothesis our group have recently demonstrated that quercetin and naringenin hamper ERα-mediated rapid activation of signaling kinases (i.e., ERK/ MAPK and PI3K/AKT) and cyclin D1 transcription only when HeLa cells, devoid of any ER isoforms, were transiently transfected with a human ERα expression vector (Virgili et al., 2004). In particular, naringenin, inducing conformational changes in ER, provokes ERα depalmitoylation faster than E2, which results in receptor rapid dissociation from caveolin-1, impairing ERα binding to molecular adaptor and signaling proteins (e.g., modulator of non genomic actions of the ER, c-Src) involved in the activation of the mitogenic signaling cascades (i.e., ERK/MAPK and PI3K/AKT) (Galluzzo et al., 2008). Moreover, naringenin induces the ERα-dependent, but palmitoylation-independent, activation of p38/MAPK, which in turn is responsible for naringenin-mediated antiproliferative effects in cancer cells. Naringenin, decoupling ERα action mechanisms, prevents the activation ERK/MAPK and PI3K/AKT signal transduction pathways thus, drives cells to apoptosis (Galluzzo et al., 2008). On the other hand, naringenin does not impair the ERα-mediated transcriptional activity of an ERE-containing promoter (Totta et al., 2004; Virgili et al., 2004). As a whole, this flavanone modulates specific ERα mechanisms and can be considered as 'mechanism-specific ligands of ER' (Totta et al., 2004).

In the same cell system, we recently demonstrated that quercetin activates the rapid ERα-dependent phosphorylation of p38/MAPK and, in turn, the induction of a proapoptotic cascade (i.e., caspase-3 activation and PARP cleavage) (Galluzzo et al., 2008a). This result proves that quercetin- and naringenin-induced apoptosis in cancer cells depends on the flavonoid interference with ERα-mediated rapid actions suggesting a role of endocrine disruptor for these flavonoids (Galluzzo et al 2008a).

As previously described, E2 mediates a wide variety of complex biological processes including skeletal muscle differentiation via ERα-dependent signals (Marino, personal communication). Our recent data show that Nar stimulation of rat skeletal muscle cells (L6), decoupling ERα mechanism of action, impedes the E2-dependent differentiation further sustaining the antiestrogenic role played by flavonoids (Marino, personal communication).

Thus, flavonoids have a very complex spectrum of activities: they can function as mechanism-specific ligands of ERα (Totta et al., 2004) due to their ability to decouple ERα activities, eliciting estrogenic or antiestrogenic effects downstream of these pathways (Galluzzo et al., 2008).

CONCLUSIONS

Interest on dietary compounds has evolved since their therapeutic properties has been discovered. Flavonoids are documented to play a major role amongst the hormonally agents in food, nonetheless the importance of their role in human health has not yet unequivocally established.

Flavonoids have a chemical structure compatible with a strong putative antioxidant. Neverthless, flavonoids antioxidant/pro-oxidant properties could be considered a simplified approach to the function of molecules of nutritional interest due to the fact that their antioxidant and/or pro-oxidant capacities are chemical properties which are not necessarily associated to an equivalent biological function (Virgili and Marino, 2008). Remarkably, flavonoids have also a strong affinity for protein so they can modulate cellular function inhibiting or modulating protein functions (Figure 3).

Normally, human flavonoid plasma concentrations are in the low nanomolar range, but upon flavonoid supplementation they may increase to the high nanomolar or low micromolar range (Boots et al., 2008).

Thus, flavonoids do not appear to be present in the circulation at high enough concentrations to contribute significantly to total antioxidant capacity (concentration of circulating endogenous antioxidant, ascorbate or urate, has been estimated to be in the range of 159-380 μmol/l for a normal individual) (Stevenson and Hurst, 2007) or inhibition kinases activity.

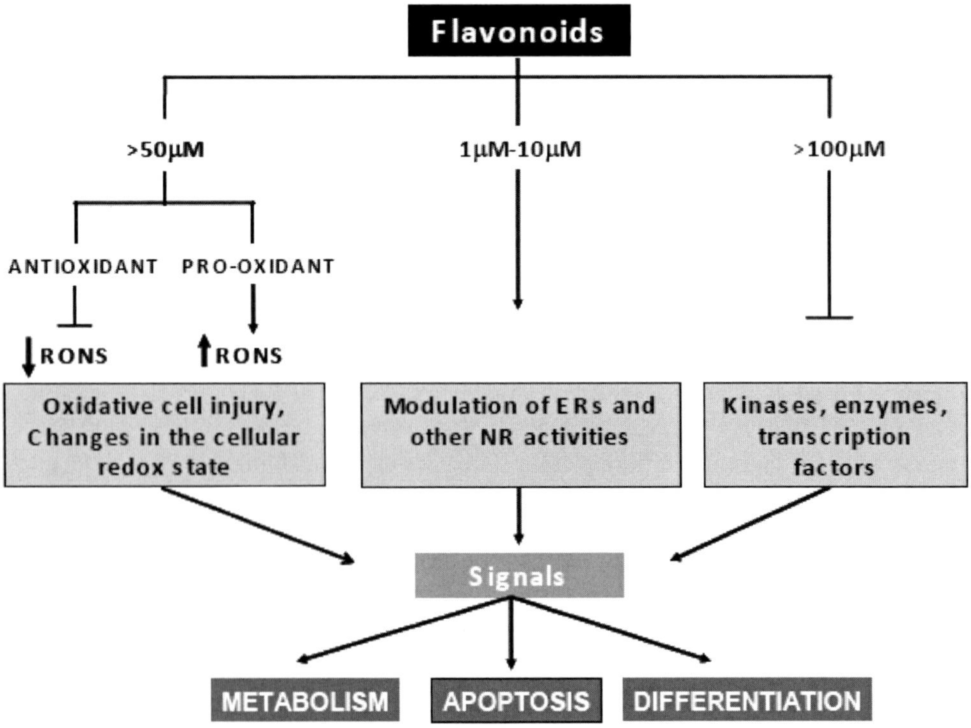

Figure 3. Schematic model illustrating the multiple effects of flavonoids on cell functions.

At concentrations more physiologically achievable in the plasma (from 0.1 μM to 10 μM) after the consumption of meals rich in flavonoids (Manach et al., 2004), these compounds can bind to and, consequently, modulate ER activities leading to estrogenic or antiestrogenic effects (Figure 3). As before reported, the long-term estrogenic effects of flavonoids have been extensively studied, whereas there is a lack of experimental data concerning the influence of natural estrogenic compounds on rapid E2-mediated mechanism (Galluzzo and Marino, 2006). Our recent data have highlighted the ability of these compounds to influence also rapid actions of E2 in both reproductive and non reproductive E2-target tissues (Totta et al., 2004; Galluzzo et al., 2008; Galluzzo et al., 2008a).

Thus more attention have to be focus on estrogenicity or antiestrogenicity of these compounds. Estrogenicity *per se* is not an adverse effect, it is a natural mechanism of hormone action controlled via homeostatic mechanisms. However, a chemical with estrogenic properties acting out of context within the endocrine system, or at a vulnerable developmental time-point may have the potential to induce an adverse effect (Fisher et al., 2004). As well as estrogenicity, compounds with antiestrogenic effects could exert both protective or adverse effects depending on cellular context (Galluzzo and Marino, 2006). A current mounting evidence also show that *in utero* and early life phytoestrogen exposure, may promote the onset of breast cancer later in life (Tomar and Shiao, 2008). Thus, more studies are necessary to assess how flavonoid effects impact the normal development and physiological properties of cells at different phases of human life (Somjen et al., 2005; Watson et al., 2005). In particular, their effects in early infant age still deserves special consideration (Virgili and Marino, 2008). Moreover, while several studies are underway to understand how these compounds modulate ER activity, flavonoid interaction and modulation of androgen receptor (AR) is poorly understood. Because of the importance of AR activity in male physiology, also flavonoid interaction and modulation of AR should be considered.

Flavonoids act trough several and distinct action mechanisms (Figure 3). Understanding the cross-talk within these different pathways and the elaborate feedback mechanisms will provide an opportunity to obtain a full picture, which may be relevant to various physiological or pathological states. Assessing phytoestrogen effects at multiple levels, both *in vitro* and *in vivo*, could represent a step towards the employ of these compounds as nutriceuticals able to exert specific responses in target cells or to modulate selectively ER activities in specific target tissues and organs (Galluzzo et al., 2008a).

ACKNOWLEDGMENTS

The Authors wish to thank past and present members of their laboratories who contributed to the ideas presented here through data and discussions.

REFERENCES

Acconcia, F., Ascenzi, P., Bocedi, A., Spisni, E., Tomasi, V., Trentalance, A., Visca, P., and Marino, M. (2005a). Palmitoylation-dependent estrogen receptor α membrane localization: regulation by 17β-estradiol. *Mol. Biol. Cell*, 16, 231-238.

Acconcia, F., Totta, P., Ogawa, S., Cardillo, I., Inoue, S., Leone, S., Trentalance, A., Muramatsu, M., and Marino, M. (2005b). Survival versus apoptotic 17β-estradiol effect: role of ERα and ERβ activated non-genomic signaling. *J. Cell. Physiol.*, 203, 193-201.

Adachi, T., Okuno, Y., Takenaka, S., Matsuda, K., Ohta, N., Takashima, K., Yamazaki, K., Nishimura, D., Miyatake, K., Mori, C., and Tsujimoto, G. (2005). Comprehensive analysis of the effect of phytoestrogen, daidzein, on a testicular cell line, using 1210 mRNA and protein expression profile. *Food Chem. Toxicol.*, 43, 529-535.

Adlercreutz, H., Heinonen, S.M., and Penalvo-Garcia, J. (2004). Phytoestrogens, cancer and coronary heart disease. *Biofactors*, 22, 229-236.

Albini, A., Tosetti, F., Benelli, R., and Noonan, D.M. (2005). Tumor inflammatory angiogenesis and its chemoprevention. *Cancer Res.*, 65, 10637-10641.

Andreadi, C. K., Howells, L.M., Atherfold, P.A., and Manson, M.M. (2006). Involvement of Nrf2, p38, B-Raf, and nuclear factor-κB, but not phosphatidylinositol 3-kinase, in induction of hemeoxygenase-1 by dietary polyphenols. *Mol. Pharmacol.*, 69, 1033-1040.

Ascenzi, P., Bocedi, A., and Marino, M. (2006). Structure-function relationship of estrogen receptor α and β: impact on human health. *Mol. Aspects Med.*, 27, 299-402.

Béliveau, R., and Gingras, D. (2007). Role of nutrition in preventing cancer. *Can. Fam. Physician*, 53, 1905-1911.

Benavente-García, O., and Castillo, J. (2008). Update on uses and properties of citrus flavonoids: new findings in anticancer, cardiovascular, and anti-inflammatory activity. *J. Agric. Food Chem.*, 56, 6185-6205.

Bennetts, H.W., Underwood, E.J., and Shier, F.L. (1946). A specific breeding problem of sheep on subterranean clover pasture in western Australia. *Austr. Vet. J.*, 22, 2-12.

Birt, D.F., Hendrich, S., and Wang, W. (2001). Dietary agents in cancer prevention: flavonoids and isoflavonoids. *Pharmacol. Ther.*, 90, 157-177.

Boots, A.W., Haenen, G.R., and Bast, A. (2008). Health effects of quercetin: from antioxidant to nutraceutical. *Eur. J. Pharmacol.*, 585, 325-337.

Caltagirone, S., Rossi, C., Poggi, A., Ranelletti, F.O., Natali, P.G., Brunetti, M., Aiello, F.B., and Piantelli, M. (2000). Flavonoids apigenin and quercetin inhibit melanoma growth and metastatic potential. *J. Cancer*, 87, 595-600.

Chambliss, K.L., Yuhanna, I.S., Anderson, R.G., Mendelsohn, M. E., and Shaul, P.W. (2002). ERbeta has nongenomic action in caveolae. *Mol. Endo.*, 16, 938-946.

Chao, S.H., Fujinaga, K., Marion, J.E., Taube, R., Sausville, E.A., Senderowicz, A.M., Peterlin B.M., and Price D.H. (2000). Flavopiridol inhibits P-TEFb and blocks HIV-1 replication. *J. Biol. Chem.*, 275, 28345-28348.

Cheynier, V. (2005). Polyphenols in foods are more complex than often thought. *Am. J. Clin. Nutr.*, 81, 223-229.

Chiang, A.N., Wu, H.L., Yeh, H.I., Chu, C.S., Lin, H.C., and Lee, W.C. (2006). Antioxidant effects of black rice extract through the induction of superoxide dismutase and catalase activities. *Lipids*, 41, 797-803.

Conney, A.H. (2003). Enzyme induction and dietary chemicals as approaches to cancer chemoprevention: the seventh DeWitt S. Goodman lecture. *Cancer Res.*, 63, 7005-7031.

Dalu, A., Haskell, J.F., Coward, L., and Lamartiniere, C.A. (1998). Genistein, a component of soy, inhibits the expression of the EGF and ErbB2/Neu receptors in the rat dorsolateral prostate. *Prostate*, 37, 36-43.

Dang, Z.C., Audinot, V., Papapoulos, S.E., Boutin, J.A., and Lowik, C.W. (2003). PPARγ as a molecular target for the soy phytoestrogen genistein. *J. Biol. Chem.*, 278, 962-967.

Dang, Z.C., and Lowik, C. (2005). Dose-dependent effects of phytoestrogens on bone. *Trends Endocrinol. Metab.*, 16, 207-213.

Delclos, K.B., Bucci, T.J., Lomax, L.G., Latendresse, J.R., Warbritton, A., Weis, C.C., and Newbold, R.R. (2001). Effects of dietary genistein exposure during development on male and female CD (Sprague–Dawley) rats. *Reprod. Toxicol.*, 15, 647-663.

Distefano, E., Marino, M., Gillette, J.A., Hanstein, B., Pallottini, V., Bruning, J., Krone, W., and Trentalance, A. (2002). Role of tyrosine kinase signaling in estrogen-induced LDL receptor gene expression in HepG2 cells. *Biochim. Biophys. Acta*, 1580, 145-149.

Doerge, D.R., Twaddle, N.C., Churchwell, M.I., Newbold, R.R., and Delclos, K.B. (2006). Lactational transfer of the soy isoflavone, genistein, in Sprague-Dawley rats consuming dietary genistein. *Reprod. Toxicol.*, 21, 307-312.

El Bedoui, J., Oak, M.H., Anglard, P., and Schini-Kerth, V.B. (2005). Catechins prevent vascular smooth muscle cell invasion by inhibiting MT1-MMP activity and MMP-2 expression. *Cardiovasc. Res.*, 67, 317-325.

Elisaf, M. (2002). Effects of fibrates on serum metabolic parameters. *Curr. Med. Res. Opin.*, 18, 269-276.

Escande, A., Pillon, A., Servant, N., Cravedi, J.P., Larrea, F., Muhn, P., Nicolas, J.C., Cavailles, V., and Balaguer, P. (2006). Evaluation of ligand selectivity using reporter cell lines stably expressing estrogen receptor alpha or beta. *Biochem. Pharmacol.*, 71, 1459-1469.

Espìn, J.C., Garcìa-Conesa, M.T., and Tomàs-Barberàn, F.A. (2007). Nutraceuticals: facts and fiction. *Phytochemistry*, 68, 2986-3008.

Farach-Carson, M.C., and Davis, P.J. (2003). Steroid hormone interactions with target cells: cross talk between membrane and nuclear pathways. *J. Pharmacol. Experimen. Ther.*, 307, 839- 845.

Fenton, J.I., and Hord, N.G. (2004). Flavonoids promote cell migration in nontumorigenic colon epithelial cells differing in Apc genotype: implications of matrix metalloproteinase activity. *Nutr. Cancer*, 48, 182-188.

Filomeni, G., Graziani, I., Rotilio, G., and Ciriolo, M.R. (2007). Trans-resveratrol induces apoptosis in human breast cancer cells MCF-7 by the activation of MAP kinases pathways. *Genes Nutr.*, 2, 295-305.

Fisher, J.S. (2004). Are all EDC effects mediated via steroid hormone receptors? *Toxicol.*, 205, 33-41.

Flynn, K.M., Ferguson, S.A., Delclos, K.B. and Newbold, R.R. (2000). Effects of genistein exposure on sexually dimorphic behaviors in rats. *Toxicol. Sci.*, 55, 311-319.

Galati, G., Moridani, M.Y., Chan, T.S., and O'Brien, P.J. (2001). Peroxidative metabolism of apigenin and naringenin versus luteolin and quercetin: glutathione oxidation and conjugation. *Free Radic. Biol. Med.*, 30, 370-382.

Galati, G., Teng, S., Moridani, M.Y., Chan, T.S., and O'Brien, P.J. (2000). Cancer chemoprevention and apoptosis mechanisms induced by dietary polyphenolics. *Drug Metabol. Drug Interact.*, 17, 311-349.

Galluzzo, P., Ascenzi, P., Bulzomi, P., and Marino, M. (2008). The nutritional flavanone naringenin triggers antiestrogenic effects by regulating estrogen receptor α-palmitoylation. *Endocrinology*, 149, 2567-2575.

Galluzzo, P., Martini, C., Bulzomi, P., Leone, S., Bolli, A., Pallottini, V., and Marino, M. (2008a). Quercitin-induced apoptotic cascade in cancer cells: antioxidant versus estrogen receptor-dependent mechanisms. *Mol. Nutr. Food Res*., In Press.

Galluzzo, P., Caiazza, F., Moreno, S., and Marino, M. (2007). Role of ERbeta palmitoylation in the inhibition of human colon cancer cell proliferation. *Endocr. Relat. Cancer,* 359, 102-107.

Galluzzo, P., and Marino, M. (2006). Nutritional flavonoid impact on nuclear and extranuclear estrogen receptor activities. *Genes Nutr.* 1, 161-176.

Gronemeyer, H., Gustafsson, J.-Å., and Laudet, V. (2004). Principles for modulation of the nuclear receptor superfamily. *Nat. Rev.,Drug Discovery*, 3, 950–964.

Guo, T.L., Germolec, D.R., Musgrove, D.L., Delclos, K.B., Newbold, R.R., Weis, C.C. and White, K.L.Jr. (2005). Myelotoxicity in genistein-, nonylphenol-, methoxychlor-, vinclozolin- or ethinyl estradiol-exposed F1 generations of Sprague-Dawley rats following developmental and adult exposures. *Toxicology,* 211, 207-219.

Hagiwara, M., Inoue, S., Tanaka, T., Nunoki, K., Ito, M., and Hidaka, H. (1988). Differential effects of flavonoids as inhibitors of tyrosine protein kinases and serine/threonine protein kinases. *Biochem. Pharmacol.*, 37, 2987-2992.

Hanasaki, Y., Ogawa, S., and Fukui, S. (1994). The correlation between active oxygens scavenging and antioxidative effects of flavonoids. *Free Rad. Biol. Med.,* 16, 845-850.

Hao, Q., Rutherford, S. A., Low, B., and Tang, H. (2006). Selective regulation of hydrogen peroxide signaling by receptor tyrosine phosphatase-α. *Free Radic. Biol. Med.,* 41, 302-310.

Hehner, S.P., Hofmann, T.G., Dienz, O., Droge, W., and Schmitz, M. L. (2000). Tyrosine-phosphorylated Vav1 as a point of integration for T-cell receptor-and CD28- mediated activation of JNK, p38, and interleukin-2 transcription. *J. Biol. Chem,*. 275, 18160–18171.

Ioannides, C., and Lewis, D. F. (2004). Cytochromes P450 in the bioactivation of chemicals. *Curr. Top. Med. Chem.,* 4, 1767-1788.

Iqbal, M. J., Yaegashi, S., Ahsan, R., Lightfoot, D.A., and Banz, W. J. (2002). Differentially abundant mRNAs in rat liver in response to diets containing soy protein isolate. *Physiol. Genomics,* 11, 219-226.

Jacobs, M.N., and Lewis, D.F. (2002). Steroid hormone receptors and dietary ligands: a selected review. *Proc. Nutr. Soc.*, 61, 105-122.

Jakobs, S., Fridrich, D., Hofem, S., Pahlke, G., and Eisenbrand, G. (2006). Natural flavonoids are potent inhibitors of glycogen phosphorylase. *Mol. Nutr. Food Res.,* 50, 52-57.

Kang Z.C., Tsai S.J., and Lee H. (1999). Quercetin inhibits benzo[*a*]pyrene-induced DNA adducts in human Hep G2 cells by altering cytochrome P-450 1A1 expression. *Nutr. Cancer*, 35, 175-179.

Karunagaran, D., Rashmi, R., and Kumar, T.R. (2005). Induction of apoptosis by curcumin and its implications for cancer therapy. *Curr. Cancer Drug Targets*, 5, 117-129.

Kim, E.J., Choi, C.H., Park, J.Y., Kang, S.K., and Kim, Y.K. (2008). Underlying mechanism of quercetin-induced cell death in human glioma cells. *Neurochem. Res*., 33, 971-979.

Kirk, E.A., Sutherland, P., Wang, S.A., Chait, A., and LeBoeuf, R.C. (1998). Dietary isoflavones reduce plasma cholesterol and atherosclerosis in C57BL/6 mice but not LDL receptor-deficient mice. *J. Nutr.,* 128, 954-959.

Kuiper, G.G., Carlsson, B., Grandien, K., Enmark, E., Häggblad, J., Nilsson. S., and Gustafsson, J.A. (1997). Comparison of the ligand binding specificity and transcript tissue distribution of estrogen receptors α and β. *Endocrinology*, 138, 863-870.

Kweon, M.H., In Park, Y., Sung, H.C., and Mukhtar, H. (2006). The novel antioxidant 3-O-caffeoyl-1-methylquinic acid induces Nrf2-dependent phase II detoxifying genes and alters intracellular glutathione redox. *Free Radic. Biol. Med.,* 40, 1349-1361.

Lee, J. S., and Surh, Y. J. (2005). Nrf2 as a novel molecular target for chemoprevention. *Cancer Lett.* 224, 171-184.

Levin, E.R. (2005). Integration of the extranuclear and nuclear actions of estrogen. *Mol. Endocrinol.*, 19, 1951-1959.

Ling, S., Dai, A., Williams, M.R., Husband, A.J., Nestel, P.J., Komesaroff, P.A., and Sudhir, K. (2004). The isoflavone metabolite cis-tetrahydrodaidzein inhibits ERK-1 activation and proliferation in human vascular smooth muscle cells. *J. Cardiovasc. Pharmacol.*, 435, 622-628.

Liu, M. M., Albanese, C., Anderson, C. M., Hilty, K., Webb, P., Uht, R. M., Price, R. H., Pestell, R. G., and Kushner, P. J. (2002). Opposing action of estrogen receptors a and b on cyclin D1 gene expression. *J. Biol. Chem.,* 277, 24353-24360.

Manach, C., Scalbert, A., Morand, C., Remesy, C., and Jimenez L. (2004). Polyphenols: food sources and bioavailability. *Am. J. Clin. Nutr.,* 79, 727-747.

Manna, S.K., Mukhopadhyay, A. and Aggarwal, B.B. (2000). Resveratrol suppresses TNFα-induced activation of nuclear transcription factors NF-κB, activator protein-1, and apoptosis: potential role of reactiveoxygen intermediates and lipid peroxidation. *J. Immunol.*, 164, 6509-6519.

Manthey, J.A. (2000). Biological properties of flavonoids pertaining to inflammation, *Microcirculation*, 6, 29-34.

Marino, M., Acconcia, F., and Ascenzi P. (2005). Estrogen receptor signalling: bases for drug actions. *Curr Drug Targets Imm. Endo. Metabol. Disorder.*, 5, 305-14.

Mezei, O., Banz, W.J., Steger, R.W., Peluso, M.R., Winters, T.A., and Shay, N. (2003). Soy isoflavones exert antidiabetic and hypolipidemic effects through the PPAR pathways in obese Zucker rats and murine RAW 264.7 cells. *J. Nutr.*, 133, 1238-1243.

Middleton, E.Jr., Kandaswami, C., and Theoharides, T.C. (2000). The effects of plant flavonoids on mammalian cells: implications for inflammation, heart disease, and cancer. *Pharmacol. Rev.*, 52, 673-751.

Miyoshi, N., Naniwa, K., Yamada, T., Osawa, T., and Nakamura, Y. (2007). Dietary flavonoid apigenin is a potential inducer of intracellular oxidative stress: The role in the interruptive apoptotic signal, *Arch. Biochem. Biophys.*, 466, 274-82.

Mnif, W., Pascussi, J. M., Pillon, A., Escande, A., Bartegi, A., Nicolas, J. C., Cavaillès, V., Duchesne, M.J., and Balaguer, P. (2007). Estrogens and antiestrogens activate hPXR. *Toxicol. Lett.,* 170, 19-29.

Moore, J.T., and Kliewer, S.A. (2000).Use of the nuclear receptor PXR to predict drug interactions. *Toxicol.,* 153, 1-10.

Morrissey C., O'Neill A., Spengler B., Christoffel V., Fitzpatrick J.M., and Watson R.W. (2005). Apigenin drives the production of reactive oxygen species and initiates a mitochondrial mediated cell death pathway in prostate epithelial cells. *Prostate,* 63, 131-142.

Moskaug, J.O., Carlsen, H., Myhrstad, M.C., and Blomhoff, R. (2005). Polyphenols and glutathione synthesis regulation. *Am. J. Clin. Nutr.*, 81, 277-283.

Mueller, S. O. (2002). Overview of in vitro tools to assess the estrogenic and antiestrogenic activity of phytoestrogens. *J. Chromatogr.*, 777, 155-165.

Mueller, S.O., Simon, S., Chae, K., Metzler, M., and Korach, K.S. (2004). Phytoestrogens and their human metabolites show distinct agonistic and antagonistic properties on estrogen receptor alpha (ERalpha) and ERbeta in human cells. *Toxicol. Sci.*, 80, 14-25.

Nilsson, S., Makela, S., Treuter, E., Tujague, M., Thomsen, J., Andersson, G., Enmark, E., Pettersson, K., Warner, M., and Gustafsson, J.-Å. (2001). Mechanism of estrogen action, *Physiol. Rev.*, 81, 1535-1565.

Nomura, M., Takahashi, T., Nagata, N., Tsutsumi, K., Kobayashi, S., Akiba, T., Yokogawa, K., Moritani, S., and Miyamoto, K. (2008). Inhibitory mechanisms of flavonoids on insulin-stimulated glucose uptake in MC3T3-G2/PA6 adipose cells. *Biol. Pharm. Bull.*, 31, 1403-9.

O'Brien P.J. (2000). Peroxidases, *Chem. Biol. Interact.*, 129, 113-139.

O'Loghlen, A., Perez-Morgado, M.I., Salinas, M., and Martin, M.E. (2003). Reversible inhibition of the protein phosphatase 1 by hydrogen peroxide: potential regulation of eIF2α phosphorylation in differentiated PC12 cells. *Arch. Biochem. Biophys.*, 417, 194-202.

Pellegatta, F., Bertelli, A.A.E., Staels, B., Duhem, C., Fulgenzi, A., and Ferrero, M.E. (2003). Different short- and long-term effects of resveratrol on nuclear factor-kappaB phosphorylation and nuclear appearance in human endothelial cells. *Am. J. Clin. Nutr.*, 77, 1220-1228.

Peterson, G., Barnes, S. (1993). Genistein and biochanin A inhibit the growth of human prostate cancer cells but not epidermal growth factor receptor tyrosine autophosphorylation. *Prostate,* 22, 335-345.

Peterson, G., Barnes, S. (1996). Genistein inhibits both estrogen and growth factor-stimulated proliferation of human breast cancer cells. *Cell Growth Differ.*, 7, 1345-1351.

Rice, S., and Whitehead, S.A. (2006). Phytoestrogens and breast cancer-promoters or protectors?, *Endocr. Relat. Cancer*, 13, 995-1015.

Ricketts, M.L., Moore, D.D., Banz, W.J., Mezei, O., and Shay, N.F. (2005). Molecular mechanisms of action of the soy isoflavones includes activation of promiscuous nuclear receptors. *J. Nutr. Biochem.*, 16, 321-330.

Saarinen, N.M., Mäkelä, S., Penttinen, P., Wärri, A., Lorenzetti, S., Virgili, F., Mortensen, A., Sørensen, I.K., Bingham, C., Valsta, L.M., Vollmer, G., and Zierau, O. (2006). Tools to evaluate estrogenic potency of dietary phytoestrogens: a consensus paper from the EU Thematic Network "Phytohealth" (QLKI-2002-2453). *Genes Nutr.,* 1, 143-158.

Shay, N. F., and Banz, W. J. (2005). Regulation of gene transcription by botanicals: novel regulatory mechanisms. *Ann. Rev. Nutr.,* 25, 297-315.

Somjen, D., Kohen, E., Lieberherr, M., Gayer, B., Schejter, E., Katzburg, S., Limor, R., Sharon, O., Knoll, E., Posner, G.H., Kaye, A.M., and Stern, N. (2005). Membranal effects of phytoestrogens and carboxy derivatives of phytoestrogens on human vascular and bone cells: new insights based on studies with carboxy-biochanin. *A. J. Steroid Biochem. Mol. Biol.,* 93, 293-303.

Spencer, J.P., Rice-Evans, C., Williams, R.J. (2003). Modulation of pro-survival Akt/protein kinase B and ERK1/2 signaling cascades by quercetin and its in vivo metabolites underlie their action on neuronal viability. *J. Biol. Chem.*, 278, 34783-34793.

Stevens, J.F., and Page, J. E. (2004). Xanthohumol and related prenylflavonoids from hops and beer: to your good health!, *Phytochem.*, 65, 1317-1330.

Stevenson, D.E., and Hurst, R.D. (2007). Polyphenolic phytochemicals-just antioxidants or much more?, *Cell Mol. Life Sci.*, 64, 2900-2916.

Stone, J.R., and Yang, S. (2006). Hydrogen peroxide: a signaling messenger. *Antioxid. Redox Signaling,* 8, 243-270.

Suetsugi, M., Su, L., Karlsberg, K., Yuan, Y.C., and Chen, S. (2003). Flavone and isoflavone phytoestrogens are agonists of estrogen-related receptors. *Mol. Cancer Res.*, 1, 981-991.

Surh, Y.J. (2003). Cancer chemoprevention with dietary phytochemicals. *Nat. Rev. Cancer,* 3, 768-780.

Terasaka, S., Aita, Y., Inoue, A., Hayashi, S., Nishigaki, M., Aoyagi, K., Sasaki, H., Wada-Kiyama, Y., Sakuma, Y., Akaba, S., Tanaka, J., Sone, H., Yonemoto, J., Tanji, M., and Kiyama, R.U. (2004). Using a customized DNA microarray for expression profiling of the estrogen-responsive genes to evaluate estrogen activity among naturalestrogens and industrial chemicals. *Environ. Health Perspect.,* 112, 773-781.

Tomar, R.S,. and Shiao, R. (2008). Early Life and Adult Exposure to Isoflavones and Breast Cancer Risk. *J. Environ. Sci. Health C. Environ. Carcinog. Ecotoxicol. Rev.*, 26, 113-73.

Totta, P., Acconcia, F., Leone, S., Cardillo, I., and Marino, M. (2004). Mechanisms of naringenin-induced apoptotic cascade in cancer cells: involvement of estrogen receptor α and β signalling. *IUBMB Life,* 56, 491-499.

Totta, P., Acconcia, F., Virgili, F., Cassidy, A., Weinberg, P.D., Rimbach, G., and Marino, M. (2005). Daidzein-sulfate metabolites affect transcriptional and antiproliferative activities of estrogen receptor-beta in cultured human cancer cells. *J. Nutr.,* 135, 2687-2693.

Ueda, S., Nakamura, H., Masutani, H., Sasada, T., Takabayashi, A., Yamaoka, Y., and Yodoi, J. (2002). Baicalin induces apoptosis via mitochondrial pathway as prooxidant, *Mol. Immunol.*, 38, 781-91.

Ursini, F., Maiorino, M., Morazzoni, P., Roveri, A., and Pifferi, G. (1994). A novel antioxidant flavonoid (IdB 1031) affecting molecular mechanisms of cellular activation. *Free Rad. Biol. Med.*, 16, 547-553.

Vargo M.A., Voss O.H., Poustka F., Cardounel A.J., Grotewold E., and Doseff A.I. (2006). Apigenin-induced-apoptosis is mediated by the activation of PKCδ and caspases in leukemia cells. *Biochem. Pharmacol.*, 72, 681-692.

Virgili, F., and Marino, M. (2008). Regulation of cellular signals from nutritional molecules: a specific role for phytochemicals, beyond antioxidant activity. *Free Radic. Biol. Med.,* 45, 1205-1216.

Virgili, F., Acconcia, F., Ambra, R., Rinna, A., Totta, P., and Marino, M. (2004). Nutritional flavonoids modulate estrogen receptor α signaling. *IUBMB Life,* 56, 145-151.

Wang I.K., Lin-Shiau S.Y., and Lin J.K. (1999). Induction of apoptosis by apigenin and related flavonoids through cytochrome c release and activation of caspase-9 and caspase-3 in leukaemia HL-60 cells. *Eur. J. Cancer*, 35, 1517-1525.

Wang, H., Huang, H., Li, H., Teotico, D.G., Sinz, M., Baker, S.D., Staudinger, J., Kalpana, G., Redinbo, M.R., and Mani, S. (2007). Activated pregnenolone X-receptor is a target for ketoconazole and its analogs. *Clin. Cancer Res.,* 13, 2488-2495.

Watson, C.S., Bulayeva, N.N., Wozniak, A.L., and Finnerty, C.C. (2005). Signaling from the membrane via membrane estrogen receptor-alpha: estrogens, xenoestrogens and phytoestrogens. *Steroids,* 70, 364-371.

Wung B.S., Hsu M.C., Wu C.C., and Hsieh C.W. (2005). Resveratrol suppresses IL-6-induced ICAM-1 gene expression in endothelial cells: Effects on the inhibition of STAT3 phosphorylation. *Life Sciences,* 78, 389-397.

Zhang, X., Shu, X.O., Gao, Y., Yang, G., Li, Q., Li, H., Jin, F., and Zheng, W. (2003). Soy food consumption is associated with lower risk of coronory heart disease in Chinese women. *J. Nutr.*, 133, 2874-2878.

In: Flavonoids: Biosynthesis, Biological Effects… ISBN: 978-1-60741-622-7
Editor: Raymond B. Keller

Chapter 8

ANTIOPHIDIAN MECHANISMS OF MEDICINAL PLANTS

Rafael da Silva Melo[1], Nicole Moreira Farrapo[1], Dimas dos Santos Rocha Junior[1,4], Magali Glauzer Silva[1], José Carlos Cogo[2], Cháriston André Dal Belo[3], Léa Rodrigues-Simioni[4], Francisco Carlos Groppo[5] and Yoko Oshima-Franco*[1,4]

[1]Universidade de Sorocaba, UNISO, Sorocaba, São Paulo, Brazil
[2]Universidade do Vale do Paraiba, UNIVAP, São José dos Campos, São Paulo, Brazil
[3]Universidade Federal do Pampa, São Gabriel, RS, Brazil
[4]Universidade Estadual de Campinas, UNICAMP, Campinas, São Paulo, Brazil
[5]Universidade Estadual de Campinas, UNICAMP, Piracicaba, São Paulo, Brazil

ABSTRACT

Vegetal extracts usually have a large diversity of bioactive compounds showing several pharmacological activities, including antiophidian properties. In this study, both coumarin and tannic acid (100 μg/mL) showed no changes in the basal response of twitches in mouse nerve phrenic diaphragm preparations. In opposite, *Crotalus durissus terrificus* (Cdt 15 μg/mL) or *Bothrops jararacussu* (Bjssu 40 μg/mL) venoms caused irreversible neuromuscular blockade. Tannic acid (preincubated with the venoms), but not coumarin, was able to significantly inhibit ($p<0.05$) the impairment of the muscle strength induced by Cdt (88 ± 8%) and Bjssu (79 ± 7.5%), respectively. A remarkable precipitation was observed when the venoms were preincubated with tannic acid, but not with coumarin. *Plathymenia reticulata* is a good source of tannins and flavonoids whereas *Mikania laevigata* contain high amounts of coumarin. *P. reticulata* (PrHE, 0.06 mg/mL) and *M. laevigata* (MlHE, 1 mg/mL) hydroalcoholic extracts were assayed with or without Bjssu or Cdt venoms. Both PrHE and MlHE showed protection against Bjssu (79.3 ± 9.5% and 65 ± 8%, respectively) and Cdt (73.2 ± 6.7% and 95 ± 7%, respectively) neuromuscular blockade. In order to observe if the protective mechanism could be induced by protein precipitation, tannins were eliminated from both extracts and

* Phone: +55 15 2101 7000 - Fax: +55 15 2101 7112, E-mail: yofranco@terra.com.br

the assay was repeated. MlHE protected against the blockade induced by Bjssu (57.2 ± 6.7%), but not against Cdt. We concluded that plants containing tannins could induce the precipitation of venoms' proteins and plants containing coumarin showed activity against *Bothrops* venoms, but not against *Crotalus* venoms. We also concluded that the use of isolated bioactive compounds could not represent the better strategy against ophidian venoms, since the purification may exclude some bioactive components resulting in a loss of antivenom activity. In addition, *M. laevigata* showed better antiophidian activity than *P. reticulata*.

Keywords: *Bothrops jararacussu*, *Crotalus durissus terrificus*, medicinal plant.

INTRODUCTION

The use of medicinal plants has been practiced for many generations. In addition, plants had contributed for the development of many valuable substances such as morphine, the principal alkaloid in opium and the prototype opiate analgesic and narcotic; vincristine, the antitumor alkaloid isolated from *Vinca Rosea*; rutin, a flavonol glycoside found in many plants, used therapeutically to decrease capillary fragility [4].

The animal kingdom constitutes another interesting source of investigation, mainly venomous animals, first due to its pathological effects caused by envenomation and second by the therapeutical possibilities of their constituents. For example, bradykinin, a nonapeptide messenger enzymatically produced from kallidin in the blood, is derived from *Bothrops jararaca* venom [21].

Many people have been seeking complementary and alternative medicines as an adjunct to conventional therapies. There is a renewed interest in the therapeutic potential of venoms from bees, snakes and scorpions or sea-anemones toxins [23]. Salmosin, a desintegrin derived from snake venom that contains the Arg-Gly-Asp (RGD) sequence, was reported to be both antiangiogenic and anti-tumorigenic [18].

The natural resources are the largest reservoir of drugs [29], and the investigation of substances with therapeutic effects has been performed by isolation, extraction and/or purification of new compounds of vegetable origin [1]. Nowadays, there are many sophisticated - but yet very expensive, laborious and long-time demanding – methods to obtain these new compounds from plant or animal origin.

One of the most used experimental models to test pharmacological and antivenom properties of new compounds is the nerve phrenic diaphragm preparations isolated from rats [3], which was also modified for mice. Anatomically and physiologically this preparation represents the nerve-muscle synapse and the muscular contraction, respectively. Pharmacological effects can be showed by blockade, facilitation or contracture, among other possibilities. *B. jararacussu* venom, for example, causes both neuromuscular blockade and severe local myonecrosis.

Mikania laevigata, popularly known as "guaco", is related to *Mikania glomerata* Sprengel, being both used to treat respiratory diseases. Both have pharmacological activities attributed to coumarin [5, 12, 20, 24]. The main difference between the two species is the flowering period: *M. laevigata* flourishes in September and *M. glomerata* in January [24].

Some authors have also attributed an antiophidian property against brazilian snake venoms to *M. glomerata* [20, 28], but this property was not studied in *M. laevigata*.

Plathymenia reticulata Benth, popularly known as "vinhático", is a plant from Brazilian "cerrado" that has anti-inflammatory properties, and a previous phytochemical study identified tannins and flavonoids as its principal constituents [11].

The aim of the present study was to investigate the neutralizing ability of two commercial phytochemicals (tannic acid and coumarin) against the neuromuscular blockade induced by two crude snake venoms - *Bothrops jararacussu* and *Crotalus durissus terrificus*. In addition, hydroalcoholic extracts from plants containing tannic acid (*Plathymenia reticulata* Benth) and coumarin (*Mikania laevigata* Schultz Bip. ex Baker) were assayed against *B. jararacussu* venom.

Materials and Methods

Animals

Male Swiss white mice (26-32 g) were supplied by Anilab - Animais de Laboratório (Paulínia, São Paulo, Brazil). The animals were housed at 25 ± 3°C on a 12-h light/dark cycle and had access to food and water *ad libitum*. This project (protocol number A078/CEP/2007) was approved by the institutional Committee for Ethics in Research of Vale do Paraiba University (UNIVAP), and the experiments were carried out according to the guidelines of the Brazilian College for Animal Experimentation.

Venoms

Crude venoms were obtained from adults *Bothrops jararacussu* (Bjssu) and *Crotalus durissus terrificus* (Cdt) snakes (Serpentário do Centro de Estudos da Natureza) and certified by Prof. Dr. José Carlos Cogo, Vale do Paraíba University (UNIVAP, São José dos Campos, SP, Brazil).

Phytochemicals

Tannic acid and coumarin were purchased from Sigma-Aldrich (USA) and used as standard phytochemicals.

M. Laevigata Extract

The leaves of *M. laevigata* (1 kg) were harvested from plants at the University of Sorocaba (UNISO) herbarium. A voucher specimen was deposited in the UNISO herbarium. The powder (1 kg) obtained from *M. laevigata* leaves were percolated during 10 days in 50% hydroalcoholic solution. After this period, the solution was dried at 40°C by using forced air circulation (dryer Marconi, São Paulo, Brazil) and crushed (10 Mesh, 1.70 mm) by using a macro mill (type Wiley, MA 340 model, Marconi, São Paulo, Brazil). After this procedure,

50% hydroalcoholic solution (Synth, São Paulo, Brazil) was added until complete extraction (when the solution was incolor). Then, the extract was evaporated until dryness by using a rotatory evaporator (Tecnal, São Paulo, Brazil) at 50 °C. The resulting powder (131.68g) was stored at room temperature and protected from light and humidity until the assays.

P. Reticulata Extract

The barks from *P. reticulata* were collected in October 2006 in Miracema city, Tocantins State, Brazil. A specimen was deposited (protocol NRHTO 3327) at the herbarium of Federal University of Tocantins (UFT). The barks were dehydrated in a stove at 37°C during 48 hours, powdered, ground in a mill, macerated with alcohol (70%) during 24 hours and percolated in order to obtain a 20% (m/v) hydroalcoholic extract [27].

Protein Precipitation Assay and Tannins Determination

The proteins in the extract solutions were precipitated [14] with 1.0 mg/mL bovine serum albumine (BSA, fraction V, Sigma) solution in 0.2 M acetate buffer (pH 4.9). After centrifugation, the precipitate was dissolved in sodium dodecyl sulfate (Sigma)/triethanolamine (Merck) solution and the tannins were complexed with $FeCl_3$. The supernatant of each extract (containing free tannins) was used for venom neutralizing assays, and the coloring complex was spectrophotometrically read at 510 nm for tannins determination [13, 14]. The tannin concentration in the samples was measured through a standard curve obtained by a polynomial regression $y=1.754x-0.1253$ ($R^2=0.9971$). Tannic acid was used for the standard curve. All solutions were analyzed in triplicate.

Thin Layer Chromatography

Aliquots of the *M. laevigata* and *P. reticulata* hydroalcoholic extracts (MlHE and PrHE, respectively) were spotted in thin-layer silica gel plates (0.3 mm thick, Merck, Germany) with appropriate standards [15, 30]. The solvent system consisted of acetone:chloroform:formic acid (10:75:8, v/v). The phytochemical groups used as standards (1% methanol - m/v, Sigma-Aldrich, USA) were coumarin and tannic acid. The separated spots were visualized with NP/PEG as following: 5% (v/v) ethanolic NP (diphenylboric acid 2-aminoethyl ester, Sigma, Switzerland) followed by 5% (v/v) ethanolic PEG 4000 (polyethylene glycol 4000, Synth, Brazil), being visualized under U.V. light at 360 nm. The retention factor (Rf) of each standard was compared with those spots exhibited by both extracts obtained from *M. laevigata* and *P. reticulata*.

Mouse Phrenic Nerve-Diaphragm Muscle (PND) Preparation

The phrenic nerve-diaphragm muscle [3] was obtained from mice previously anesthetized with halotane and sacrificed by exsanguination. The diaphragm was removed and mounted under a tension of 5 g in a 5 mL organ bath containing aerated Tyrode solution (control).

After equalization with 95% O_2 and 5% CO_2, the pH of this solution was 7.0. The preparations were indirectly stimulated with supramaximal stimuli (4 x threshold, 0.06 Hz, 0.2 ms) delivered from a stimulator (model ESF-15D, Ribeirão Preto, Brazil) to the nerve by bipolar electrodes. Isometric twitch tension was recorded with a force displacement transducer (cat. 7003, Ugo Basile), coupled to a 2-Channel Recorder Gemini physiograph device (cat. 7070, Ugo Basile) via a Basic Preamplifier (cat. 7080, Ugo Basile). PND preparations were allowed to stabilize for at least 20 min before the addition of one of the following solutions: Tyrode solution (control, n=7); phytochemicals (tannic acid or coumarin, 100 mg/mL, n=6 each); venoms (Bjssu 40 µg/mL, n=10; Cdt 15 µg/mL, n=7); *P. reticulata* hydroalcoholic extract (PrHE, 0.06 mg/mL, n=8) or *M. laevigata* hydroalcoholic extract (MlHE, 1 mg/mL, n=5). The neutralization assays were carried out after preincubating the PND preparations with the Tyrode solution during 30 min. After preincubation, the following substances were added to the bath: phytochemicals + Cdt or Bjssu (n=6, each); MlHE + Bjssu ou Cdt venoms (n=19 and 6, respectively); PrHE + Bjssu or Cdt venoms (n=8 and 5, respectively). In order to verify the influence of tannins on the venoms neutralization, extracts free of tannins (-) were also assayed against the crude venoms.

Experimental Design

The rationale experimental design is bellow presented (Figure 1).

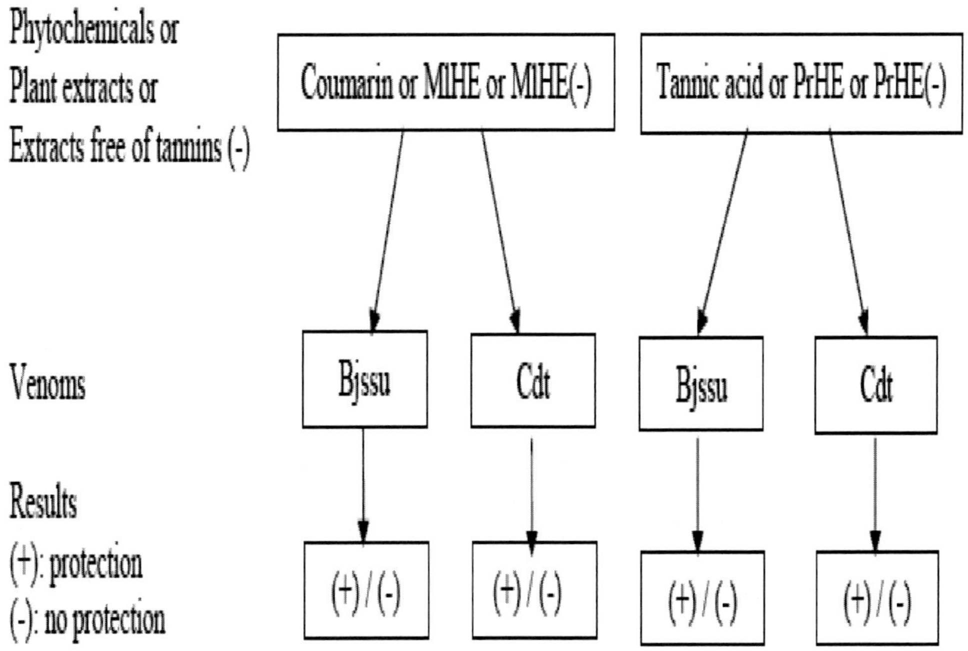

Figure 1. Experimental design showing the rationale steps of the study on the isolated preparation.

Statistical Analysis

Each pharmacological protocol was repeated at least five times. The results were expressed as the mean ± S.E.M. Student's *t*-test was used for statistical comparison of the data and the significance level was set at 5%.

Results and Discussion

Medicinal plants with inhibitory properties against snake venoms have been extensively studied and excellent reviews have been published [19, 32]. Searches focusing the source (leaves, branches, stems, roots, rhizomes, seeds, barks, aerial parts or whole) that concentrates the major bioactive compound, which is able to neutralizing the toxicological effects of venomous snake, have been received special attention [10, 25, 33].

The isolation of bioactive compound usually involves extensive and laborious work using high amount of solvents and expensive techniques such as nuclear magnetic resonance coupled to mass spectrum that is only available in big research facilities.

When a plant extract shows some pharmacological action, it has been required the same evidence by its bioactive compound. Cintra-Francischinelli et al. [8] showed that the methanolic extract from Casearia sylvestris Sw. has inhibitory effect against the in vitro neurotoxicity and myotoxicity of Bothrops jararacussu venom and its major toxin, bothropstoxin-I. Although the authors showed rutin as an important component in the methanol extract of C. sylvestris, the isolated rutin in its commercial form did not protect against the toxic effects of both venom and toxin.

Based on these observations, a reverse strategy was hypothesized using initially two commercial phytochemical standards (tannic acid and coumarin) against two snake venoms: *Bothrops jararacussu* (Bjssu) and *Crotalus durissus terrificus* (Cdt). The same protocol was also repeated with selected hydroalcoholic extracts from *Plathymenia reticulata*, which has tannins and flavonoids [11], and *Mikania laevigata*, which has coumarin [9]. The standard phytochemicals at concentration of 100 μg/mL caused no change on the basal response of neuromuscular preparation, and this concentration was chosen for further neutralization assays against the characteristic blockade induced by Bjssu (Figure 2A) and Cdt (Figure 2B) venoms.

Only tannic acid was able to neutralizing the paralysis of both venoms ($^*p<0.05$, compared to the respective venoms). During the incubation time only tannic acid showed a precipitate formation (Figure 3), which was more intense when incubated with Cdt than with Bjssu venom, which in turn showed a certain turbidity level. The formation of a precipitate due to a protein complex formation caused by tannic acid maybe could cause loss of venom toxicity. Kuppusamy and Das [17] also found evidences of the protective effects of tannic acid, when injected subcutaneously, against lethal activity, haemorrhage and creatine kinase release that are induced in mice submitted to poisoning with *Crotalus adamanteus* venom. Pithayanakul et al. [26] investigated the *in vitro* venom neutralizing capacity of tannic acid against the activities of *Naja kaouthia* (*Naja naja kaouthia* Lesson - Elapidae).

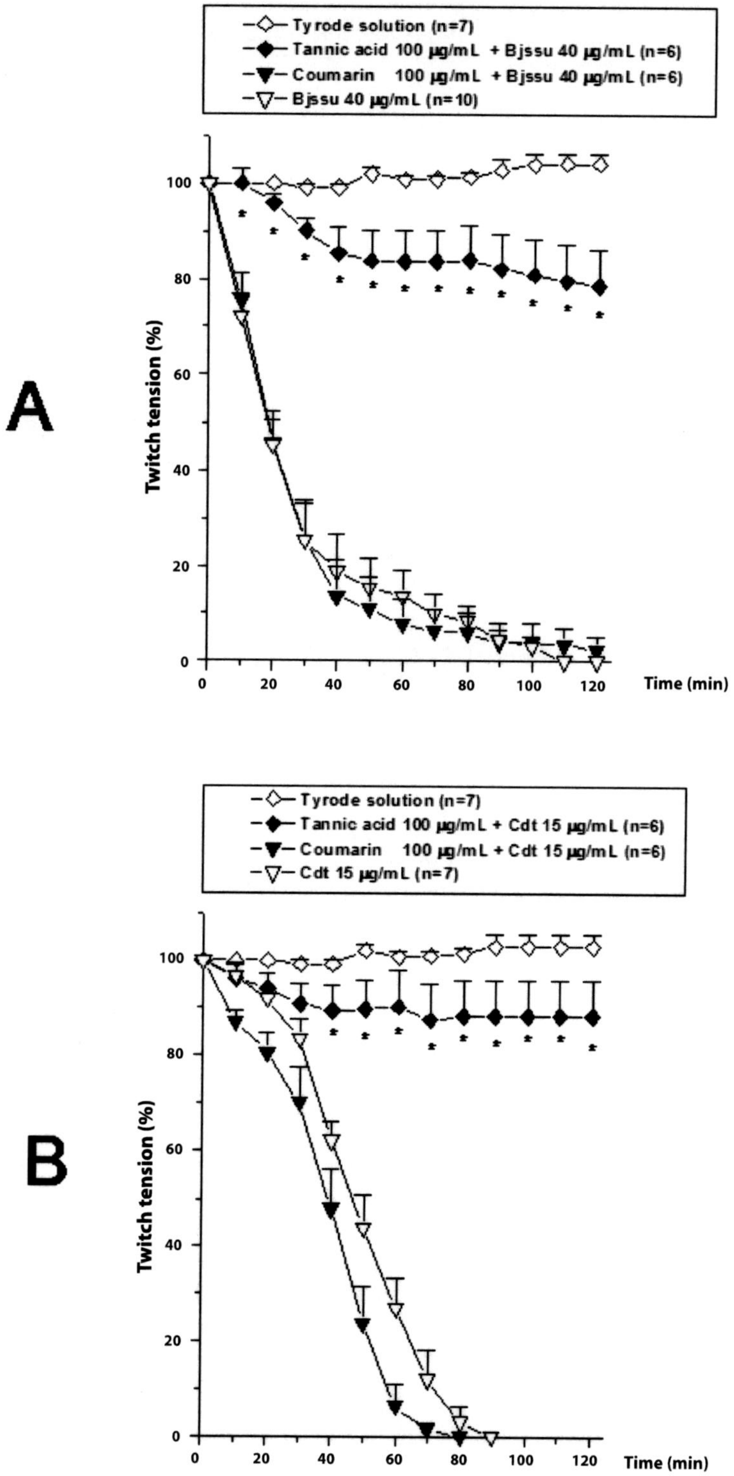

Figure 2. Pharmacological assays on mouse phrenic nerve-diaphragm preparations (indirect stimuli). Neutralization of *Bothrops jararacussu* venom (A, Bjssu), and *Crotalus durissus terrificus* venom (B, Cdt) by tannic acid and coumarin. Each point represents the mean ± S.E.M. of the number of experiments (n) showed in the legend. **p*<0.05 compared to venom.

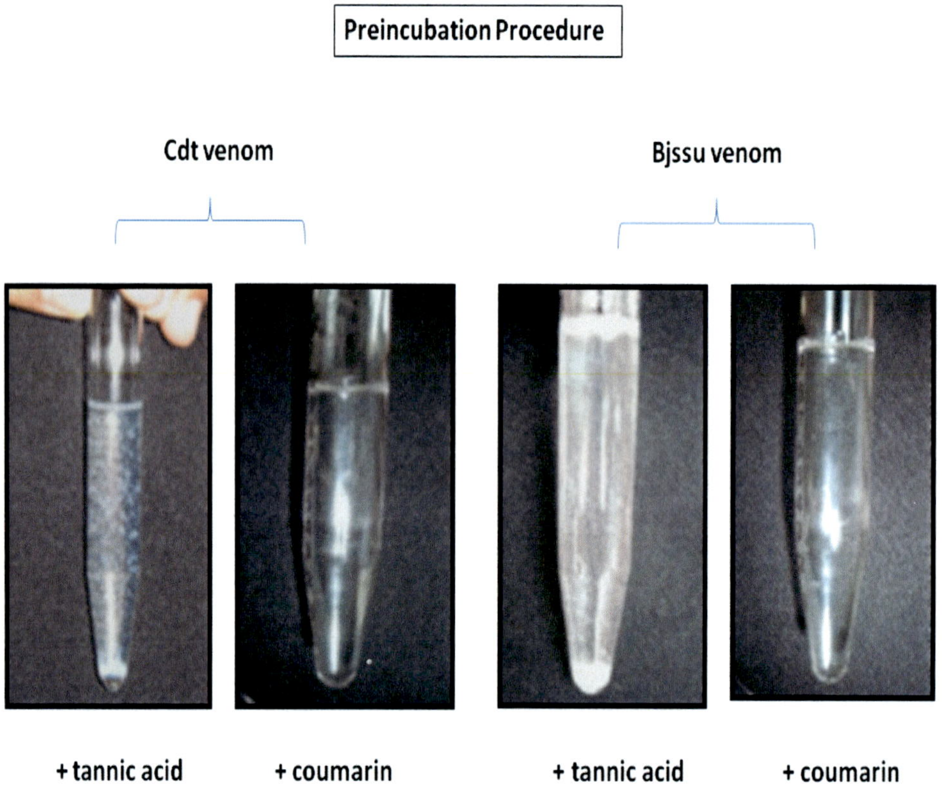

Figure 3. Preincubation procedure. *Crotalus durissus terrificus* venom (Cdt) or *Bothrops jararacussu* venom (Bjssu) were preincubated with tannic acid or coumarin, 30 min prior the pharmacological assays. Note that tannic acid causes a visible protein precipitation, but not coumarin.

PrHE (1) showed two different substances with retention factor (Rf) of 1.8 cm and 5.2 cm. Tannic acid (2) showed substances with Rf of 1.9 cm and 4.5 cm. MlHE (6) showed four substances with Rf 4.3 cm, 5.5 cm, 8.5 cm and 9.0 cm. Under the solvent and revelator systems used, commercial coumarin was not visualized (5). When tannins were complexed with bovine serum albumin (BSA), no substance was visualized in 3, 4 and 7, respectively free of tannins (-), PrHE (-) and MlHE (-).

The pharmacological results using extracts free of tannins (-) are showed in Figure 6. Note that only MlHE (-) partially protected against the paralysis of Bjssu venom (Figure 6A), but not against Cdt venom (Figure 6B). It is known that *in vivo* Cdt venom triggers different mechanism of action than Bjssu. The neurotoxicity induced by the *Crotalus* genus is attributed to crotoxin, the main toxin from this venom [2, 7, 31], whereas the *Bothrops* genus is mainly myotoxic [22], due its main toxin, bothropstoxin-I [16]. Maybe plants having coumarin could inhibit phospholipases with no catalytic activity (Lys49PLA$_2$), as those found in Bjssu venom, but they are not able to avoid the action of Asp49PLA$_2$ triggered by Cdt venom. Similar understanding was related by Cavalcante et al. [6] regarding to the ability of aqueous extract of *Casearia sylvestris* against snake venoms phospholipase A$_2$ toxins.

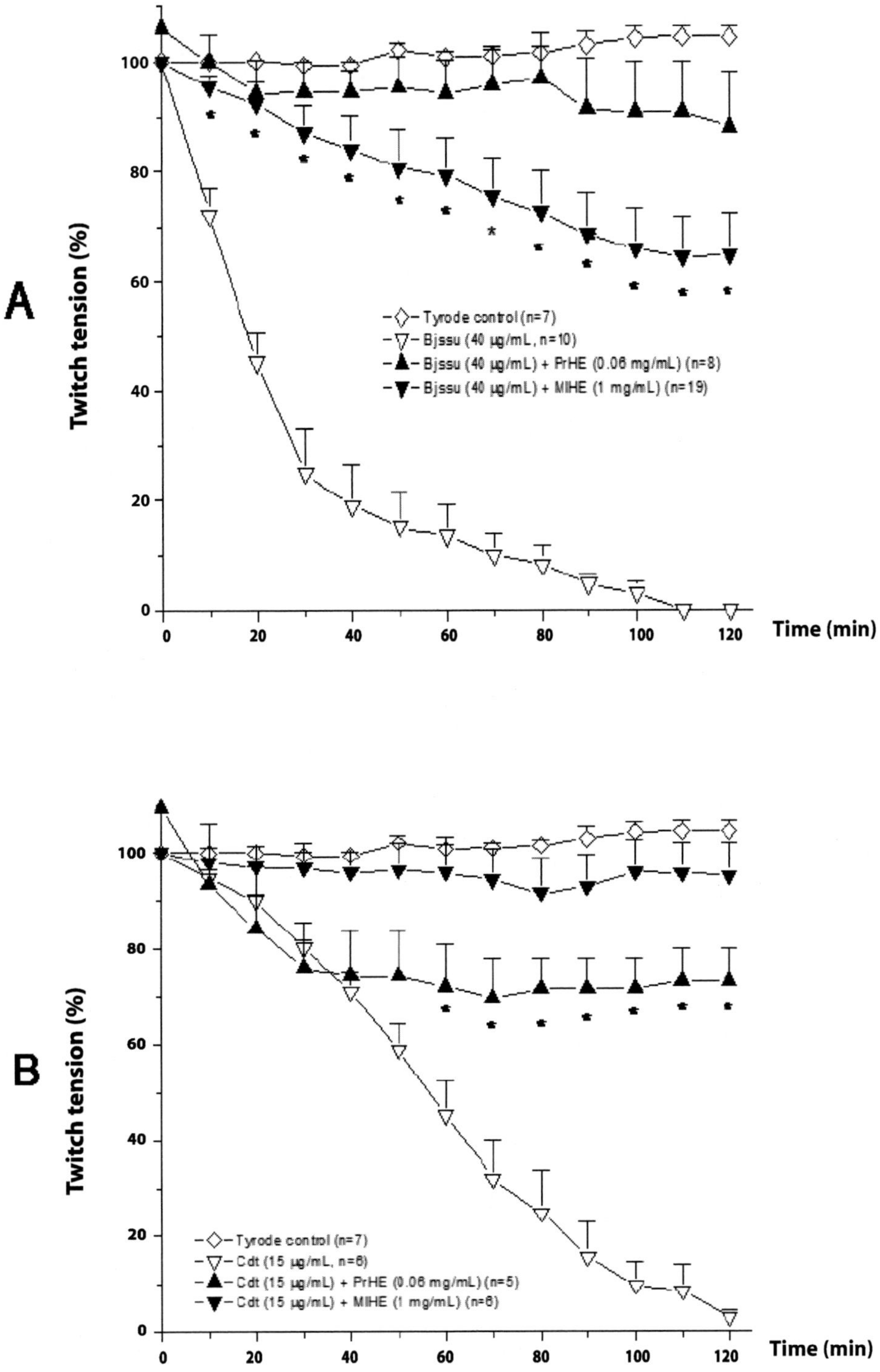

Figure 4. Pharmacological assays on mouse phrenic nerve-diaphragm preparations (indirect stimuli). Neutralization of Bothrops jararacussu venom (A, Bjssu), and Crotalus durissus terrificus venom (B, Cdt) by P. reticulata (PrHE) and M. laevigata (MlHE) hydroalcoholic extracts. Each point represents the mean ± S.E.M. of the number of experiments (n) showed in legend. *$p<0.05$ compared to venom.

The isolation of substances from potential medicinal plants, even at high costs, to try to keep their pharmacological effect at the end of the process is a modern tendency. We presented a rationale experimental design, which tests probably phytochemicals before their commercial availability. Our results showed that isolated compounds not always preserve the same pharmacological efficacy as that seen with total extract.The results allowed proposing the following different mechanisms by which plants can neutralize crude venoms: 1) complexing proteins *in vitro* (as verified in tannic acid) or 2) mechanistically by a phytocomplex formation.

We also observed the interference of phytochemicals free of tannins (-) such as the ones showed in the chromatoplaque (Figure 5).

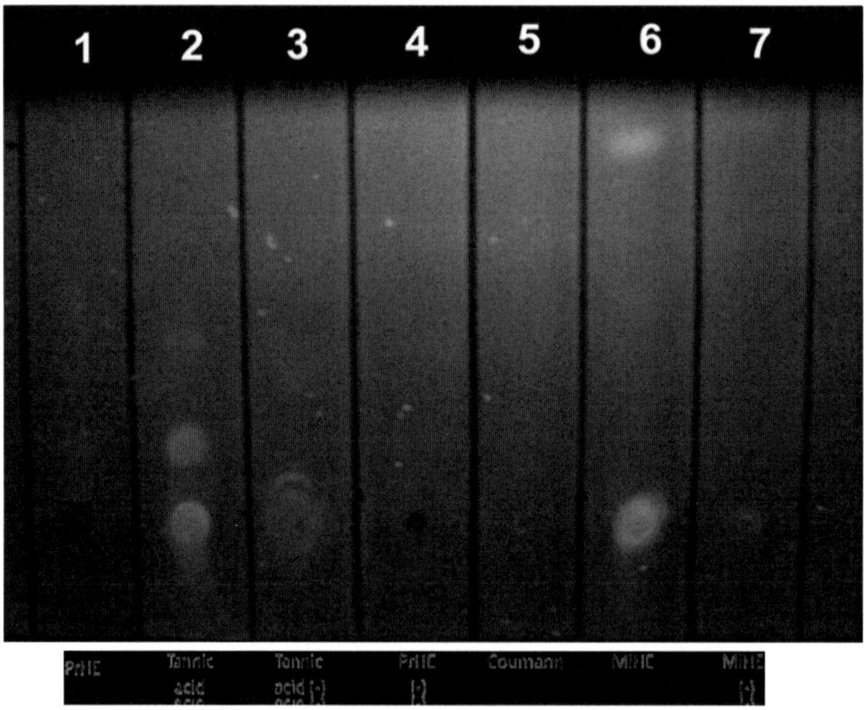

Figure 5. Thin layer chromatography. Extracts + phytochemicals with ou without tannins (-). Chromatographic profile of (1) or *M. laevigata* (6) hydroalcoholic extracts. Phytochemicals are showed in 2 (tannic acid) and 5 (coumarin). The withdrawal of tannins (-) from the tannic acid and *P. reticulata* and *M. laevigata* hydroalcoholic extracts and are showed in 3, 4 and 7, respectively.

The isolation of substances from potential medicinal plants, even at high costs, to try to keep their pharmacological effect at the end of the process is a modern tendency. We presented a rationale experimental design, which tests probably phytochemicals before their commercial availability. Our results showed that isolated compounds not always preserve the same pharmacological efficacy as that seen with total extract.The results allowed proposing the following different mechanisms by which plants can neutralize crude venoms: 1) complexing proteins *in vitro* (as verified in tannic acid) or 2) mechanistically by a phytocomplex formation.

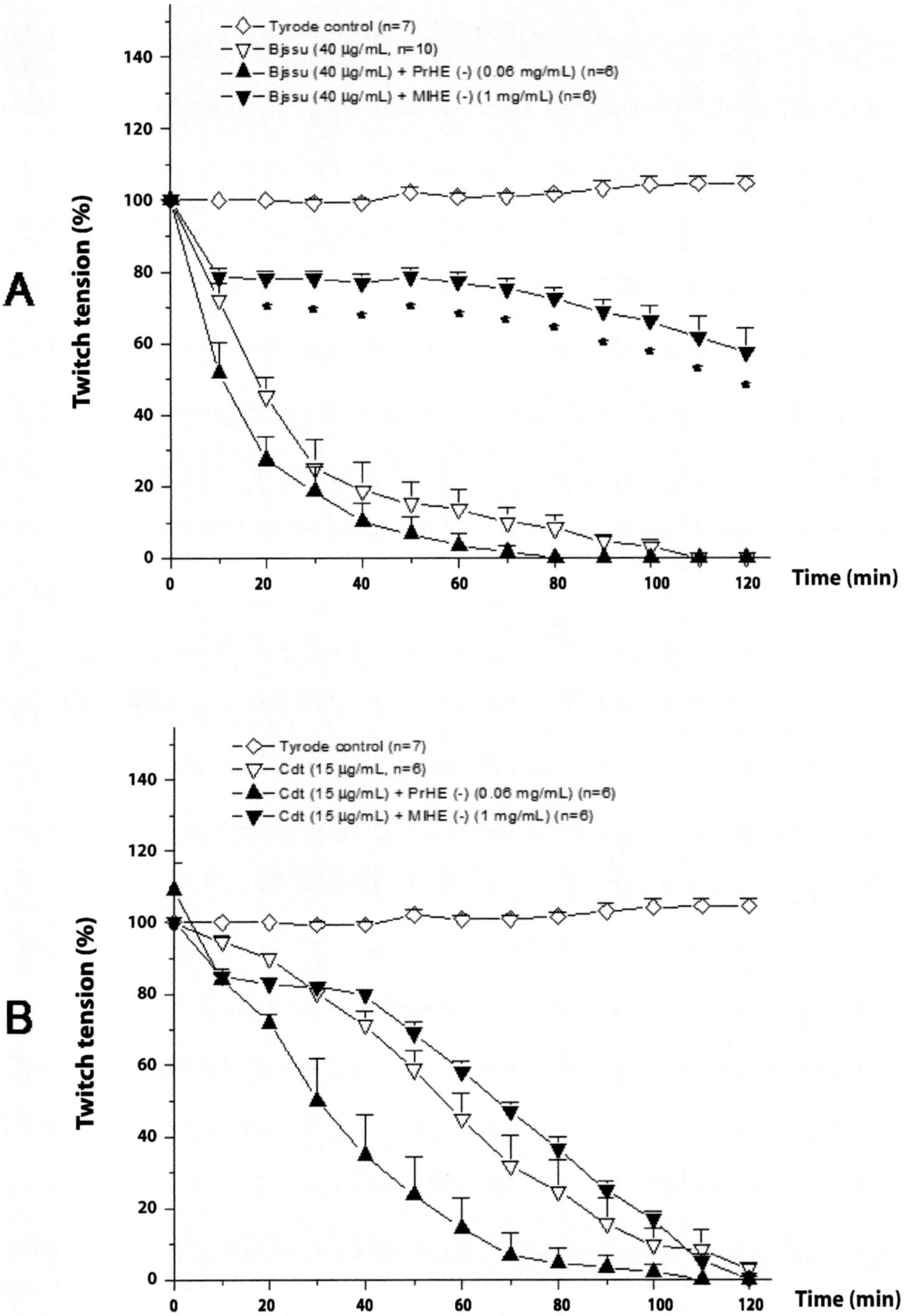

Figure 6. Pharmacological assays on mouse phrenic nerve-diaphragm preparations (indirect stimuli). Neutralization of *Bothrops jararacussu* venom (A, Bjssu), and *Crotalus durissus terrificus* venom (B, Cdt) by *P. reticulata* free of tannins [PrHE (-)] and *M. laevigata* free of tannins [MlHE (-)] hydroalcoholic extracts. Each point represents the mean ± S.E.M. of the number of experiments (n) showed in legend. **p*<0.05 compared to venom.

Acknowledgments

This work was supported by a research grant from Fundação de Amparo à Pesquisa do Estado de São Paulo (Proc. FAPESP 04/09705-8) and PROBIC/UNISO. R.M.S. was granted a scholarship (I.C.) from PIBIC/CNPq.

References

[1] Bezerra, JA; Campos, AC; Vasconcelos, PR; Nicareta, JR; Ribeiro, ER; Sebastião, AP; Urdiales, AI; Moreira, M; Borges, AM. Extract of *Passiflora edulis* in the healing of colonic anastomosis in rats: tensiometric and morphologic study. *Acta Cir. Bras*. 2006, 21, 16-25.

[2] Bon, C. Multicomponent neurotoxic phospholipases A_2. In: Kini RM editor. *Venom phospholipase A_2 enzymes: structure, function and mechanism.* Chichester, England: John Wiley and Sons; 1997; 269-285.

[3] Bülbring, E. Observation on the isolated phrenic nerve diaphragm preparation of the rat. *Br. J. Pharmacol.* 1946, 1, 38-61.

[4] Calixto, JB; Beirith, A; Ferreira, J; Santos, AR; Filho, VC; Yunes, RA. Naturally occurring antinociceptive substances from plants. *Phytother. Res*. 2000, 14, 401-418.

[5] Castro, EV de; Pinto, JEBP; Bertolucci, SKV; Malta, MR; Cardoso, M das G; , FA de M; Coumarin contents in young *Mikania glomerata* plants (guaco) under different radiation levels and photoperiod. *Acta Farm. Bonaerense* 2006, 25, 387-392.

[6] Cavalcante, WLG; Campos, TO; Dal Pai-Silva, MD; Pereira, OS; Oliveira, CZ; Soares, AM; Gallaci M. Neutralization of snake venom phospholipase A_2 toxins by aqueous extract of *Casearia sylvestris* (Flacourtiaceae) in mouse neuromuscular preparation. *J. Ethnopharmacol.* 2007, 112, 490-497.

[7] Chang, CC; Lee, JD. Crotoxin, the neurotoxin of South American rattlesnake venom, is a presynaptic toxin acting like beta-bungarotoxin. *Naunyn Schmiedebergs Arch. Pharmacol.* 1977, 296, 159-168.

[8] Cintra-Francischinelli, M; Silva, MG; Andréo-Filho, N; Gerenutti, M; Cintra, ACO; Giglio, JR; Leite, GB; Cruz-Höfling, MA; Rodrigues-Simioni, L; Oshima-Franco, Y. *Phytother. Res*. 2008, 6, 784-790.

[9] Dos Santos, SC; Krueger, CL; Steil, AA; Kreuger, MR; Biavatti, MW; Wisniewski Junior, A. LC characterisation of guaco medicinal extracts, *Mikania laevigata* and *M. glomerata*, and their effects on allergic pneumonits. *Planta Med.* 2006, 72, 679-684.

[10] Esmeraldino, LE; Souza, AM; Sampaio, SV. Evaluation of the effect of aqueous extract of *Croton urucurana* Baillon (Euphorbiaceae) on the hemorrhagic activity induced by the venom of *Bothrops jararaca*, using new techniques to quantify hemorrhagic activity in rat skin. *Phytomedicine* 2005, 12, 570-576.

[11] Fernandes, TT; Fernandes, ATS; Pimenta, SC. Atividade antimicrobiana das plantas *Plathymenia reticulata*, *Hymenea courbaril* e *Guazuma ulmifolia*. *Rev. Patol. Trop.* 2005, 34, 113-122.

[12] Fierro, IM; da Silva, AC; Lopes, C da S; de Moura, RS; Barja-Fidalgo, C. Studies on the anti-allergic activity of *Mikania glomerata*. *J. Ethnopharmacol*. 1999, 66, 19-24.

[13] Hagerman, AE; Butler, LG. Choosing appropriate methods and standards for assaying tannins. *J. Chem. Ecol.* 1989, 15, 1795-1810.

[14] Hagerman, AE; Butler, LG. Protein precipitation method for the quantitative determination of tannins. *J. Agr. Food Chem.* 1978, 26, 809-812.

[15] Harborne, JB. *Phytochemical Methods: A Guide to Modern Techniques of Plants Analysis*, 3rd Edition, London: Chapman and Hall, 1998.

[16] Homsi-Brandeburgo, MI; Queiroz, LS; Santo-Neto, H; Rodrigues-Simioni, L; Giglio, JR. Fractionation of *Bothrops jararacussu* snake venom: partial chemical characterization and biological activity of bothropstoxin. *Toxicon* 1988, 26, 615-627.

[17] Kuppusamy, UR; Das, NP. Protective effects of tannic acid and related natural compounds on *Crotalus adamanteus* subcutaneous poisoning in mice. *Pharmacol. Toxicol.* 1993, 72, 290-295.

[18] Kim, SI; Kim, KS; Kim, HS; Choi, MM; Kim, DS; Chung, KH; Park, YS. Inhibition of angiogenesis by salmosin expressed *in vitro*. *Oncol. Res.* 2004, 14, 227-233.

[19] Lizano, S; Domont, G; Perales, J. Natural phospholipase A(2) myotoxin inhibitor proteins from snakes, mammals and plants. *Toxicon* 2003, 42, 963-977.

[20] Maiorano, VA; Marcussi, S; Daher, MAF; Oliveira, CZ; Couto, LB; Gomes, AO; França, SZ; Soares, AM; Pereira, PS. Antiophidian properties of the aqueos extract of *Mikania glomerata*. *J. Ethnopharmacol.* 2005, 102, 364-370.

[21] MeSH – Medical Subject Headings (2008) Bradykinin. Available in: <http://www.ncbi.nlm.nih.gov/entrez/query.fcgi?CMD=searchandDB=mesh>, Pubmed, 25 June 2008.

[22] Ministério da Saúde do Brasil. *Manual de diagnóstico e tratamento de acidentes por animais peçonhentos*, 2nd Edition, Brasília: Fundação Nacional da Saúde; 2001.

[23] Mirshafiey, A. Venom therapy in multiple sclerosis. *Neuropharmacology* 2007, 53, 353-361.

[24] Moraes, MD. *A família* Asteraceae *na planície litorânea de Picinguaba* – Município de Ubatuba (master thesis), São Paulo, Brazil: Universidade Estadual de Campinas, 1997.

[25] Mors, WB; Nascimento, MC; Pereira, BM; Pereira, NA. Plant natural products active against sanke bite – the molecular approach. *Phytochemistry* 2000, 55, 627-642.

[26] Pithayanukul, P; Ruenraroengsak, P; Bavovada, R; Pakmanee, N; Suttisri, R. *In vitro* investigation of the protective effects of tannic acid against the activities of *Naja kaouthia* venom. *Pharmaceutical Biol.* 2007, 45, 94-97.

[27] Portuguese Farmacopeia. Instituto Nacional da Farmácia e do Medicamento. 7th Edition, Lisboa: Infarmed, 2002, 2792p.

[28] Ruppelt, BM; Pereira, EF; Gonçalves, LC; Pereira, NA. Pharmacological screening of plants recommended by folk medicine as anti-snake venom--I. Analgesic and anti-inflammatory activities. *Mem. Inst. Oswaldo Cruz* 1991, 86, 203-205.

[29] Sévenet, T. Looking for new drugs: what criteria? *J. Ethnopharmacol.* 1991, 32, 83-90.

[30] Simões, CMO; Schenkel, EP; Gosmann, G; Mello, JCP; Mentz, LA; Petrovick, PR. *Farmacognosia: da Planta ao Medicamento*, 5th Edition, Porto Alegre/Florianópolis: UFRGS/UFSC, 2004.

[31] Slotta, KH; Fraenkel-Conrat, H. Schlangengiffe, III: Mitteilung Reiningung und crystallization des klappershclangengiffes. *Ber. Dtsch. Chem. Ges.* 1938, 71, 1076-1081.

[32] Soares, AM; Ticli, FK; Marcussi, S; Lourenço, MV; Januário, AH; Sampaio, SV; Giglio, JR; Lomonte, B; Pereira, PS. Medicinal plants with inhibitory properties against snake venoms. *Curr. Med. Chem.* 2005, 12, 2625-2641.

[33] Veronese, EL; Esmeraldino, LE; Trombone, AP; Santana, AE; Bechara, GH; Kettelhut, I; Cintra, AC; Giglio, JR; Sampaio, SV. Inhibition of the myotoxic activity of *Bothrops jararacussu* venom and its two major myotoxins, BthTX-I and BthTX-II, by the aqueous extract of *Tabernaemontana catharinensis* A. DC. (Apocynaceae). *Phytomedicine* 2005, 12, 123-130.

In: Flavonoids: Biosynthesis, Biological Effects...
Editor: Raymond B. Keller
ISBN: 978-1-60741-622-7

Chapter 9

Molecular Targets of Flavonoids during Apoptosis in Cancer Cells

Kenichi Yoshida*

Department of Life Sciences, Meiji University, 1-1-1 Higashimita, Tama-ku, Kawasaki, Kanagawa 214-8571, Japan

Abstract

There are serious concerns about the increasing global cancer incidence. As currently used chemotherapeutics agents often show severe toxicity in normal cells, anti-carcinogenic compounds included in the dietary intakes of natural foods are expected to be applicable to a novel approach to preventing certain types of cancer without side effects. Polyphenolic compounds, such as flavonoids, are ubiquitous in plants and are presently considered to be the most promising in terms of having anti-carcinogenic properties probably due to their antioxidant effect. To gain further insights into how flavonoids exert anti-carcinogenic actions on cancer cells at the molecular level, many intensive investigations have been performed. Currently, the common signaling pathways elicited by flavonoids are recognized as tumor suppressor p53 and survival factor AKT. These factors are potential effectors of flavonoid-induced apoptosis via activation of Bax and caspase family genes. The present chapter emphasizes pivotal molecular mechanisms underlying flavonoid-induced apoptosis in human cancer cells. In particular, this chapter focuses on representative flavonoids such as soy isoflavone, green tea catechin, quercetin, and anthocyanin.

Introduction

A major part of cancer incidence is thought to be related to life style factors such as dietary intake tendencies. Considerable attention has been paid to bioactive polyphenols, especially flavonoids, in dietary intake of many fruits and vegetables for the sake of cancer prevention, because human population or epidemiologic studies have suggested that flavonoid

* Tel. and Fax.: +81-44-934-7107, e-mail: yoshida@isc.meiji.ac.jp

intake may reduce the risk of specific types of cancer [1-3]. Flavonoids have been extensively investigated in terms of how they act on various signal transduction pathways and their influences on the processes of cell fate determination [4, 5]. Induction of apoptosis in cancer cells by flavonoids is one of the most promising lines of evidence. Apoptosis induced by flavonoids usually involves modulating p53, nuclear factor-kappaB (NF-kappaB), activator protein-1 (AP-1), or mitogen-activated protein kinases (MAPK) [6-8]. Natural products are being investigated that can antagonize the anti-apoptotic effects of Bcl-2 family proteins such as Bcl-xL and Bcl-2 [9].

The changes which transform normal cells into cancer cells have been characterized as successive molecular events including activation of oncogenes and inactivation of antioncogenes, and all of these genes are known to be essential components of cellular signal transduction pathways and effectors of the cell cycle and apoptosis control. Basically, loss of anti-oncogenes results in the fragility of chromosomes and oncogenic activation renders cells more resistant to apoptosis and metastatic phenotypes. Needless to say, in considering cancer cell control via inhibition of metastasis and angiogenesis, inducing immune response and inflammatory cascade specific for cancer cells, and modulation of drug resistance are all promising approaches. In this chapter, we summarize recent progress in molecular studies of major flavonoids acting on apoptotic cancer cells.

1. Tea Polyphenol Catechins

Polyphenolic compounds contained in tea leaves are called as catechins, the most abundant of which is (-)-epigallocatechin-3-gallate (EGCG). EGCG has been known to regulate the cell cycle and apoptosis, and this is achieved in part by modulating the RAS/RAF/MAPK, phosphoinositide 3-kinase (PI3-K)/AKT, protein kinase C (PKC), NF-kappaB, AP-1 signaling pathways, and ubiquitin/proteasome degradation pathways [10-21]. Among these, inhibition of AKT signaling and modulation of pro-apoptotic factors by EGCG are well known. For example, EGCG has been shown to increase Bax and decrease Bcl-2 and AKT Ser473 phosphorylation in MDA-MB-231 human breast cancer cells [22]. Induction of pro-apoptotic proteins such as Bax, Bid and Bad, and suppression of Bcl-xL and Bcl-2 by EGCG in human gastric cancer cells MKN45 has also been described [23]. In hepatocellular carcinoma cells HLE, EGCG-induced apoptosis down-regulated Bcl-xL and Bcl-2 via inactivation of NF-kappaB [24]. These line of evidence suggest a mitochondrial-dependent pathway to be pivotal for EGCG-induced apoptosis. EGCG-induced apoptosis in MCF-7 breast cancer cells involves down-regulation of surviving expression via suppression of the AKT signaling pathway [25]. In MCF-7 breast cancer cells as well, JNK activation and Bax expression were reported in EGCG-induced apoptosis [26]. In human bladder cancer cells T24, inhibition of PI3-K/AKT activation and the resultant modulation of Bcl-2 family proteins during EGCG-induced apoptosis has been reported [27].

EGCG can affect two important transcription factors, p53 and NF-kappaB, during apoptosis in cancer cells. Involvement of the NF-kappaB pathway has been shown in EGCG-mediated apoptosis of human epidermoid carcinoma cells, A431 [28, 29]. EGCG can stabilize p53 and inhibit NF-kappaB, and this leads to a change in the ratio of Bax/Bcl-2 in a manner that favors apoptosis in human prostate carcinoma cells, LNCaP [30]. The importance of p53 and Bax during EGCG-induced apoptosis has also been shown in human breast cancer cells MDA-MB-468 [31]. Using different prostate cancer cell lines, p53 downstream targets p21 and Bax have been shown to be essential for EGCG-induced apoptosis [32]. There is also a controversial report about p53, but this is not the case for p21, being dispensable for apoptosis in human prostate carcinoma cells [33]. Other than p53, EGCG has been shown to affect many cell cycle regulators such as the cyclin-dependent kinase (CDK) inhibitor and the retinoblastoma gene product (pRb)-E2F in different cancer cells [34-37]. Recent findings on EGCG-induced apoptosis in cancer cells favor an essential role of p53 in EGCG-induced apoptosis. Additionally, survival factor AKT tends to be suppressed by EGCG in many cancer cells. These two pathways appear to synergistically induce cell cycle deregulation and alteration of Bcl-2/Bax balance, thereby leading to the induction of apoptosis in cancer cells.

2. Soy Isoflavones

Genistein, which is structurally related to 17beta-estradiol, is one of the predominant soybean isoflavones. Genistein has been shown to inhibit protein tyrosine kinase activity, especially those of epidermal growth factor receptor and Src tyrosine kinase [38, 39], and is implicated in protection against different cancers [40]. By regulating a wide array of genes, genistein regulates the cell cycle and apoptosis. The common signaling pathways inhibited by genistein for the prevention of cancer have been extensively examined and are known as the NF-kappaB and AKT signaling pathways [41-45]. For example, apoptosis in many cancer cells including the breast cancer cell line MDA-MB-231, prostate cancer cell line PC3, and head and neck cancer cells treated with genistein has been shown to be executed partly through the down-regulation of NF-kappaB and AKT pathways [46-48].

In contrast to apoptosis induced by EGCG in cancer cells, accumulating evidence suggests that p53 does not appear to play a significant role during apoptosis in cancer cells. Genistein induced apoptosis in a variety of human cancer cells regardless of p53 status [49]. A p53-independent pathway of genistein-induced apoptosis in non-small cell lung cancer cells H460 has also been reported [50]. Although Puma, a p53-induced apoptosis regulator, has been identified as an up-regulated gene in genistein-induced apoptosis of A549 cells, its down-regulation had no effects on genistein-induced apoptosis [51]. p21, p53-target gene, has been shown to be an important candidate molecule in determining the sensitivity of normal and malignant breast epithelial cells to genistein and also in genistein-induced apoptosis in prostate adenocarcinoma and non-small lung cancer cell line H460 [52-55]. Notably, p21 induction by genistein was reported to function in a p53-independent manner in human breast carcinoma cells and prostate carcinoma cells [56, 57]. Genistein-induced apoptosis in primary gastric cancer cells is partly explained by down-regulation of Bcl-2 and up-regulation of Bax [58]. Along with p21, Bax was detected in genistein-induced apoptosis of the breast cancer cell line MDA-MB-231 through a p53-independent pathway [59]. Taken together, these observations indicate that genistein induces apoptosis in variety of cancer cells largely via inhibition of AKT and NF-kappaB pathways, and that p53 involvement in genistein-induced apoptosis may well be minor while p21 and Bax play certain roles in genistein-induced apoptosis.

3. QUERCETIN

Quercetin is a ubiquitous bioactive plant flavonoid found in onions, grapes, green vegetables, etc., which has been shown to inhibit the proliferation of a variety of human cancer cells. Quercetin is thought to induce apoptosis possibly through regulating MAPK such as by suppressing extracellular signal-regulated kinase (ERK) and c-Jun N-terminal kinase (JNK) phosphorylation [60]. Tumor necrosis factor (TNF) alpha-induced apoptosis in osteoblastic cells, MC3T3-E1, was shown to be promoted by quercetin when JNK and AP-1 were activated [61]. TNF-related apoptosis-inducing ligand (TRAIL)-induced apoptosis and the resultant caspase activation was also promoted by quercetin in human prostate cancer cells with accompanying suppression of AKT phosphorylation [62]. In human prostate cancer cells, LNCaP, quercetin-induced apoptosis was accompanied by a decrease in the inhibitory AKT Ser473 phosphorylation and its downstream Bad Ser136 phosphorylation. These processes can promote dissociation of Bax from Bcl-xL and then Bax translocation to the mitochondrial membrane, and induce activation of caspase family genes [63]. In a human hepatoma cell line HepG2, quercetin induced apoptosis possibly by direct activation of the caspase cascade and by inhibiting survival signaling such as AKT [64]. These results indicate that quercetin-directed suppression of AKT phosphorylation could be the major molecular axis for quercetin-induced apoptosis in cancer cells.

p53 has been thought to have an important role in apoptosis in quercetin-treated=cells [65]; however, there is a discrepancy regarding the p53 requirement in quercetin-induced apoptosis. Regardless of p53 status, quercetin was able to induce Bad and caspase family genes and this resulted in apoptosis of nasopharyngeal carcinoma cell lines [66]. Quercetin induced apoptosis in the human prostate cancer cell line PC-3 with increased levels of insulin-like growth factor-binding protein-3 (IGFBP-3), Bax, and p21 protein and with decreased levels of Bcl-xL and Bcl-2 proteins, suggesting that quercetin-induced apoptosis may occur in a p53-independent manner because PC-3 lack p53 [67, 68]. In contrast to the above reports, quercetin has been shown to induce cell cycle arrest and apoptosis in human hepatoma cells, HepG2, in a p53-dependent manner, and this resulted in an increased ratio of Bax/Bcl-2 [69]. Moreover, p53-dependent up-regulation of p21 has been shown to attenuate apoptosis in quercetin-treated A549 and H1299 lung carcinoma cells [70]. An important role of p21 in quercetin-induced apoptosis of MCF-7 human breast cancer cells has been reported [71]. Taken together, these findings indicate that quercetin-induced apoptosis in cancer cells requires both inactivation of survival factor AKT and modulation of the expression of the Bcl-2 family of proteins, especially for Bax activation. Recent findings suggest that quercetin-induced apoptosis does not apparently requir p53, though more extensive studies are needed. Results obtained to date indicate that quercetin can be applied to a wide variety of cancer cells that lack p53.

4. ANTHOCYANINS

Anthocyanins, reddish pigments, are abundant in many fruits and vegetables such as blueberries and red cabbage. As is well known for other flavonoids, anthocyanins have the ability to act as antioxidants and are expected to be of potential clinical relevance as evidenced by animal models [72]. Moreover, berry phenolics, in which the major components are anthocyanins, have been known to show anti-carcinogenic properties mainly through the induction of apoptosis in multiple types of cancer cells [73-76]. Among anthocyanins, malvidin, has been shown to be the most potent apoptosis inducer by modulating specifically MAPK in the human gastric adenocarcinoma cell line AGS [77]. Anthocyanins, derived from potato, induced apoptosis in the prostate cancer cell line LNCaP and PC-3 accompanied by MAPK and JNK activation, but caspase-dependent apoptosis was observed only in LNCaP cells [78]. Hibiscus anthocyanins induced apoptosis in human promyelocytic leukemia cells, HL-60, and this was critically regulated specifically by p38 kinase in MAPK and PI3-K [79]. In the human hepatoma cell line HepG2, delphinidin, components of anthocyanins induced apoptosis with increased JNK phosphorylation and Bax and decreased Bcl-2 protein [80]. Molecular targets of anthocyanins likely include two regulatory axes: 1) MAPK activation followed by JUN phosphorylation and 2) p53 activation followed by Bax protein activation. These two pathways are known to contribute equally to apoptosis in normal cells [81]. The contribution of p53 status in anthocyanin-induced apoptosis should be further verified by studying a series of cancer cells.

CONCLUSION

Flavonoids are rich sources of potentially useful medical compounds, because they have been well characterized as reducing cancer risk. Indeed, flavonoids are known to exhibit antioxidant and anti-inflammatory actions as well as anti-carcinogenic effects on many types of cancer cells. Cell culture-based experiments have revealed numerous candidate molecules for development of flavonoids for drug targeting; however, the results of assays with very high concentrations of flavonoids do not necessarily support the adaptablility of these compounds to clinical treatments. The results cell culture-based experiments should be verified and confirmed first using animal models and then in epidemiological studies. Molecular mechanisms of flavonoid actions on cellular targets are not fully characterized and many features remain to be elucidated. For example, the synergistic actions of flavonoids should be carefully investigated, because we usually ingest multiple flavonoids simultaneously from dietary sources, such as fruits, and beverages. Moreover, combination effects between flavonoids and cancer preventive chemotherapeutic agents are a promising approach to reducing side effects. Exploring the actual molecular targets of flavonoids would presumably be a very promising road to the control cancer cells.

REFERENCES

[1] Neuhouser ML. Dietary flavonoids and cancer risk: evidence from human population studies. *Nutr. Cancer*. 2004. 50 (1): 1-7.

[2] Schabath MB, Hernandez LM, Wu X, Pillow PC, Spitz MR. Dietary phytoestrogens and lung cancer risk. *JAMA*. 2005. 294 (12): 1493-1504.

[3] Theodoratou E, Kyle J, Cetnarskyj R, Farrington SM, Tenesa A, Barnetson R, Porteous M, Dunlop M, Campbell H. Dietary flavonoids and the risk of colorectal cancer. *Cancer Epidemiol Biomarkers Prev*. 2007. 16 (4): 684-693.
[4] Ramos S. Effects of dietary flavonoids on apoptotic pathways related to cancer chemoprevention. *J. Nutr. Biochem*. 2007. 18 (7): 427-442.
[5] Ramos S. Cancer chemoprevention and chemotherapy: dietary polyphenols and signalling pathways. *Mol. Nutr. Food Res*. 2008. 52 (5): 507-526.
[6] Dong Z. Effects of food factors on signal transduction pathways. *Biofactors*. 2000. 12 (1-4): 17-28.
[7] Kong AN, Yu R, Chen C, Mandlekar S, Primiano T. Signal transduction events elicited by natural products: role of MAPK and caspase pathways in homeostatic response and induction of apoptosis. *Arch. Pharm. Res*. 2000. 23 (1): 1-16.
[8] Fresco P, Borges F, Diniz C, Marques MP. New insights on the anticancer properties of dietary polyphenols. *Med. Res. Rev*. 2006. 26 (6): 747-766.
[9] Pellecchia M, Reed JC. Inhibition of anti-apoptotic Bcl-2 family proteins by natural polyphenols: new avenues for cancer chemoprevention and chemotherapy. *Curr. Pharm. Des*. 2004. 10 (12): 1387-1398.
[10] Yang CS, Chung JY, Yang GY, Li C, Meng X, Lee MJ. Mechanisms of inhibition of carcinogenesis by tea. *Biofactors*. 2000. 13 (1-4): 73-79.
[11] Lin JK. Cancer chemoprevention by tea polyphenols through modulating signal transduction pathways. *Arch Pharm Res*. 2002. 25 (5): 561-571.
[12] Lambert JD, Yang CS. Mechanisms of cancer prevention by tea constituents. *J. Nutr*. 2003. 133 (10): 3262S-3267S.
[13] Park AM, Dong Z. Signal transduction pathways: targets for green and black tea polyphenols. *J. Biochem. Mol. Biol*. 2003. 36 (1): 66-77.
[14] Chen D, Daniel KG, Kuhn DJ, Kazi A, Bhuiyan M, Li L, Wang Z, Wan SB, Lam WH, Chan TH, Dou QP. Green tea and tea polyphenols in cancer prevention. *Front Biosci*. 2004. 9: 2618-2631.
[15] Beltz LA, Bayer DK, Moss AL, Simet IM. Mechanisms of cancer prevention by green and black tea polyphenols. *Anticancer Agents Med. Chem*. 2006. 6 (5): 389-406.
[16] Khan N, Afaq F, Saleem M, Ahmad N, Mukhtar H. Targeting multiple signaling pathways by green tea polyphenol (-)-epigallocatechin-3-gallate. *Cancer Res*. 2006. 66 (5): 2500-2505.
[17] Na HK, Surh YJ. Intracellular signaling network as a prime chemopreventive target of (-)-epigallocatechin gallate. *Mol. Nutr. Food Res*. 2006. 50 (2): 152-159.
[18] Chen L, Zhang HY. Cancer preventive mechanisms of the green tea polyphenol (-)-epigallocatechin-3-gallate. *Molecules*. 2007. 12 (5): 946-957.
[19] Shankar S, Ganapathy S, Srivastava RK. Green tea polyphenols: biology and therapeutic implications in cancer. *Front Biosci*. 2007. 12: 4881-4899.
[20] Shukla Y. Tea and cancer chemoprevention: a comprehensive review. *Asian Pac. J. Cancer Prev*. 2007. 8 (2): 155-166.
[21] Chen D, Milacic V, Chen MS, Wan SB, Lam WH, Huo C, Landis-Piwowar KR, Cui QC, Wali A, Chan TH, Dou QP. Tea polyphenols, their biological effects and potential molecular targets. *Histol Histopathol*. 2008. 23 (4): 487-496.

[22] Thangapazham RL, Passi N, Maheshwari RK. Green tea polyphenol and epigallocatechin gallate induce apoptosis and inhibit invasion in human breast cancer cells. *Cancer Biol. Ther.* 2007. 6 (12): 1938-1943.

[23] Ran ZH, Xu Q, Tong JL, Xiao SD. Apoptotic effect of Epigallocatechin-3-gallate on the human gastric cancer cell line MKN45 via activation of the mitochondrial pathway. *World J. Gastroenterol.* 2007. 13 (31): 4255-4259.

[24] Nishikawa T, Nakajima T, Moriguchi M, Jo M, Sekoguchi S, Ishii M, Takashima H, Katagishi T, Kimura H, Minami M, Itoh Y, Kagawa K, Okanoue T. A green tea polyphenol, epigalocatechin-3-gallate, induces apoptosis of human hepatocellular carcinoma, possibly through inhibition of Bcl-2 family proteins. *J. Hepatol.* 2006. 44 (6): 1074-1082.

[25] Tang Y, Zhao DY, Elliott S, Zhao W, Curiel TJ, Beckman BS, Burow ME. Epigallocatechin-3 gallate induces growth inhibition and apoptosis in human breast cancer cells through survivin suppression. *Int. J. Oncol.* 2007. 31 (4): 705-711.

[26] Hsuuw YD, Chan WH. Epigallocatechin gallate dose-dependently induces apoptosis or necrosis in human MCF-7 cells. *Ann. N Y Acad Sci.* 2007. 1095: 428-440.

[27] Qin J, Xie LP, Zheng XY, Wang YB, Bai Y, Shen HF, Li LC, Dahiya R. A component of green tea, (-)-epigallocatechin-3-gallate, promotes apoptosis in T24 human bladder cancer cells via modulation of the PI3K/Akt pathway and Bcl-2 family proteins. *Bioche.m Biophys Res. Commun.* 2007. 354 (4): 852-857.

[28] Ahmad N, Gupta S, Mukhtar H. Green tea polyphenol epigallocatechin-3-gallate differentially modulates nuclear factor kappaB in cancer cells versus normal cells. *Arch. Biochem. Biophys.* 2000. 376 (2): 338-346.

[29] Gupta S, Hastak K, Afaq F, Ahmad N, Mukhtar H. Essential role of caspases in epigallocatechin-3-gallate-mediated inhibition of nuclear factor kappa B and induction of apoptosis. *Oncogene.* 2004. 23 (14): 2507-2522.

[30] Hastak K, Gupta S, Ahmad N, Agarwal MK, Agarwal ML, Mukhtar H. Role of p53 and NF-kappaB in epigallocatechin-3-gallate-induced apoptosis of LNCaP cells. *Oncogene.* 2003. 22 (31): 4851-4859.

[31] Roy AM, Baliga MS, Katiyar SK. Epigallocatechin-3-gallate induces apoptosis in estrogen receptor-negative human breast carcinoma cells via modulation in protein expression of p53 and Bax and caspase-3 activation. *Mol. Cancer Ther.* 2005. 4 (1): 81-90.

[32] Hastak K, Agarwal MK, Mukhtar H, Agarwal ML. Ablation of either p21 or Bax prevents p53-dependent apoptosis induced by green tea polyphenol epigallocatechin-3-gallate. *FASEB J.* 2005. 19 (7): 789-791.

[33] Gupta S, Ahmad N, Nieminen AL, Mukhtar H. Growth inhibition, cell-cycle dysregulation, and induction of apoptosis by green tea constituent (-)-epigallocatechin-3-gallate in androgen-sensitive and androgen-insensitive human prostate carcinoma cells. *Toxicol Appl. Pharmacol.* 2000. 164 (1): 82-90.

[34] Ahmad N, Cheng P, Mukhtar H. Cell cycle dysregulation by green tea polyphenol epigallocatechin-3-gallate. *Biochem. Biophys Res. Commun.* 2000. 275 (2): 328-334.

[35] Masuda M, Suzui M, Weinstein IB. Effects of epigallocatechin-3-gallate on growth, epidermal growth factor receptor signaling pathways, gene expression, and chemosensitivity in human head and neck squamous cell carcinoma cell lines. *Clin. Cancer Res.* 2001. 7 (12): 4220-4229.

[36] Ahmad N, Adhami VM, Gupta S, Cheng P, Mukhtar H. Role of the retinoblastoma (pRb)-E2F/DP pathway in cancer chemopreventive effects of green tea polyphenol epigallocatechin-3-gallate. *Arch. Biochem. Biophys*. 2002. 398 (1): 125-131.

[37] Gupta S, Hussain T, Mukhtar H. Molecular pathway for (-)-epigallocatechin-3-gallate-induced cell cycle arrest and apoptosis of human prostate carcinoma cells. *Arch. Biochem. Biophys*. 2003. 410 (1): 177-185.

[38] Peterson G. Evaluation of the biochemical targets of genistein in tumor cells. *J. Nutr.*. 1995. 125 (3 Suppl): 784S-789S.

[39] Bektic J, Guggenberger R, Eder IE, Pelzer AE, Berger AP, Bartsch G, Klocker H. Molecular effects of the isoflavonoid genistein in prostate cancer. *Clin. Prostate Cancer*. 2005. 4 (2): 124-129.

[40] Valachovicova T, Slivova V, Sliva D. Cellular and physiological effects of soy flavonoids. *Mini Rev. Med. Chem*. 2004. 4 (8): 881-887.

[41] Sarkar FH, Li Y. Mechanisms of cancer chemoprevention by soy isoflavone genistein. *Cancer Metastasis Rev*. 2002. 21 (3-4): 265-280.

[42] Sarkar FH, Li Y. Soy isoflavones and cancer prevention. *Cancer Invest*. 2003. 21 (5): 744-757.

[43] Sarkar FH, Li Y. The role of isoflavones in cancer chemoprevention. *Front Biosci*. 2004. 9: 2714-2724.

[44] Li Y, Ahmed F, Ali S, Philip PA, Kucuk O, Sarkar FH. Inactivation of nuclear factor kappaB by soy isoflavone genistein contributes to increased apoptosis induced by chemotherapeutic agents in human cancer cells. *Cancer Res*. 2005. 65 (15): 6934-6942.

[45] Sarkar FH, Adsule S, Padhye S, Kulkarni S, Li Y. The role of genistein and synthetic derivatives of isoflavone in cancer prevention and therapy. *Mini. Rev. Med. Chem*. 2006. 6 (4): 401-407.

[46] Gong L, Li Y, Nedeljkovic-Kurepa A, Sarkar FH. Inactivation of NF-kappaB by genistein is mediated via Akt signaling pathway in breast cancer cells. *Oncogene*. 2003. 22 (30): 4702-4709.

[47] Li Y, Sarkar FH. Inhibition of nuclear factor kappaB activation in PC3 cells by genistein is mediated via Akt signaling pathway. *Clin. Cancer Res*. 2002. 8 (7): 2369-2377.

[48] Alhasan SA, Aranha O, Sarkar FH. Genistein elicits pleiotropic molecular effects on head and neck cancer cells. *Clin. Cancer Res*. 2001. 7 (12): 4174-4181.

[49] Li M, Zhang Z, Hill DL, Chen X, Wang H, Zhang R. Genistein, a dietary isoflavone, down-regulates the MDM2 oncogene at both transcriptional and posttranslational levels. *Cancer Res*. 2005. 65 (18): 8200-8208.

[50] Lian F, Li Y, Bhuiyan M, Sarkar FH. p53-independent apoptosis induced by genistein in lung cancer cells. *Nutr. Cancer*. 1999. 33 (2): 125-131.

[51] Tategu M, Arauchi T, Tanaka R, Nakagawa H, Yoshida K. Puma is a novel target of soy isoflavone genistein but is dispensable for genistein-induced cell fate determination. *Mol. Nutr. Food Res*. 2008. 52 (4): 439-446.

[52] Davis JN, Singh B, Bhuiyan M, Sarkar FH. Genistein-induced upregulation of p21WAF1, downregulation of cyclin B, and induction of apoptosis in prostate cancer cells. *Nutr. Cancer*. 1998. 32 (3): 123-131.

[53] Lian F, Bhuiyan M, Li YW, Wall N, Kraut M, Sarkar FH. Genistein-induced G2-M arrest, p21WAF1 upregulation, and apoptosis in a non-small-cell lung cancer cell line. *Nutr. Cancer*. 1998. 31 (3): 184-191.

[54] Shao ZM, Wu J, Shen ZZ, Barsky SH. Genistein exerts multiple suppressive effects on human breast carcinoma cells. *Cancer Res*. 1998. 58 (21): 4851-4857.

[55] Upadhyay S, Neburi M, Chinni SR, Alhasan S, Miller F, Sarkar FH. Differential sensitivity of normal and malignant breast epithelial cells to genistein is partly mediated by p21(WAF1). *Clin. Cancer Res*. 2001. 7 (6): 1782-1789.

[56] Shao ZM, Alpaugh ML, Fontana JA, Barsky SH. Genistein inhibits proliferation similarly in estrogen receptor-positive and negative human breast carcinoma cell lines characterized by P21WAF1/CIP1 induction, G2/M arrest, and apoptosis. *J. Cell Biochem*. 1998. 69 (1): 44-54.

[57] Choi YH, Lee WH, Park KY, Zhang L. p53-independent induction of p21 (WAF1/CIP1), reduction of cyclin B1 and G2/M arrest by the isoflavone genistein in human prostate carcinoma cells. *Jpn J. Cancer Res*. 2000. 91 (2): 164-173.

[58] Zhou HB, Chen JJ, Wang WX, Cai JT, Du Q. Apoptosis of human primary gastric carcinoma cells induced by genistein. *World J. Gastroenterol*. 2004. 10 (12): 1822-1825.

[59] Li Y, Upadhyay S, Bhuiyan M, Sarkar FH. Induction of apoptosis in breast cancer cells MDA-MB-231 by genistein. *Oncogene*. 1999. 18 (20): 3166-3172.

[60] Ahn J, Lee H, Kim S, Park J, Ha T. The anti-obesity effect of quercetin is mediated by the AMPK and MAPK signaling pathways. *Biochem. Biophys Res. Commun*. 2008. 373 (4): 545-549.

[61] Son YO, Kook SH, Choi KC, Jang YS, Choi YS, Jeon YM, Kim JG, Hwang HS, Lee JC. Quercetin accelerates TNF-alpha-induced apoptosis of MC3T3-E1 osteoblastic cells through caspase-dependent and JNK-mediated pathways. *Eur. J. Pharmacol*. 2008. 579 (1-3): 26-33.

[62] Kim YH, Lee YJ. TRAIL apoptosis is enhanced by quercetin through Akt dephosphorylation. *J. Cell Biochem*. 2007. 100 (4): 998-1009.

[63] Lee DH, Szczepanski M, Lee YJ. Role of Bax in quercetin-induced apoptosis in human prostate cancer cells. *Biochem. Pharmacol*. 2008. 75 (12): 2345-2355.

[64] Granado-Serrano AB, Martín MA, Bravo L, Goya L, Ramos S. Quercetin induces apoptosis via caspase activation, regulation of Bcl-2, and inhibition of PI-3-kinase/Akt and ERK pathways in a human hepatoma cell line (HepG2). *J. Nutr*. 2006. 136 (11): 2715-2721.

[65] Plaumann B, Fritsche M, Rimpler H, Brandner G, Hess RD. Flavonoids activate wild-type p53. *Oncogene*. 1996. 13 (8): 1605-1614.

[66] Ong CS, Tran E, Nguyen TT, Ong CK, Lee SK, Lee JJ, Ng CP, Leong C, Huynh H. Quercetin-induced growth inhibition and cell death in nasopharyngeal carcinoma cells are associated with increase in Bad and hypophosphorylated retinoblastoma expressions. *Oncol Rep*. 2004. 11 (3): 727-733.

[67] Vijayababu MR, Kanagaraj P, Arunkumar A, Ilangovan R, Dharmarajan A, Arunakaran J. Quercetin induces p53-independent apoptosis in human prostate cancer cells by modulating Bcl-2-related proteins: a possible mediation by IGFBP-3. *Oncol Res*. 2006. 16 (2): 67-74.

[68] Vijayababu MR, Kanagaraj P, Arunkumar A, Ilangovan R, Aruldhas MM, Arunakaran J. Quercetin-induced growth inhibition and cell death in prostatic carcinoma cells (PC-3) are associated with increase in p21 and hypophosphorylated retinoblastoma proteins expression. *J. Cancer Res. Clin. Oncol.* 2005. 131 (11): 765-771.

[69] Tanigawa S, Fujii M, Hou DX. Stabilization of p53 is involved in quercetin-induced cell cycle arrest and apoptosis in HepG2 cells. *Biosci. Biotechnol. Biochem.* 2008. 72 (3): 797-804.

[70] Kuo PC, Liu HF, Chao JI. Survivin and p53 modulate quercetin-induced cell growth inhibition and apoptosis in human lung carcinoma cells. *J. Biol. Chem.* 2004. 279 (53): 55875-55885.

[71] Choi JA, Kim JY, Lee JY, Kang CM, Kwon HJ, Yoo YD, Kim TW, Lee YS, Lee SJ. Induction of cell cycle arrest and apoptosis in human breast cancer cells by quercetin. *Int. J. Oncol.* 2001. 19 (4): 837-844.

[72] Fimognari C, Lenzi M, Hrelia P. Chemoprevention of cancer by isothiocyanates and anthocyanins: mechanisms of action and structure-activity relationship. *Curr. Med. Chem.* 2008. 15 (5): 440-447.

[73] Hou DX. Potential mechanisms of cancer chemoprevention by anthocyanins. *Curr. Mol. Med.* 2003. 3 (2): 149-159.

[74] Yi W, Fischer J, Krewer G, Akoh CC. Phenolic compounds from blueberries can inhibit colon cancer cell proliferation and induce apoptosis. *J. Agric. Food Chem.* 2005. 53 (18): 7320-7329.

[75] Seeram NP, Adams LS, Zhang Y, Lee R, Sand D, Scheuller HS, Heber D. Blackberry, black raspberry, blueberry, cranberry, red raspberry, and strawberry extracts inhibit growth and stimulate apoptosis of human cancer cells in vitro. *J. Agric. Food Chem.* 2006. 54 (25): 9329-9339.

[76] Neto CC. Cranberry and its phytochemicals: a review of in vitro anticancer studies. *J. Nutr.* 2007. 137 (1 Suppl): 186S-193S.

[77] Shih PH, Yeh CT, Yen GC. Effects of anthocyanidin on the inhibition of proliferation and induction of apoptosis in human gastric adenocarcinoma cells. *Food Chem. Toxicol.* 2005. 43 (10): 1557-1566.

[78] Reddivari L, Vanamala J, Chintharlapalli S, Safe SH, Miller JC Jr. Anthocyanin fraction from potato extracts is cytotoxic to prostate cancer cells through activation of caspase-dependent and caspase-independent pathways. *Carcinogenesis.* 2007. 28 (10): 2227-2235.

[79] Chang YC, Huang HP, Hsu JD, Yang SF, Wang CJ. Hibiscus anthocyanins rich extract-induced apoptotic cell death in human promyelocytic leukemia cells. *Toxicol Appl. Pharmacol.* 2005. 205 (3): 201-212.

[80] Yeh CT, Yen GC. Induction of apoptosis by the Anthocyanidins through regulation of Bcl-2 gene and activation of c-Jun N-terminal kinase cascade in hepatoma cells. *J. Agric Food Chem.* 2005. 53 (5): 1740-1749.

[81] Lo CW, Huang HP, Lin HM, Chien CT, Wang CJ. Effect of Hibiscus anthocyanins-rich extract induces apoptosis of proliferating smooth muscle cell via activation of P38 MAPK and p53 pathway. *Mol. Nutr. Food Res.* 2007. 51 (12): 1452-1460.

In: Flavonoids: Biosynthesis, Biological Effects...
Editor: Raymond B. Keller
ISBN: 978-1-60741-622-7

Chapter 10

FLAVAN-3-OL MONOMERS AND CONDENSED TANNINS IN DIETARY AND MEDICINAL PLANTS

Chao-Mei Ma* and Masao Hattori*

Institute of Natural Medicine, University of Toyama, 2630 Sugitani,
Toyama 930-0194, Japan

ABSTRACT

Flavan-3-ols with the most well known members being catechin and epicatechin are a group of phenolic compounds widely distributed in nature. The oligomers and polymers of flavan-3-ols are known as condensed tannins which used to be considered as anti-nutritional components. In recent years, more and more evidences proved that these compounds were beneficial to human health as nutrition and lifestyle have fundamentally changed in modern society. These phenolic compounds showed great potential for the treatment of lifestyle related diseases, such as type 2 diabetes, obesity, and metabolic syndrome. They were also reported to have effects on slowing down the aging progress as well as on prevention of Alzheimer's disease, cardiovascular disease, and cancer. This chapter describes the structures, chemical properties, isolation and identification methods, bioactivity and distribution of flavan-3-ol monomers and condensed tannins in dietary sources and medicinal plants. Case studies such as the chemical and biological investigations of tannins in the stems of *Cynomorium songaricum* (a well known tonic in China) and in other plants are provided.

INTRODUCTION

Flavan-3-ols with the most well known members being catechin and epicatechin are a group of phenolic compounds widely distributed in nature. The oligomers and polymers are known as proanthocyanidins or in another word, condensed tannins, characterized by their

---

* Corresponding authors: Phone: (81)-76-4347633. Fax: (81)-76-4345060. Email: saibo421@inm.u-toyama.ac.jp (M. Hattori); ma@inm.u-toyama.ac.jp or mchaomei@hotmail.com (CM. Ma).

typical astringency taste. This sensory property causes the dry and puchery feeling in the mouth following the consumption of tea, red wine and some unripened fruits (http://en.wikipedia.org/wiki/Tannin). Tannins used to be considered as anti-nutritional components due to their ability to bind with proteins. However, as nutrition and lifestyle have fundamentally changed in modern society, more and more evidences proved that these compounds have beneficial effects to human health (Ren and Chen, 2007; Shahidi, 1997). As polyphenol compounds with potent anti-oxidative activity, they showed effects on slowing down the aging progress as well as on prevention of Alzheimer's disease, cardiovascular disease, and cancer. These phenolic compounds also showed potential for the treatment of lifestyle-related diseases, such as type 2 diabetes, obesity, and metabolic syndrome. There is an excellent review well discussed the bioactivities of tannins from edible sources, especially their antioxidant and radical scavenging activities, their prevention effects of cancer and cardiovascular diseases, inhibition of LDL oxidation and platelet aggregation effects (Santos-Buelga and Scalbert, 2000). The present chapter describes more about the chemical aspect of these compounds, including the structures, chemical properties, isolation and identification methods of flavan-3-ol monomers and condensed tannins in dietary sources. Their updated bioactivities will also be discussed. Case studies such as the chemistry and bioactivity of tannins in teas, peanut skins, grapes, wine and in the stems of *Cynomorium songaricum* (a well known tonic in China) are presented.

Chemical Structures of Flavan-3-ol Monomers

The most widely spread flavan-3-ols, (-)-epicatechin and (+)-catechin, are a pair of epimers, both possessing a catechol group in their structures with the difference only on the stereo chemistry of C-3. Other flavan-3-ol monomers include epigallocatechin/gallocatechin and epiafzelechin/afzelechin, each pair of them having the same stereo-chemical difference as that of epicatechin/catechin. Epigallocatechin/gallocatechin have a galloyl group (one more hydroxyl group in the structure of catechol) in their structures while epiafzelechin/afzelechin have one less phenolic hydroxyl group in the structures of catechol (Figure 1).

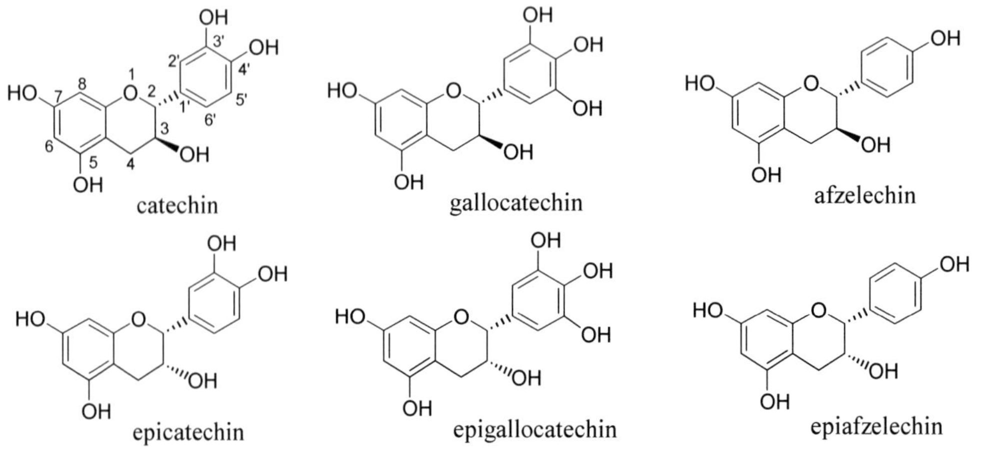

Figure 1. Structures of flavan-3-ol monomers.

Flavan-3-ol monomers are the basic component units of oligomers and polymers (often called condensed tannin). Epicatechin/catechin are the most frequently used extending flavan-3-ol units in tannin structures. Sometimes epicallocatechin/gallocatechin and epiafzelechin/afzelechin are also found as the extending flavan-3-ol units.

Oligomers of Flavan-3-ols (Harborne FRS JB and Baxter H, 1999)

Dimers of flavan-3-ols linked through one C-C bond are named as procyanidin Bs. There are many isomers of procyanidin Bs differed by the nature of their component monomer units, order of the monomers, configurations of the linkage bonds and the linkage positions. The most common linkages are C4→C8 (such as procyanidins B_1-B_4, figure 2) or C4→C6 (such as procyanidins B_5 and B_6, figure 2). Most prodelphinidins are flavan 3-ol dimers using one or two gallocatechin/epigallocatechin as their monomer unit(s), such as prodephinidin B_1. A-type procyanidins are flavan-3-ol dimers linked through one ether bond in addition to a C-C bond. The most common procyanidin As are procyanidins A_2 and A_1 (Figure 3). Procyanidin Cs are flavan-3-ol trimers (Figure 4). The following figures show the structures of some representative flavan-3-ol oligomers. Please note that though in most cases procyanidin Bx is the same compound of proanthocyanidin Bx (where x is a certain number), sometimes they are different compounds. For example, procyanidin B_6 and proanthocyanidin B_6 are different, the former being a catechin (4→6) catechin dimer while the latter containing a galloyl group conjugated with an epicatechin dimer (Scifinder). Most flavan 3-ols link with C4→C8/C4→C6 bonds in larger oligomers and polymers (Figure 5). Some times procyanidin A units can also be found in the structures of oligomers and polymers of condensed tannins.

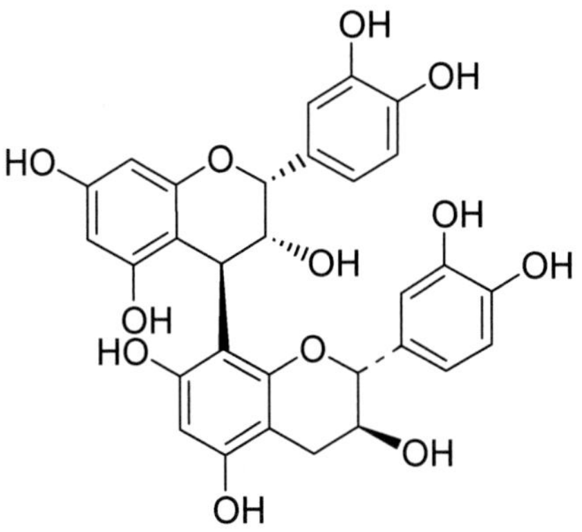

Procyanidin B_1
Epicatechin-(4β-8)-catechin
Proanthocyanidin B1
Procyanidol B1

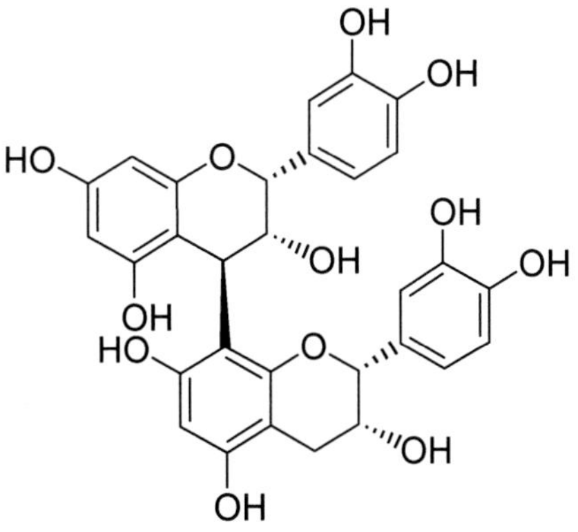

Procyanidin B_2
Epicatechin-(4β-8)-epicatechin
Proanthocyanidin B2
Procyanidol B2

Figure 2. (Continued).

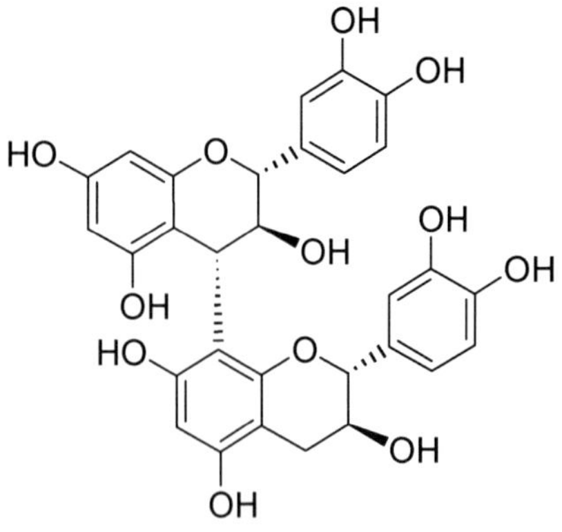

Procyanidin B_3
Catechin-(4α-8)-catechin
Proanthocyanidin B3
Procyanidol B3

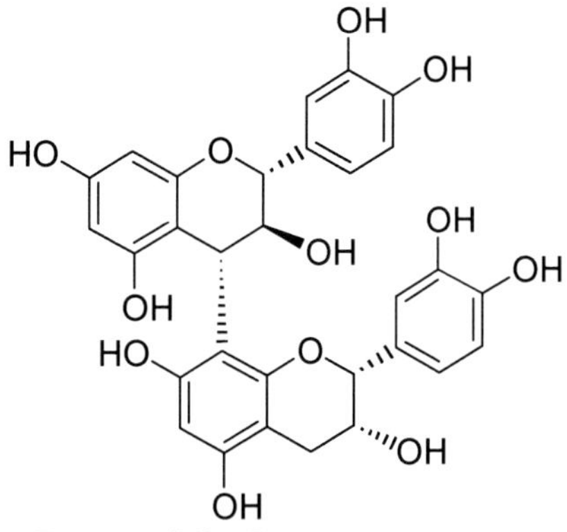

Procyanidin B_4
Catechin-(4α-8)-epicatechin
(-)-Procyanidin B4
Procyanidol B4

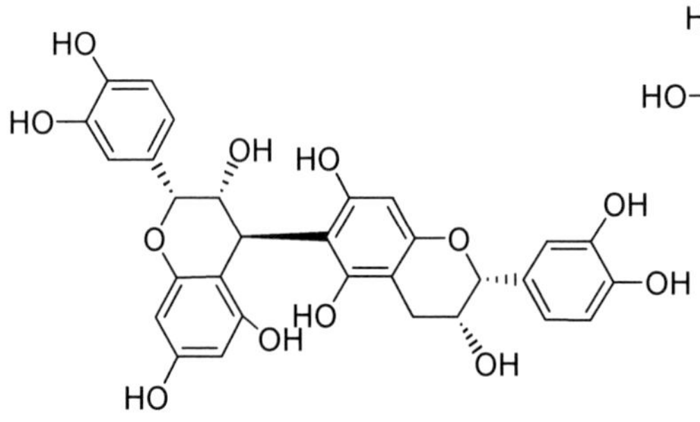

Procyanidin B_5
Epicatechin-(4β-6)-epicatechin
Proanthocyanidin B5
Procyanidol B5

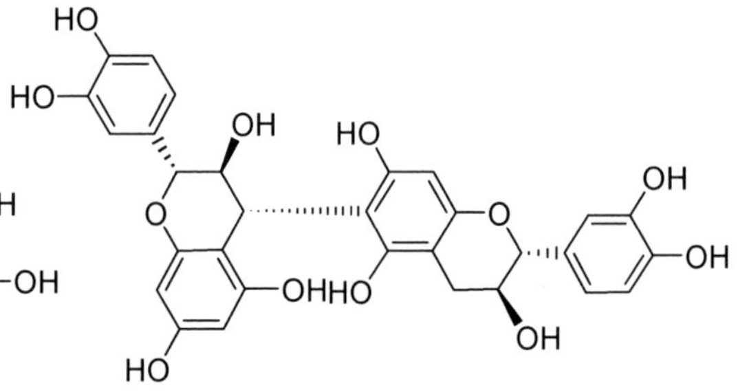

Procyanidin B_6
Catechin-(4α-6)-catechin
Procyanidol B6

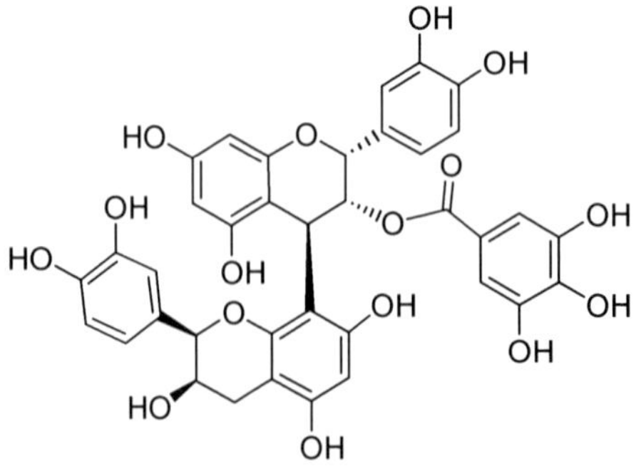

Proanthocyanidin B_6

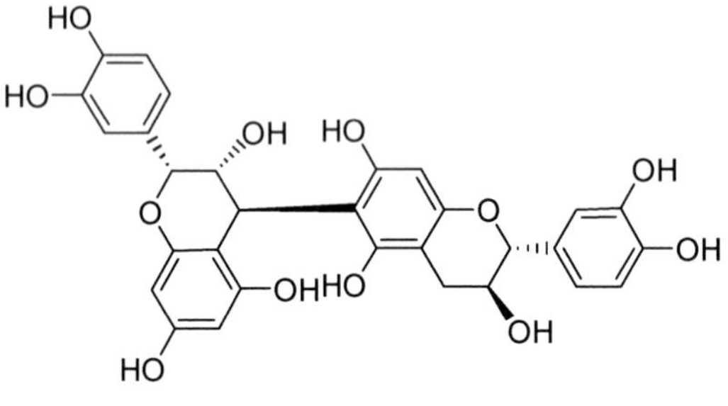

Procyanidin B_7
Epicatechin-(4β-6)-catechin
Proanthocyanidin B7

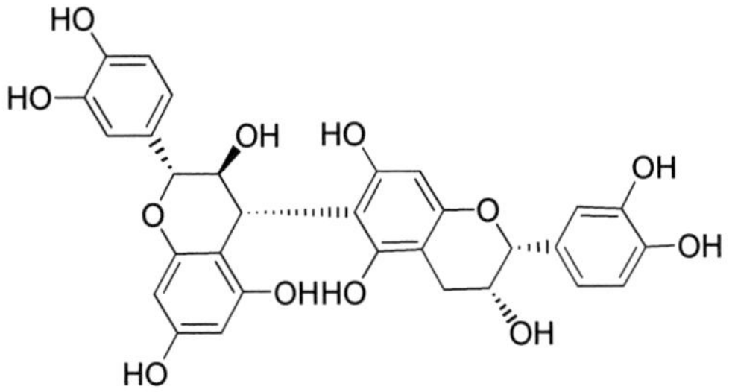

Procyanidin B_8
Catechin-(4α-6)-epicatechin
Procyanidol B_8

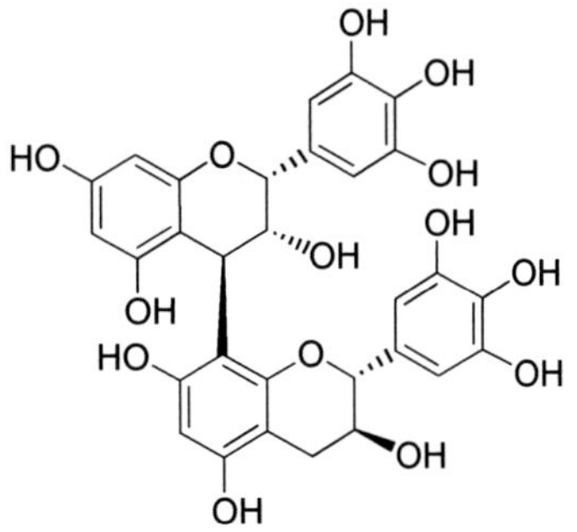

Prodelphinidin B_1
Epigallocatechin-(4β-8)-gallocatechin

Figure 2. Structures of some procyanidin Bs and prodelphinidin B_1.

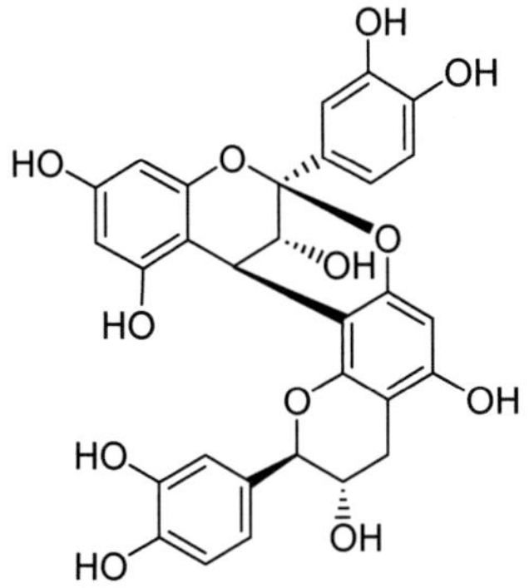

Proanthocyanidin A_1
Epicatechin-(2β-O-7, 4β-8)-catechin

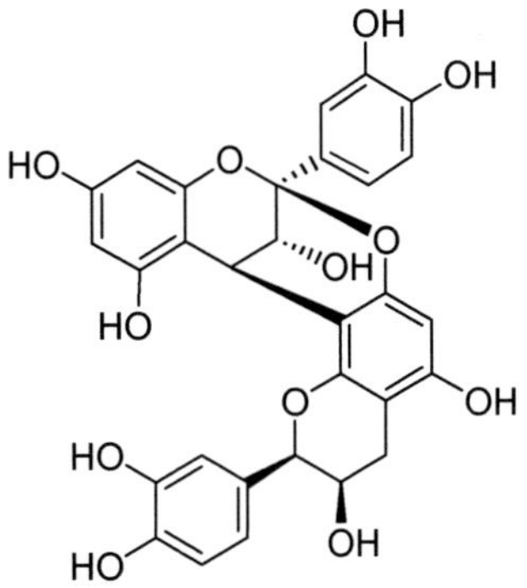

Proanthocyanidin A_2
Epicatechin-(2β-O-7, 4β-8)-epicatechin

Figure 3. Structures of two representative procyanidin As.

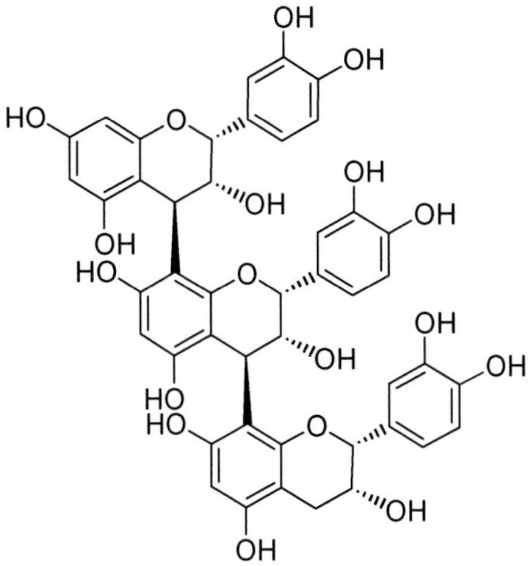

Procyanidin C1

Figure 4. Structures of one representative procyanidin Cs.

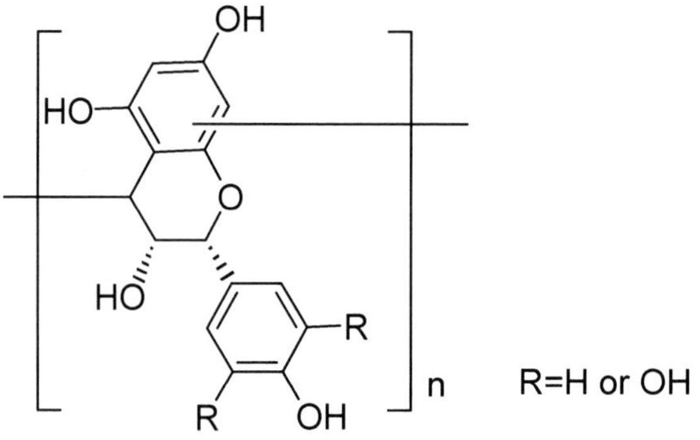

Figure 5. Structures of flavan-3-ol oligomers and polymers.

Astringency and Bitterness

Astringency and bitterness are the characteristic tastes of tannins. A study has showed that these sensory properties are related to the structures especially for flavan-3-ol monomers, dimers and trimers. The monomers were significantly higher in bitterness than the dimers, which were significantly higher than the trimers. Astringency of the monomers was lower than the dimers or trimers. The linkages between the monomeric units also influence both of the sensory properties. Catechin-(4→6)-catechin was more bitter than catechin-(4→8)-catechin/epicatechin. Astringency was affected by both the linkage and the identity of the monomeric units. Catechin-(4→8)-catechin had lower astringency than either catechin-(4→6)-catechin or catechin-(4→8)-epicatechin (Peleg *et al.*, 1999).

Chemical Properties

Flavan-3-ols are chemically unstable, being especially liable to undergoing numerous enzymatic and chemical oxidation or condensation. Adequate use of the oxidation and condensation process can produce foods of special color and taste. For example, oolong tea (semi-fermented), and black tea (fermented) can be produced by controlling the fermentation degree catalyzed by the enzyme. Due to the phenolic hydroxyl and ether groups in the para and ortho-positions, C8 and C6 are highly nucleophilic. In the contrast, C4 is electrophilic due to its aliphatic nature and near to some eletro-withdraw groups. As a result, the linkages between monomers in condensed tannins are usually C4→C8 or C4→C6. These linkage bonds are sensitive to acids and alkaline and this property can be used to induce degradation of the oligomers and polymers to study their monomer components. This property can also be used to produce water soluble smaller oligomers or their derivatives by acid treatment of the insoluble polymers in the presence of other reagents. A successful example is the preparation of oligomeric proanthocyanidin-cysteine complexes (Figure 6) which showed higher bioavailability and antioxidant capacity and prolonged survival time in the animal test groups (Fujii *et al.*, 2007). Other interesting bioactive compounds can also be synthesized using flavan-3-ols as starting materials. For example, under acid catalyst, catechin reacts with ketone compounds via an Oxa-Pictet-Spengler reaction to yield planer derivatives with a bridge between the 3-*O* group on ring C and C6′ on ring B (Figure 6). The planer catechin derivatives showed potent anti-oxidative activity and strong α-glucosidase inhibitory activity, suggesting the potential of using these planer catechin derivatives as lead compounds for the development of anti-diabetic agents [Hakamata *et al.*, 2006; Fukuhara *et al.*, 2002]. The highly nucleophilic C-8 position makes it possible to react with some electrophilic reagents to yield the C-8 substituted catechin derivatives (Figure 6). These compounds were synthesized upon protection of the phenolic OH groups with benzyl groups and de-protection with hydrogenation after the reaction finished (Nour-Eddine *et al.*, 2007).

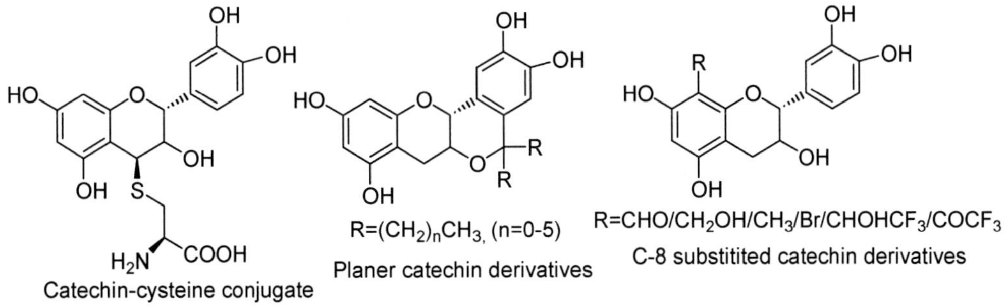

Figure 6. Structures of some synthesized catechin derivatives.

Isolation and Identification Methods

Acetone-water 7:3 is an effective solvent to extract flavan-3-ol monomers and oligomers. The procedure is usually carried out at room temperature and ultrasound can improve the extraction rate. After evaporation of the acetone under reduced pressure, the residual aqueous phase is extracted with ethyl acetate to eliminate some lipophilic non-tannin compounds. The aqueous solution containing tannin is applied to a Sephadex LH_{20} column, eluted with water containing increasing amount of methanol/ethanol to separate the flavan 3-ol oligomers. To obtain pure flavan 3-ol oligomers, repeated chromatography on Sephadex LH_{20} and in combination with Diaion HP-20 column chromatography are needed. Thin-layer chromatography on SiO_2 gel with an acidic solvent system gives better separation than on ODS. Benzene-ethyl formate-formic acid (2/1:7:1), chloroform-ethyl acetate-formic acid (1:7:1) and chloroform-ethyl acetate-formic acid-isopropanol (1:7:1:1) are some examples of the solvent systems used for separation of these compounds on normal phase TLC (Ezaki-Furuichi *et al.*, 1986). In the case of HPLC, normal-phase is better than ODS in separation and purification of flavan 3-ol oligomers. One example of the mobile phase for normal-phase HPLC composed of A: chloromethane/methanol/water (42:7:1) and B: dichloromethane/methanol/water (5:44:1). The elution program was set by slowly increasing solvent B from 0% to100% in 5 h (Hellström *et al.*, 2007).

The structures of flavan 3-ol monomers and oligomers are usually determined by careful analysis of their NMR and MS data and by comparing with reported data. Sometimes chemical degradation is needed to determine the structures of new flavan 3-ol oligomers. Professor Nishioka and his group in Japan have isolated and determined the structures of many new flavan 3-ol oligomers from various plants. Their published papers displayed detailed spectral data of the condensed tannins. These spectral data can be used to assistant structure determination of pure tannin compounds isolated from other plant sources (Hwang *et al.*, 1989; Morimoto *et al.*, 1987; Morimoto *et al.*, 1988; Kashiwada *et al.*, 1986; Hsu *et al.*, 1985).

Determination of Polyphenol Contents

Flavan-3-ol oligomers of low molecular weight can be detected and estimated by chromatographic techniques. As the polymerization degree increases, the number of isomers increases rapidly, which result in a broad peak for the complex mixture of isomers. For this reason, some non-chromatographic methods were developed for measuring total phenolic compounds, total tannins, or condensed tannins. Non-extractable tannin are measured by degradation of the polymers to monomers first.

Folin-Ciocalteu colorimetric method or its modified method relies on the property that phenolic compounds inhibit the oxidation of the reagent. As a result, the method is not specific for tannins but for all reducing substances. This method is used to determine the total reducing capacity of the samples and sometimes used to estimate the contents of total phenolic compounds. Briefly, 50 μl of sample solution, 250 μl of Folin-Diocalteu's reagent and 750 μl of 10% Na_2CO_3 were mixed and incubated at rt for 2 h. The absorbance at 756 nm was measured and the results were expressed as milligrams of catechin (or gallic acid equivalent or other compounds) equivalent per gram of dry plant (Mai *et al.*, 2007).

Aromatic aldehydes, such as vanillin or 4-dimethylaminocinnamaldehyde (DMACA) method is based on the property that tannins react with aldehyde compound to form colored products. This method is more specific to condensed tannins than the Folin-Ciocalteu method, but some other phenolic compounds may also react with the reagent (Herderich *et al.*, 2008).

The n-BuOH-HCl-Fe^{III} method is to de-polymerize condensed tannins and oxidize the released units to colored anthocyanidins under the strong reaction condition. The reaction mixture consists of a methanol solution of tested sample, n-BuOH-conc.HCl (95:5, v/v) and the ferric reagent (2% of $NH_4Fe(SO_4)_2$ $12H_2O$ in 2M HCl) in a ratio of 1:6:0.2. The solution is thoroughly mixed and the container is tightly closed before being heated at 95° C for 40 min. Absorbance at 520-580 nm (560 nm for example) is measured and the content is calculated by comparing with catechin solutions of known concentrations underwent the same reaction. The results are expressed as catechin equivalent (Porter LJ *et al.*, 1986.)

Protein precipitate assay can be used to estimate the amount of total tannins. Other compounds that precipitate with proteins such as, hydrolysable tannins and some other phenolic compounds will be included. The degree of polymerization and the number and position of phenolic hydroxyl groups influence the precipitate ability. The results are usually expressed as tannic acid equivalent. Using the property that tannin-protein complexes dissolve in sodium dodecylsulfate solution to liberate the proteins and tannins. A dot-blot assay for protein determination based on the reversible binding of benzoxanthene yellow to the protein spots can be used for the quantification (Hoffmann *et al.*, 2002.).

Thiolysis de-polymerization of condensed tannins in the presence of benzylmercaptan releases monomer derivatives such as benzylthioepicatechin. HPLC analysis of the degradation products could qualitatively and quantitatively determine the extender units of condensed tannins (Matthews *et al.*, 1997; Santos-Buelga and Scalbert 2000).

ESI and API-MS are also used to study flavan-3-ol oligomers. TOFMS can be used to analyze flavan-3-ol oligomers/polymers with higher molecular weights. The MS method can provide information about the polymerization degree and the type of the component monomer units. However, it is hard to determine the exact structures of these condensed tannins only by MS and accurate quantification of these compounds by MS is difficult to achieve, especially for larger oligomers or polymers.

TANNINS IN SOME DIETARY MATERIALS

Peanut Skins

Peanut skins are used to treat chronic haemorrhage and bronchitis in Chinese traditional medicine. The skins contain both B-type and A-type proanthocyanidins. The B-type dimers include B2, B3 and B4.

The A-type dimers, with one C-C bond and one ether bond linkages, include proanthocyanidin A_1 (p1), proanthocyanidine A_2 (p2), epicatechin-(2β-*O*-7, 4β-8)-*ent*-epicatechin (p3), epicatechin-(2β-*O*-7, 4β-6)-catechin (p4), epicatechin-(2β-*O*-7, 4β-6)-*ent*-catechin (p5) and epicatechin-(2β-*O*-7, 4β-6)-*ent*-epicatechin (p6). Peanut skins also contain some oligomers having A-type proanthocyanidin unit, such as p7 and p8 (Figure 7). These compounds may be responsible for the bitter taste of the peanut skins. Like other phenolic compounds, these compounds showed free radical-scavenging effects, which could protect the fatty acids in the peanut seeds from oxidation (Lou *et al.*, 2004; Lou *et al.*,1999).

Tea Polyphenols

Teas contain large quantity of polyphenols with gallocatechins and their gallate esters being among the main constituents. During fermentation process, the colorless (gallo) catechins in fresh tea leaves are oxidized to theaflavins and thearubigins in the presence of tea polyphenol oxidase and peroxidase and under the influence of pH. Theaflavins display a bright orange-red color and thearubigins display a red-brown or dark-brown color in solution. The chemical structures of theaflavins contain a substituted benzotropolone moiety formed from two flavan 3-ol units (Figure 8). Thearubigins are heterogeneous polymers whose chemical structures have not yet been completely characterized (Davis *et al.*, 1997; Takino *et al.*, 1965).

Tea flavan 3-ols exhibited a wide range of health beneficial effects. Professor Yokozawa and her group in University of Toyama, Japan, have worked on pharmacological evaluation of green teas and the components for decades. Their research group proved that the flavan-3-ols had effects on scavenging of nitric oxide and superoxide and that gallic acid conjugates of flavan-3-ols were more active than the un-conjugated ones. (-)-Epigallocatechin 3-*O*-gallate, (-)-gallocatechin 3-*O*-gallate and (-)-epicatechin 3-*O*-gallate exhibited higher scavenging activity on both nitric oxide and superoxide than (-)-epigallocatechin, (+)-gallocatechin, (-)-epicatechin and (+)-catechin did (Nakagawa and Yokozawa, 2002). These compounds

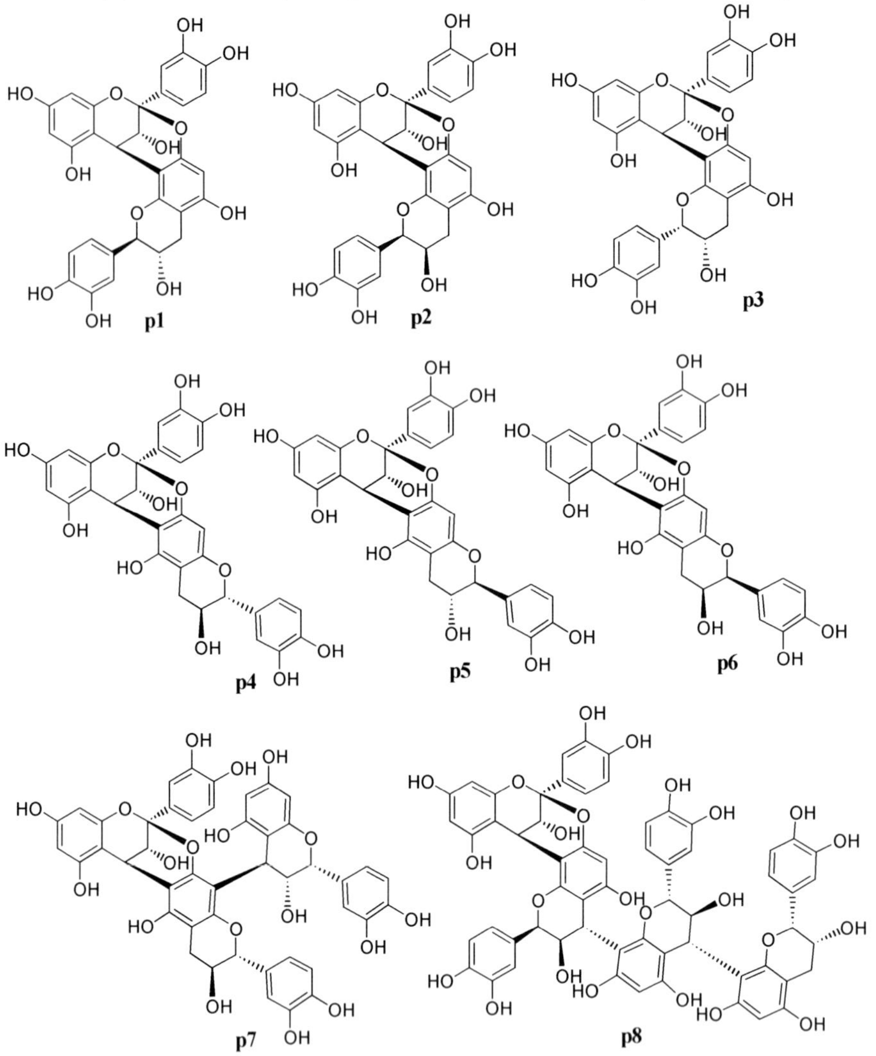

Figure 7. Structures of some flavan-3-ol dimers and trimers isolated from peanut skins.

also showed protective effect on 2,2'-azobis(2-amidinopropane) dihydrochloride (AAPH)-induced cellular damage. Again, the gallic acid conjugates of flavan-3-ols were more effective than the un-conjugated ones (Yokozawa *et al.*, 2000).This group also examined the effect of green tea polyphenols on diabetic nephropathy, using rats that had been subjected to subtotal nephrectomy and injection of streptozotocin. After 50 days administration of the tea polyphenols, improved kidney function was observed in the rats with diabetic nephropathy by measuring the following parameters: urinary protein excretion, kidney weight, morphological changes, serum levels of urea nitrogen, creatinine clearance and hyperglycaemia. Administration of tea polyphenols also increased the activity of superoxide dismutase in the kidney to a significant extent. Based on these results, the researchers suggested that tea polyphenols may be beneficial for patients with diabetic nephropathy (Yokozawa *et al.*,

2005). In addition, oral administration of (-)-epigallocatechin 3-*O*-gallate, one of the major constituents of teas, had protective effect for rats with chronic renal failure (Nakagawa *et al.*, 2004).

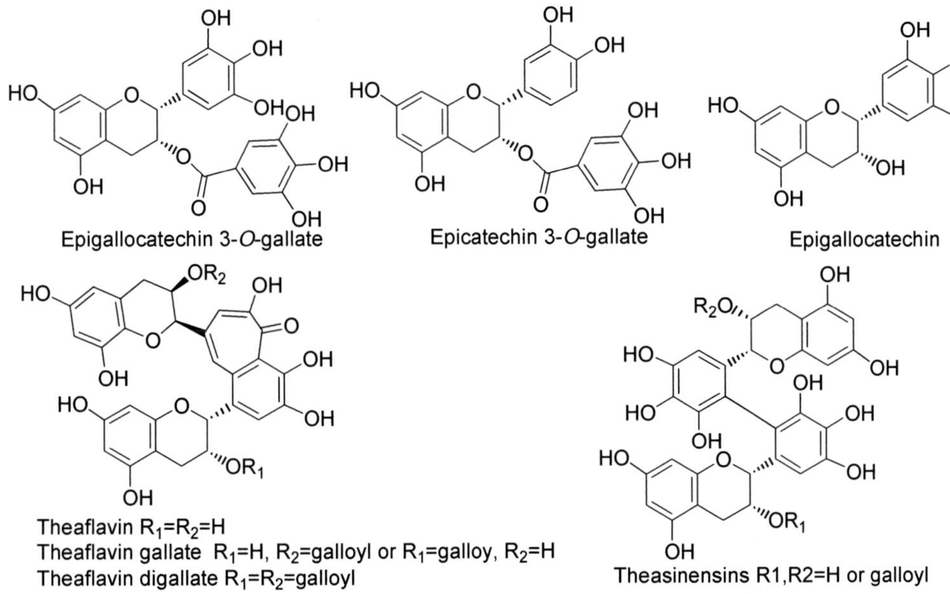

Figure 8. Structures of some phenolic compounds in teas.

Flavan-3-ols in Wine

Phenolic compounds, mainly flavan-3-ols and anthocyanins play important roles in the quality of wines. Their structures and amounts affect the color and sensory property such as astringency of the wines. The type and quantity of flavan-3-ols in wines depend not only on the kinds of the original fruits but also on the manufacture method, storage time and storage temperature. Due to their high chemical reactivity, the phenolic compounds polymerize and condense with other compounds in the wine solution to produce some special compounds for individual wines. The condensation causes a change of color from light to dark during the storage and aging process. The reaction of catechin condensed with glyoxylic acid, a compound may be derived from tartaric acid, is such an example (Figure 9). This reaction is generally observed during the aging of wines and other grape-derived foods (Es-Safi *et al.*, 2000.)

Flavan-3-ol related compounds, anthocyanins (Figure 10), can also undergo similar condensation, such as with pyruvic acid, an end-product of the glycolysis cycle during fermentation, to form stable red pigments as shown in Figure 11. Other yeast metabolites other than pyruvic acid were also found to react with grape anthocyanins, suggesting that this type of condensation may be an important route of conversion grape anthocyanins into stable pigments during the maturation and ageing of wine, thus increase the color stability of aged wines (Fulcrand *et al.*,1998).

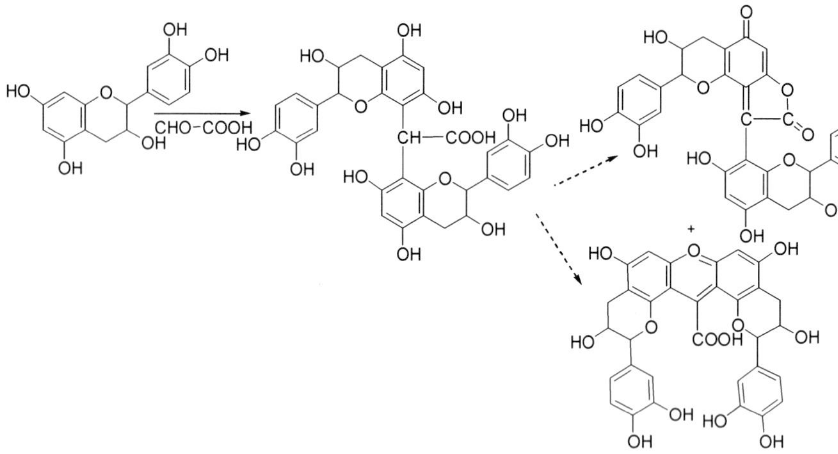

Figure 9. Proposed products for the condensation of flavan-3-ol with glyoxylic acid.

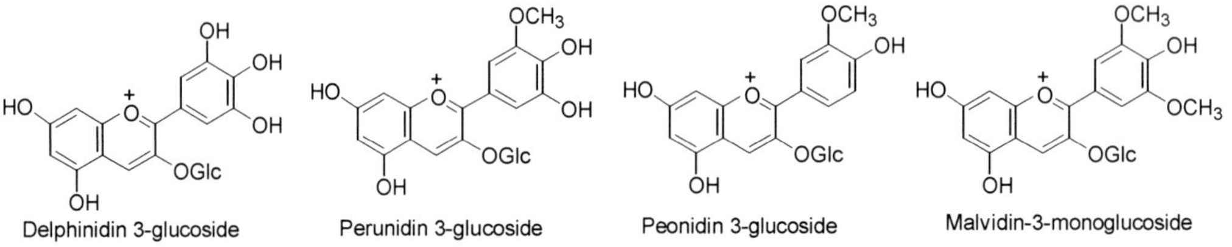

Figure 10. Some anthocyanins in grape.

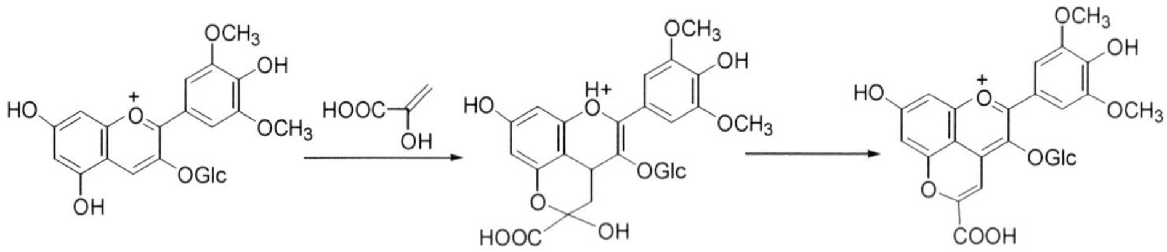

Figure 11. Reaction between pyruvic acid and malvidin 3-monoglucoside.

Grape Tannins

Recent years have witnessed increasing interest in using grape seed extracts as active ingredients in health promotion products. Grape seed tannins are a complex mixture of oligomers and polymers composed of catechin, epicatechin and epicatechin-3-gallate. Oligomers are mainly B-type linked through the C4→C6 or C4→C8 bond (Núñez *et al.*, 2006). Epicatechin was the major component in the extended chain while catechin was more abundant in terminal units than in extension units. The proportion of galloyllated units varied from 13% to 29% as the M_r, increased. Degrees of polymerization ranged from 2.3 to 15.1 or from 2.4 to 16.7 as measured by two different methods (Prieur *et al.*, 1994).

Grape skins also contain tannins with epicatechin representing 60% of the extension units, whereas 67% of the terminal units consisting of catechin. The degree of polymerization ranged from 3 to 80. The proportion of galloyllated units was 3% to 6% (Souquet *et al.*, 1996).

Tannins in grape seeds are shorter and have more epicatechin gallate as the monomer units. Tannins in grapes skin are generally larger and comprise more epigallocatechin as the monomer units (Herderich and Smith, 2008).

Cynomorium Tannins

Cynomorium songaricum Rupr (Cynomoriaceae) (Figure 12) is a parasitic plant living on the roots of *Nitraria sibirica,* mainly growing in the northern part of China, such as Inner Mongolia Autonomous Region. The stems of *C. Songaricum* is a well known traditional Chinese medicine reputed to have tonic effect. In addition to medicinal applications, extracts of this plant are frequently added to wines and teas. The fresh stems are also consumed by the local people as food or vegetable. Our research results showed that this plant contained large amount of condensed tannins (in catechin equivalent: nearly 20% of the dried stems).

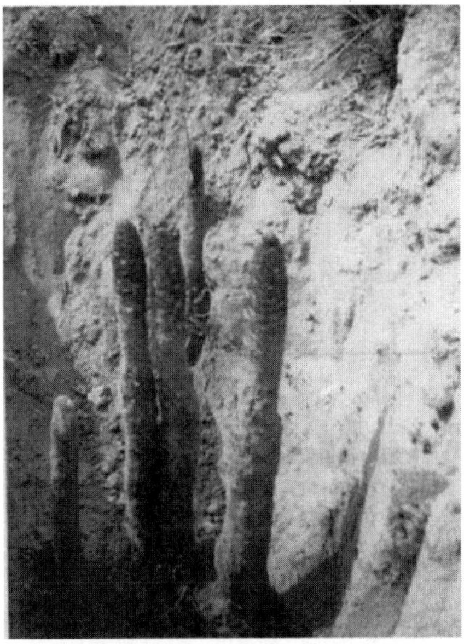

Figure 12. *C. songaricum* growing in the half-deserted areas of Inner Mongolia, China.

By separating the tannin fractions on Sephadex LH-20 and MCI gel CHP20P columns, both with H_2O-MeOH as mobile phases, we isolated procyanidins B_1 and B_6, flavan 3-ol trimers, tetramers, pentamers and a mixture of higher oligomers and polymers. The two isomers (procyanidins B_1 and B_6) of dimeric flavan 3-ols were separated as pure compounds. The trimers, tetramers and pentamers were obtained as mixtures of isomers containing epicatechin/catechin as the flavan 3-ol unit as indicated by their API-MS spectra. The polymer fraction was further divided to sub-fractions by ultrafiltration using centripre-10, centriprep-30 and cintricon plus-20 biomax-100, corresponding to 10, 30 and 100 kDa molecular-weight cutoffs. Although, for tannin, these cutoffs may not reflect the molecular sizes accurately, they may reflect the correct order of molecular sizes. Thiolytic degradation of the tannin polymers yielded benzylthioepicatechin as the predominant product, indicating that the extender flavan unit of the polymers in *C. songaricum* is mainly epicatechin. The *C. songaricum* tannins showed inhibitory activity on HIV-1 protease and the potency increased as the molecular sizes increased. The most potent activity was found in the sub-fraction with the largest molecular weights (IC_{50}=2 μg/ml) (Ma *et al.*, 1999).

Our recent study demonstrated that the methanol extract of this herb had potent anti-oxidative activity and moderate α-glucosidase inhibitory activity. Flavan-3-ol monomer and oligomers were found to be the active components by activity guided fractionation and isolation. The results suggested that that *C. songaricum* might be beneficial for patients with lifestyle related diseases, such as type 2 diabetes, obesity, and metabolic syndrome (Ma *et al.*, 2009).

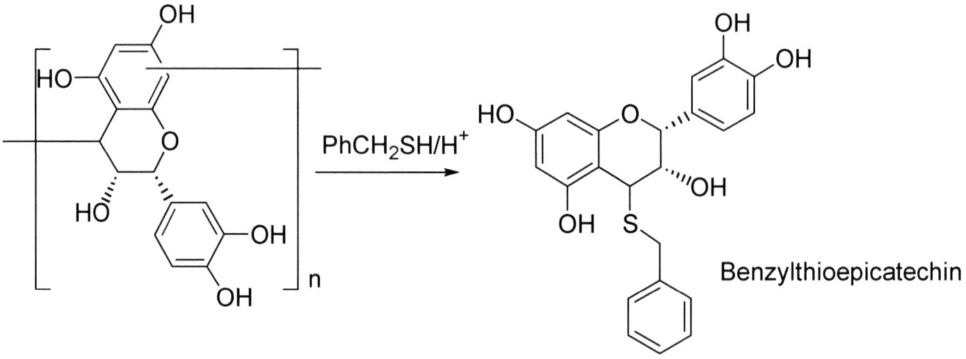

Figure 13. Thiolytic degradation of *C. songaricum* tannins.

Distribution in Other Dietary Sources

The contents of the phenolic compounds play important role in the antioxidant activity and other related bioactivities of fruits and vegetables. Cai et al. have studied a large number of plants about the relationship between their antioxidant activity and the contents of phenolic compounds. It was found that the antioxidant activity and the total phenolic contents for the tested herbs (112 species) were positively and significantly linearly correlated (methanolic/aqueous: R^2 = 0.964/0.953). Plants with higher total phenolic contents showed higher antioxidant capacity. The study showed that the contents of phenolic compounds in common fruits and vegetables were in the order of followings (from high to low phenolic contents): eggplant, spinach, Chinese lettuce, Washington red apple, broccoli, orange, Fuji apple, tomato, spring onion, kiwifruit, carrot, garlic, cucumber and pear. Tannins are among the main components of the phenolic compounds in these plants (Cai *et al.*, 2004).

Mai et al. investigated the α-glucosidase inhibitory and antioxidant activities of Vietnamese edible plants and discussed their relationships with the polyphenol contents. The results showed that the extracts from plants used for making drinks showed the highest activities, followed by edible wild vegetables, herbs, and dark green vegetables. Positive relationships among α-glucosidase inhibitory activities, antioxidant activities and polyphenol contents of these plants were found. All the 5 plants (*Camellia sinensis* (Che Xanh), *Cleistocalyx operculatus* (Voi), *Psidium guajava* (Oi), *Nelumbo nucifera* (Sen), *Sophora japonica* (Hoe)) used for making drinks had high enzyme inhibitory activities and high antioxidant activities (Mai *et al.*, 2007).

CONCLUSION

Flavan 3-ols consumed in our daily foods and beverages play important roles in helping us to keep healthy. As potent antioxidants, they have effects on slowing down the aging progress as well as on prevention of Alzheimer's disease, cardiovascular disease, and cancer. These compounds also have inhibitory activity on α-glucosidase, suggesting they may have effect to prevent some modern diseases, such as type 2 diabetes, obesity, and metabolic syndrome.

Chemically, these compounds are unstable. Their C8 and C6 are highly nucleophilic, while C4 is electrophilic. Due to these chemical properties, these compounds are easy to polymerize and to condense with other compounds co-existing in the dietary materials. Specific controls of these reactions can produce dietary materials with special color, sensory property and biological activity.

Separation and identification work for the flavan 3-ol conjugates are considerably more difficult than for other types of small natural products, and thus the identification and biological activity of pure tannin compounds have not been fully investigated.

While the healthy beneficial effects of tannins are emphasized in this paper and in many other articles in recent years, caution will also be taken not to consume too much tannin mixtures as the non-specific interactions of tannin mixtures with proteins may cause some adverse effects. However, the current situation is that people, especially those in developed countries, do not take enough phenolic compounds, which lead to increasing cases of obesity and other modern diseases, thus, higher intake of tannin-containing vegetables and fruits in daily diets is recommended.

REFERENCES

Cai Y, Luo Q, Sun M, Corke H. 2004. Antioxidant activity and phenolic compounds of 112 traditional Chinese medicinal plants associated with anticancer. *Life Sci* 74: 2157-2184.

Davis AL, Lewis JR, Cai Y, Powell C, Davies AP, Wilkins JPG, Pudney P, Clifford MN. 1997. A polyphenolic pigment from black tea. *Phytochemistry* 46:1397-1402.

Es-Safi N-E, Le Guerneve C, Cheynier V, Moutounet M. 2000. New phenolic compounds formed by evolution of (+)-catechin and glyoxylic acid in hydroalcoholic solution and their implication in changes of grape-derived foods. *J Agric Food Chem* 48: 4233-4240.

Ezaki-Furuichi E, Nonaka G, Nishioka I, Hayashi K. 1986. Tannins and related compounds. Part XLIII. Isolation and structures of procyanidins (condensed tannins) from Rhaphiolepis umbellata. *Agric Biol Chem* 50: 2061-2067.

Fujii H, Nakagawa T, Nishioka H, Sato E, Hirose A, Ueno Y, Sun B, Yokozawa T, Nonaka G. 2007. Preparation, characterization, and antioxidative effects of oligomeric proanthocyanidin−l-cysteine complexes. *J Agric Food Chem* 55: 1525-1531.

Fukuhara K, Nakanishi I, Kansui H, Sugiyama E, Kimura M, Shimada T, Urano S, Yamaguchi K, Miyata N. 2002. Enhanced radical-scavenging activity of a planar catechin analogue. *J Am Chem Soc* 124: 5952-5953.

Fulcrand H, Benabdeljalil C, Rigaud J, Cheynier V, Moutounet M. 1998. A new class of wine pigments generated by reaction between pyruvic acid and grape anthocyanins. *Phytochemistry*: 47: 1401-1407.

Hakamata W, Nakanishi I, Masuda Y, Shimizu T, Higuchi H, Nakamura Y, Saito S, Urano S, Oku T, Ozawa T, Ikota N, Miyata N, Okuda H, Fukuhara K. 2006. Planar catechin analogues with alkyl side chains: a potent antioxidant and an α-glucosidase inhibitor. *J Am Chem Soc* 128: 6524 -6525.

Harborne FRS JB, Baxter H. 1999. The handbook of natural flavonoids. 2: 2016-2067.

Hellström J, Sinkkonen J, Karonen M, Mattila P. 2007. Isolation and structure elucidation of procyanidin oligomers from Saskatoon berries (*Amelanchier alnifolia*). *J Agric Food Chem* 55: 157–164.

Herderich MJ, Smith PA. 2008. Analysis of grape and wine tannins: Methods, applications and challenges. *Aust J Grape Wine Res* 11: 205-214.

Hoffmann E M, Muetzel S, Becker K. 2002. A modified dot-blot method of protein determination applied in the tannin-protein precipitation assay to facilitate the evaluation of tannin activity in animal feeds. *Br J Nutr* 87: 421–426.

Hsu FL, Nonaka G, Nishioka I. 1985. Tannins and related compounds. XXXI. Isolation and characterization of proanthocyanidins in Kandelia candel (L.) Druce. *Chem Pharm Bul* 33: 3142-3152.

http://en.wikipedia.org/wiki/Tannin. access date: Nov 25, 2008.

Hwang T H, Kashiwada Y, Nonaka G, Nishioka I. 1989. Tannins and related compounds. Part 74. Flavan-3-ol and proanthocyanidin allosides from Davallia divaricata. *Phytochemistry* 28: 891-896.

Kashiwada Y, Nonaka G, Nishioka I. 1986. Tannins and related compounds. XLVIII. Rhubarb. (7). Isolation and characterization of new dimeric and trimeric procyanidins. *Chem Pharm Bull* 34: 4083-4091.

Lou H, Yamazaki Y, Sasaki T, Uchida M, Tanaka H, Oka S. 1999. A-type proanthocyanidins from peanut skins. *Phytochemistry* 51: 297-308.

Lou H, Yuan H, Ma B, Ren D, Ji M, Oka S. 2004. Polyphenols from peanut skins and their free radical-scavenging effects. *Phytochemistry* 65: 2391-2399.

Ma CM, Nakamura N, Miyashiro H, Hattori M, Shimotohno K. 1999. Inhibitory effects of constituents from *Cynomorium songaricum* and related triterpene derivatives on HIV-1 protease. *Chem Pharm Bull* 47: 141-145.

Ma CM, Sato N, Li XY. Nakamura N, Hattori M. 2009. Flavan-3-ol contents, anti-oxidative and α-glucosidase inhibitory activities of *Cynomorium songaricum. Food Chem* in press, *Available online 4 May 2009.*

Mai TT, Thu NN, Tien PG , Chuyen NV. 2007. alpha-glucosidase inhibitory and antioxidant activities of Vietnamese edible plants and their relationships with polyphenol contents. *J Nutr Sci Vitaminol* 53: 267-276.

Matthews S, Mila I, Scalbert A, Pollet B, Lapierre C, HerveÂ duPenhoat CLM, Rolando C, Donnelly DMX. 1997. Method for estimation of proanthocyanidins based on their acid depolymerization in the presence of nucleophiles. *J Agric Food Chem* 45:1195-1201.

Morimoto S, Nonaka G, Nishioka I. 1987. Tannins and related compounds. LIX. Aesculitannins, novel proanthocyanidins with doubly-bonded structures from Aesculus hippocastanum L. *Chem Pharm Bull* 35: 4717-29.

Morimoto S, Nonaka G, Nishioka I. 1988. Tannins and related compounds. LX. Isolation and characterization of proanthocyanidins with a doubly-linked unit from Vaccinium vitis-idaea L. *Chem Pharm Bull* 36: 33-38.

Nakagawa T, Yokozawa T. 2002. Direct scavenging of nitric oxide and superoxide by green tea. *Food Chem Toxicol* 40: 1745-1750.

Nakagawa T, Yokozawa T, Sano M, Takeuchi S, Kim Mujo, Minamoto S. 2004. Activity of (-)-Epigallocatechin 3-O-Gallate against Oxidative Stress in Rats with Adenine-Induced Renal Failure. *J Agric Food Chem* 52: 2103-2107.

Nour-Eddine E, Souhila G, Henri D P. 2007. Flavonoids: hemisynthesis, reactivity, characterization and free radical scavenging activity. *Molecules* 12: 2228-58.

Nu□n□ez V, Go□mez-Cordove□s C, Bartolome□B, Hong Y-J, Mitchell A E. 2006. Non-galloylated and galloylated proanthocyanidin oligomers in grape seeds from *Vitus vinifera* L. cv. Graciano, Tempranillo and Cabernet Sauvignon. *J Sci Food Agric* 86:915–921.

Peleg H, Gacon K, Schlich P, Noble AC. 1999. Bitterness and astringency of flavan-3-ol monomers, dimers and trimers. *J Sci Food Agric* 79:1123-1128.

Porter LJ, Hrstich LN, Chan BG. 1986. The conversion of procyanidins and prodelphinidins to cyanidin and delphinidin. *Phytochemistry* 25:223-230.

Prieur C, Rigaud J, Cheynier V, Moutounet M. 1994. Oligomeric and polymeric procyanidins from grape seeds. *Phytochemistry* 36, 781–784.

Ren Y, Chen X. 2007. Distribution, Bioactivities and therapeutical potentials of pentagalloylglucopyranose. *Curr Bioact Compd* 3: 81-88.

Santos-Buelga C, Scalbert A. 2000. Proanthocyanidins and tannin-like compounds– nature, occurrence, dietary intake effects on nutrition and health. *J Sci Food Agric* 80:1094-1117.

Scifinder, access date: Dec.7, 2008.

Shahidi F. 1997. Beneficial health effects and drawbacks of antinutrients and phytochemicals in foods. In F. Shahidi, *Antinutrients and phytochemicals in food (ACS symposium series 662)* (pp. 1-9). American Chemical Society, Washington, D.C.

Souquet JM, Cheynier V, Brossaud F, Moutounet M. 1996. Polymeric proanthocyanidins from grape skins. *Phytochemistry* 43: 509–512.

Takino Y, Ferretti A, Flanagan V, Gianturco M, Vogel M. 1965. Structure of theaflavin, a polyphenol of black tea. *Tetrahedron Lett* 6: 4019±4025.

Yokozawa T, Cho E, Hara Y, Kitani K. 2000. Antioxidative Activity of Green Tea Treated with Radical Initiator 2,2'-Azobis(2-amidinopropane) Dihydrochloride. *J Agric Food Chem* 48: 5068-5073.

Yokozawa T, Nakagawa T, Oya T, Okubo T, Juneja LR. 2005. Green tea polyphenols and dietary fibre protect against kidney damage in rats with diabetic nephropathy. *J Pharm Pharmac* 57: 773-780.

In: Flavonoids: Biosynthesis, Biological Effects...
Editor: Raymond B. Keller
ISBN: 978-1-60741-622-7

Chapter 11

Chemotaxonomic Applications of Flavonoids

Jacqui M. McRae[1,2], Qi Yang[2], Russell J. Crawford[1] and Enzo A. Palombo[1]***

[1] Environment and Biotechnology Centre, Faculty of Life and Social Sciences, Swinburne University of Technology, Hawthorn, VIC,
[2] CSIRO Molecular and Health Technologies, Clayton, VIC

Abstract

Accurate taxonomic groupings are important for many applications, especially for medicinal plants. For example, structural analogues of the antitumour agent, paclitaxel, found in common *Taxus* species have increased the availability of this life-saving medicine without relying on the slow growing and comparatively uncommon, *T. brevifolia* [1]. Flavonoids have a long history of use as chemotaxonomic markers and have assisted in resolving many taxonomic disputes that have arisen as a result of morphological classification. In recent times, there has been increased interest in using molecular systematics and bioinformatics as alternatives to traditional chemotaxonomic techniques, however the investigation of the types flavonoids present in plants is still a useful technique to rapidly assess plant taxonomy.

Planchonia careya is a medicinal plant that contains a range of antibacterial compounds. Species of this genus are morphologically related to *Barringtonia* and *Careya* species and there have been several changes of nomenclature to reflect the uncertainty of these relationships.

Our recent investigation of some of the comprising flavonoids from *Planchonia careya* has revealed similar distinctive compounds to those found in *Planchonia grandis* that are notably absent from *Barringtonia* and *Careya* taxa. Therefore the comparatively simple analysis of the flavonoid component of plant extracts can confirm or contest phenetic groupings to help resolve taxonomic discrepancies.

1. Introduction

Current taxonomic classifications group species into genera or families based on morphological similarities. Although this method has proven to be satisfactory in most cases, multiple revisions in the classification of many species highlight the inadequacies of phenetic taxonomy [2]. A more precise method of classification is often required to accurately group species, and molecular systematics and chemical taxonomy (also referred to as chemotaxonomy or biochemical systematics) have been used in these applications. Molecular systematics, including bioinformatics and DNA barcoding, is used to detect the presence of certain genetic markers in related plant species, while chemotaxonomy focuses on the similarities of compounds produced when a particular gene is expressed in related taxa [3, 4]. The utilization of both taxonomic methods can therefore provide a great deal of data for understanding the functions of secondary metabolites in plants [2, 5].

Secondary metabolites commonly have restricted distribution patterns in plants, with many occurring only in particular families or within species of a particular genus [1]. Morphologically-related plants are known to produce similar secondary metabolites and this observation led to the development of chemotaxonomy. This concept was in its infancy in the 1950s and grew in prominence over the following two decades [6, 7]. The advent of DNA sequencing technology in the 1990s eclipsed the enthusiasm for chemotaxonomy for a time, however it has since been shown that both techniques are required to provide adequate data for the phenetic and classification of a plant species [5, 7].

Chemotaxonomy ideally relies on the systematic analysis of particular phytochemicals in all known species of each family or genus. Specific types of compounds that are present in members of a particular genus and absent from representatives of a related genus (referred to as chemotaxonomic indicators or markers), can be used to prove if the morphological grouping is accurate. These compounds can also assist in the classification of new species. Chemotaxonomic markers must have particular characteristics to be of value in systematic investigations, including chemical complexity and structural variability, stability, and widespread distribution in plant species [6].

Alkaloids are a structurally diverse class of compounds and have therefore been used as chemotaxonomic markers [8, 9]. However, this class is limited in this application since these compounds occur in less than 20% of angiosperm families [10]. Flavonoids are less diverse than the alkaloids, with over 8 150 known structures reported up to the year 2006 [2] compared with the 12 000 known alkaloids, although they appear to be almost universally distributed among plant families. This makes them more widespread than other classes of secondary metabolites and therefore flavonoids have been used extensively as chemotaxonomic markers [2, 11].

Distribution patterns of flavonoid glycosylation and acylation in plant species have shown strong correlations with morphologically related species. Chemotaxonomic investigations of flavonoid glycosides have demonstrated that complex glycosidic patterns occur in many plant families and these usually correlate with morphological classifications [12]. For example, investigations of the flavonol tri- and tetraglycosides of *Styphnolobium* and *Cladrastis* genera indicated that the morphological sub-grouping of some species may be

* Email: epalombo@swin.edu.au

inaccurate [13]. Further, the closely related genera, *Pergularia* and *Gomphocarpus* (Asclepiadaceae), were confirmed as being distinct based on the presence or absence of certain quercetin O-diglycosides and acylated kaempferol glycosides [14].

Chemotaxonomy has also resolved some issues that had arisen due to the difficulty of morphological classifications. The controversial distinction between the genera *Malus* (apple) and *Pyrus* (pear) was resolved by the presence of dihydrochalcones in all known species of *Malus*, and the absence of such compounds from *Pyrus* species [6]. Further, the recent creation of a separate grouping for some *Ateleia* species (Leguminosae) has been supported by the discovery of unusual flavonoid glycosides in only some of these species. This study also confirmed the placement of the *Ateleia* genus in the subfamily Papilionoideae, based on the glycosylation pattern of the comprising flavonols, thus validating the morphological classification [15]. Chemotaxonomic investigations of the types of anthocyanins present in certain species of Lecythidaceae and Myrtiflorae have also supported the morphological division of these families [16].

These correlations validate the use of phytochemicals in plant taxonomy and also the use of flavonoids as chemotaxonomic indicators. In addition, the ongoing discovery of novel flavonoid glycosides is a testament to their structural diversity and may yet reveal many novel compounds.

2. Extraction and Analysis of Flavonoid Glycosides for Chemotaxonomy

Current phytochemical investigations of flavonoid distribution in plant samples often utilizes liquid chromatography-mass spectrometry (LC-MS) and ultraviolet (UV) spectroscopy with photodiode array (PDA) detection [17, 18]. Previous investigations often used thin layer chromatography (TLC) and spot tests, which could not fully characterize the compound structure [19]. Further investigation of unknown flavonoids requires high performance liquid chromatography (HPLC)-piloted separation and isolation of the compounds of interest for structural elucidation.

Flavonoid glycosides and conjugates are water soluble and therefore can be extracted from the plant material with aqueous solutions [20]. Initial separation of the flavonoids from the hydrophilic carbohydrates and proteins present in the crude extract is best achieved with a polymeric chromatographic media such as Amberlite^{TM} XAD resin. This media adsorbs relatively hydrophobic compounds and is particularly useful in capturing phenolic compounds from aqueous solutions [21]. Further HPLC-piloted separation and isolation is best achieved with reversed phase C18 media and size-exclusion chromatography, generally with Sephadex^{TM} LH20 gel, using the distinctive UV profiles produced by flavonoids and their conjugates as a separation guide [20].

Identification of an isolated flavonoid may involve infra-red (IR) spectroscopy to determine the functional groups present, and MS for determining the molecular weight and the distinctive fragmentation patterns of the compound [22, 23]. The most commonly used technique for structural elucidation of unknown isolated compounds is nuclear magnetic resonance (NMR) spectroscopy. This is the most powerful tool available to natural products chemists as it allows the characterization of an unknown compound without destroying the sample. Improvements in the sensitivity of the instrument (greater than 500 MHz) as well as the development of multibond heteronuclear experiments have enabled the complete characterization of complex compound structures with less than one milligram of sample [24].

NMR technology is continually being improved and recent developments include the use of cryoprobes, which greatly increase the signal to noise ratio and therefore reduce the experiment time or the amount of sample [25]. The use of submicro-inverse-detection gradient NMR probes and other inverse detection techniques has also led to increases in the sensitivity of NMR spectroscopy enabling the elucidation of compounds of less than 0.05 μmol [26]. The use of NMR spectroscopy has enabled the full structural elucidation of many thousands of novel flavonoid glycosides that may have otherwise remained only partially characterized.

3. APPLICATION OF CHEMOTAXONOMIC TECHNIQUES

This laboratory recently investigated the presence of potential chemotaxonomic indicators in the tropical Australian tree, *Planchonia careya* (F. Muell) R. Knuth (Lecythidaceae) [27]. The morphological similarities of *P. careya* with many *Barringtonia* species (Figure 1) resulted in the original classification of *P. careya* as *Barringtonia careya* F. Muell. (Barringtonaceae) (1866). This classification was later changed to *Careya arborea* Roxb. var. *australis* Benth. (alternatively referred to as *C. australis* F. Muell.) in 1882, due to the morphological similarities with the *Careya* genus, also of the Lecythidaceae family [28].

The leaves and bark of *P. careya* are used medicinally in the treatment of sores and skin infections. For cleaning a wound and preventing infection, an infusion was made from the inner bark of *P. careya*, and this was used to bathe the affected area, before applying a bandage made from the fibrous root bark [29]. Alternatively, the leaves of *P. careya* were crushed and applied directly to wounds and ulcers to prevent or treat infections [30, 31]. This traditional medicinal use has been validated by the isolation of several antibacterial compounds from the leaves [32].

Approximately 14 *Planchonia* species are found across Australasia from the Andaman Islands to Papua New Guinea and Australia [28].

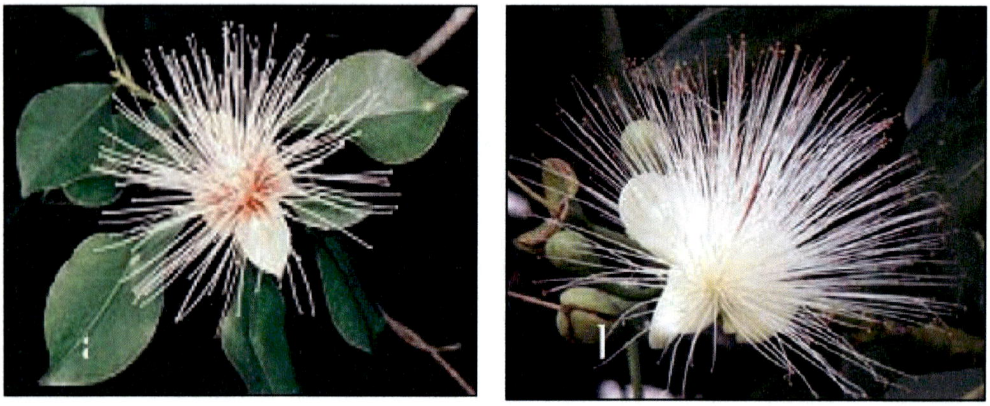

Figure 1. Comparison of the flowers from *Planchonia careya* and *Barringtonia racemosa* [39, 40].

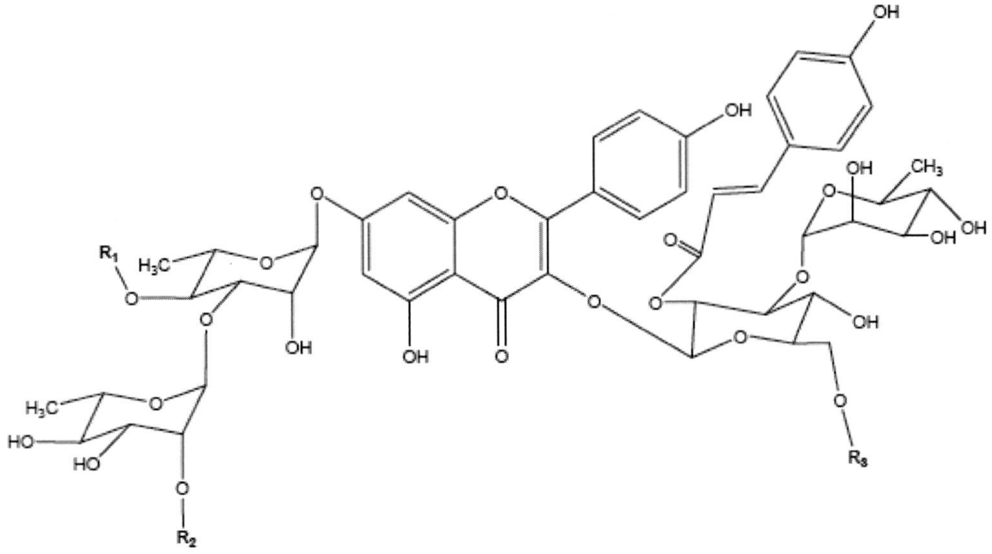

	R_1	R_2	R_3
1	*trans-p*-Coumaroyl	α-L-Rhamnosyl	β-D-Glucosyl
2	*cis-p*-Coumaroyl	α-L-Rhamnosyl	β-D-Glucosyl
3	*trans-p*-Coumaroyl	α-L-Rhamnosyl	α-L-Rhamnosyl
4	*trans-p*-Coumaroyl	H	H

Figure 2. Compounds isolated from *Planchonia* sp.: 1-3, Acylated kaempferol hexaglycosides isolated from *P. grandis*; 4, Acylated kaempferol tetraglycoside isolated from *P. careya.*

Many of these species have experienced similar taxonomic contention to *P. careya* so the exact number of species remains uncertain. Chemotaxonomy is therefore a more useful method of clarifying the classification of *Planchonia* taxa as distinct from other species. Crublet et al. [33] isolated three novel acylated kaempferol hexaglycosides from the leaves of *P. grandis* (1-3, Figure 2), yet no similar compounds have been isolated from *Careya* or *Barringtonia* species. The presence of related compounds in *P. careya* would indicate that acylated flavonol polyglycosides were effective chemotaxonomic markers for the *Planchonia* genus [27].

To assess this premise, a collection of fresh *P. careya* leaves were crushed and extracted with water by immersion in the solvent. After a total of three 24 hour extractions, the flavonoid component of the crude aqueous extract was concentrated on XAD-16 resin and eluted with methanol. Separation was achieved with reversed phase C18 (100-200 mesh) media followed by Medium Pressure C18 (15 μm) media and isolation with preparative reversed phase HPLC (5 μm) gave the novel acylated flavonol tetraglycoside, kaempferol 3-*O*-[α-rhamnopyranosyl(1→3)-(2-*O*-*p*-coumaroyl)]-β-glucopyranoside, 7-*O*-[α-rhamnopyranosyl-(1→3)-(4-*O*-*p*-coumaroyl)]-α-rhamnopyranoside (4, Figure 2). Structural elucidation was achieved with 1D and 2D (homonuclear and heteronuclear) NMR experiments and mass spectrometry, and TLC of the acid hydrolysis products enabled the verification of the comprising sugar units [34, 35].

Other acylated kaempferol glycosides, such as a 3-*O*-coumaroylglucopyranoside from the leaf hairs of *Quercus ilex* (Fagaceae), reportedly have a strong UV-B absorbing capacity, a property that is attributable to many flavonoids although stronger in those with acylating acids [36, 37]. This and the possible regulation of plant growth may the reasons for the biosynthesis of such large molecules in the leaves of plants [37, 38].

The similarity in structure and glycosylation pattern of the compounds isolated from two *Planchonia* taxa suggest that other derivatives are likely to be found in related taxa. The presence of these acylated kaempferol polyglycosides can thus be considered as a reliable taxonomic indicator for members of the *Planchonia* genus and can therefore prevent taxonomic disputes based on morphological assessment.

Conclusion

The advent of molecular systematics techniques has led to a significant reduction in chemotaxonomic investigations in recent years. However, the capacity of chemotaxonomy as a comparatively simple and reliable method of plant classification ensures the continued validity of this technique.

Acknowledgments

The authors would like to thank the Sunshine Foundation for providing financial support for this research and Andrew Ford of the CSIRO Tropical Rainforest Centre for collecting the plant material. We also thank Dr. Noel Hart for his expertise in methods of compound separation and Dr. Roger Mulder for assistance with the NMR elucidation.

References

[1] Wildman, H. G. In *Pharmaceutical bioprospecting and its relationship to the conservation and utilization of bioresources*, International conference on biodiversity and bioresources: Conservation and utilization, 1997, Phuket, Thailand, 1999; IUPAC, Ed. Phuket, Thailand, 1999.

[2] Williams, C. A., Flavone and flavonol *O*-glycosides. In: *Flavonoids: Chemistry, biochemistry and applications*, Andersen, O. M.; Markham, K. R., Eds. Taylor and Francis Group: Florida, USA, 2006; pp 749-855.

[3] Kress, W. J.; Wurdack, K. J.; Zimmer, E. A.; Weigt, L. A.; Janzen, D. H., Use of DNA barcodes to identify flowering plants. *Proceedings of the National Academy of Science*, 2005, 105, (23), 8369–8374.

[4] Lahaye, R.; van der Bank, M.; Bogarin, D.; Warner, J.; Pupulin, F.; Gigot, G.; Maurin, O.; Duthoit, S.; Barraclough, T. G.; Savolainen, V., DNA barcoding the floras of biodiversity hotspots. *Proceedings of the National Academy of Science*, 2008, 105, (8), 2923–2928.

[5] Albach, D. C.; Grayer, R. J.; Kite, G. C.; Jensen, S. R., *Veronica*: Acylated flavone glycosides as chemosystematic markers. *Biochemical Systematics and Ecology*, 2005, 33, 1167-1177.

[6] Harborne, J. B., *Comparative biochemistry of the flavonoids*. Academic Press Inc Ltd.: London, England, 1967; p 304-314.

[7] Waterman, P. G., The current status of chemical systematics. *Phytochemistry*, 2007, 68, 2896-2903.

[8] Ober, D., Chemical ecology of alkaloids exemplified with the pyrrolizidines. In: *Recent advances in phytochemistry, Volume 37: Intergrative phytochemistry from ethnobotany to molecular ecology*, Romeo, J. T., Ed. Pergamon (Elsevier Science Ltd): Oxford, England, 2003; pp 204-206.

[9] Waterman, P. G., The chemical systematics of alkaloids: A review emphasising the contribution of Robert Hegnauer. *Biochemical Systematics and Ecology*, 1999, 27, 395-406.

[10] Facchini, P. J.; Bird, D. A.; MacLeod, B. P.; Park, S.; Samanani, N., Multiple levels of control in the regulation of alkaloid biosynthesis. In: *Recent advances in phytochemistry, Volume 37: Intergrative phytochemistry from ethnobotany to molecular ecology*, Romeo, J. T., Ed. Pergamon (Elsevier Science Ltd): Oxford, England, 2003; pp 144-145.

[11] Ibrahim, R. K.; Anzellotti, D., The enzymatic basis of flavonoid biodiversity. In: *Recent advances in phytochemistry, Volume 37: Intergrative phytochemistry from ethnobotany to molecular ecology*, Romeo, J. T., Ed. Pergamon (Elsevier Science Ltd): Oxford, England, 2003; pp 2-12.

[12] Harborne, J. B.; Williams, C. A., Flavone and flavonol glycosides. In: *The flavonoids: Advances in research*, Harborne, J. B.; Mabry, T. J., Eds. Chapman and Hall Ltd: London, UK, 1982; pp 261-311.

[13] Kite, G. C.; Stoneham, C. A.; Veitch, N. C., Flavonoid tetraglycosides and other constituents from the leaves of *Styphynolobium japonicum* (Leguminosae) and related taxa. *Phytochemistry*, 2007, 68, 1407-1416.

[14] Heneidak, S.; Grayer, R. J.; Kite, G. C.; Simmonds, M. S. J., Flavonoid glycosides from Egyptian species of the tribe Ascelpiadaceae (Apocynaceae, subfamily Asclepiadoideae). *Biochemical Systematics and Ecology*, 2006, 34, 575-584.

[15] Veitch, N. C.; Tibbles, L. L.; Kite, G. C.; Ireland, H. E., Flavonol tetraglycosides from *Atelia chicoasinensis* (Leguminosae). *Biochemical Systematics and Ecology*, 2005, 33, 1274-1279.

[16] Lowry, J. B., Anthocyanins of the Melastomataceae, Myrtaceae and some allied families. *Phytochemistry*, 1976, 15, (4), 513-516.

[17] de Rijke, E.; Out, P.; Niessen, W. M. A.; Ariese, F.; Gooijer, C.; Brinkman, U. A. T., Analytical separation and detection methods for flavonoids. *Journal of Chromatography A*, 2006, 1112, 31-63.

[18] Mabry, T. J.; Markham, K. R.; Thomas, M. B., *The systematic identification of the flavonoids*. Springer-Verlag New York Inc: Berlin, Germany, 1970.

[19] Gluchoff-Fiasson, K. G.; Fiasson, J. L.; Waton, H., Quercetin glycosides from European aquatic *Ranunculus* species of subgenus *Batrachium*. *Phytochemistry*, 1997, 45, (5), 1063-1067.

[20] Marsten, A.; Hostettmann, K., Separation and quantification of flavonoids. In: *Flavonoids: Chemistry, biochemistry and applications*, Andersen, O. M.; Markham, K. R., Eds. Taylor and Francis Group: Florida, USA, 2006; pp 8-31.

[21] Hostettmann, K.; Hostettmann, M., Isolation techniques for flavonoids. In: *The flavonoids: Advances in research*, Harborne, J. B.; Mabry, T. J., Eds. Chapman and Hall Ltd: London, UK, 1982; pp 6-10.

[22] Foo, L. Y., Proanthocyanidins: Gross chemical structures by infra-red spectra. *Phytochemistry*, 1981, 20, (6), 1397-1402.

[23] Ajees, A. A.; Balakrishna, K., Arjunolic acid. *Acta Crystallographica*, 2002, E58, o682-o684.

[24] Breitmeyer, E., *Structure elucidation by NMR in organic chemistry*. 3rd ed.; John Wiley and Sons, LTD: West Sussex, England, 2002.

[25] Fossen, T.; Andersen, O. M., Spectroscopic techniques applied to flavonoids. In: *Flavonoids: Chemistry, biochemistry and applications*, Andersen, O. M.; Markham, K. R., Eds. Taylor and Francis Group: Florida, USA, 2006; pp 40-98.

[26] Martin, G. E.; Guido, J. E.; Robins, R. H.; Sharaf, M. H. M.; Schiff, J., P.L.; Tackie, A. N., Submicro Inverse-detection gradient NMR: A powerful new way of conducting structure elucidation studies with <0.05 μmol samples. *Journal of Natural Products*, 1998, 61, (5), 555-559.

[27] McRae, J. M.; Yang, Q.; Crawford, R. J.; Palombo, E. A., Acylated flavonoid tetraglycoside from Planchonia careya leaves. *Phytochemistry Letters*, 2008, 1, 99-102.

[28] Barrett, R. L., A review of Planchonia (Lecythidaceae) in Australia. *Australian Systematic Botany*, 2006, 19, 147-153.

[29] Barr, A.; Chapman, J.; Smith, N.; Beveridge, M., *Traditional bush medicines: An Aboriginal pharmacopoeia*. Greenhouse Publications Pty Ltd: Northern Territory, Australia, 1988; p 178-179.

[30] Cribb, A. B.; Cribb, J. W., *Wild medicine in Australia*. William Collins Pty Ltd.: Sydney, Australia, 1983.

[31] Lassak, E. V.; McCarthy, T., *Australian medicinal plants*. Reed New Holland Publishers (Australia) Pty Ltd: Sydney, Australia, 2001.

[32] McRae, J. M.; Yang, Q.; Crawford, R. J.; Palombo, E. A., Antibacterial compounds from *Planchonia careya* leaf extracts. *Journal of Ethnopharmacology*, 2008, 116, 554-560.

[33] Crublet, M. L.; Long, C.; Sevenet, T.; Hadi, H. A.; Lavaud, C., Acylated flavonol glycosides from leaves of *Planchonia grandis*. *Phytochemistry*, 2003, 64, 589-594.

[34] Brasseur, T.; Angenot, L., Six flavonol glycosides from leaves of *Strychnos variabilis*. *Phytochemistry*, 1988, 27, (5), 1487-1490.

[35] Malhorta, O. P.; Dey, P. M., Specificity of sweet-almond α-galactose. *Biochemistry Journal*, 1967, 103, (3), 739-743.

[36] Skaltsa, H., UV-B protective potential and flavonoids content of leaf hairs of *Quercus ilex*. *Phytochemistry*, 1994, 37, 987.

[37] Gould, K. S.; Lister, C., Flavonoids function in plants. In: *Flavonoids: Chemistry, biochemistry and applications*, Andersen, O. M.; Markham, K. R., Eds. Taylor and Francis Group: Florida, USA, 2006; pp 397-425.

[38] Furuya, M.; Galston, A. W., Flavonoid complexes in Pisum sativum L. - I: Nature and distribution of the major components *Phytochemistry*, 1965, 4, 285-296.

[39] van Heygen, G. http://www.vanheygen.com/Silhouette/images/baringtonia.jpg.

[40] TSOE Townsville city council state of the environment report. http://www.soe-townsville.org/nat_days/tree_day/images/PlanchoniaCareyaFlower.jpg.

In: Flavonoids: Biosynthesis, Biological Effects...
Editor: Raymond B. Keller
ISBN: 978-1-60741-622-7

Chapter 12

BIOANALYSIS OF THE FLAVONOID COMPOSITION OF HERBAL EXTRACTS AND DIETARY SUPPLEMENTS

Shujing Ding[1] and Ed Dudley[2]
[1]MRC Human Nutrition Research,
Elsie Widdowson Laboratory,
Fulbourn Road, Cambridge CB1 9NL, UK
[2]Biochemistry and Biomolecular Mass Spectrometry,
Swansea University, Singleton Park, Swansea, SA2 8PP, UK

ABSTRACT

Flavonoids are one of the most diverse and widespread groups of natural products. They ubiquitously occur in all parts of plants including the fruit, pollen, roots and heartwood. Plant extracts rich in flavonoids such as: Ginkgo biloba extract, soy bean extract and green tea extract are popular dietary supplements. Numerous physiological activities have been attributed to them and their potential roles in the prevention of hormone-dependent cancers have been investigated. Over 5000 different flavonoids have been described to date and they are classified into at least 10 chemical groups. Flavonoid compounds usually occur in plants as glycosides in which one or more of the phenolic hydroxyl groups are combined with sugar residues.

Quality control of these plant-extract products is problematic due to the many varying factors in herbal medicine. Unlike synthetic drugs (in which the concentration and activity of a single known bio-molecule is monitored), there are many uncertainties in terms of species variation, geographical source, cultivation, harvest, storage and processing techniques which may lead to a product of different quality and efficacy. To evaluate the quality of flavonoids contained within plant extracts it is therefore very important to develop an analytical method which can monitor the quantity and variety of flavonoids efficiently. Also the study of the absorption and retention of these compounds within individuals is more problematic as more than one active compound is ingested from the plant extracts.

The challenge presented by such extracts is therefore to determine the different flavonoid species present in any given extract and also to determine any modification or fortification of the extract. Furthermore, Administration, Distribution, Metabolism and Excretion (ADME) studies require the quantitative analysis of multiple components rather than a single drug compound. The increase in the number of new flavonoid reports is due to two main factors: the advances in methods of separation and the rapid development and application of modern mass spectrometry (MS). Mass spectrometry proved to be the most effective technique in flavonoids research both in plant extract and in biological samples. In this expert commentary we will review the methods available for studying this wide-ranging class of compounds and also how modern techniques have been applied in order to "mine" the data obtained for flavonoid specific information from a complex metabolomic analysis.

FLAVONOIDS: SOURCE, CLINICAL PROPERTIES AND STRUCTURES

The flavonoids represent a very diverse group of natural products with more than 6500 known flavonoid structures having been identified [1]. They ubiquitously occur in all parts of plants and plant extracts rich in flavonoids such as *Ginkgo biloba* extracts are among the most popular dietary supplements taken by the general public. The flavonoids are structurally similar to steroid hormones, particularly estrogens, and have been studied extensively. These studies have shown that flavonoids exhibit many biological activities, including anti-allergenic, anti-viral, anti-inflammatory and vasodilating actions. Numerous physiological activities have also been attributed to these compounds and their potential role in the prevention of hormone-dependent cancers has also been investigated [2]. A summary of some of the herbal remedies that contain flavonoids and the benefits associated with them is shown in Table 1. Flavonoids are largely planar molecules and their structural variation arises in part from the pattern of substitutions within this basic molecule such as: hydroxylation, methoxylation, prenylation or glycosylation.

Table 1. Herbal extracts, their flavonoid content and medical proterties

Plant name	Flavonoid content	Major flavonoids	Medical properties	Ref
Lycium Barbarum	0.16% wt/vol	myricetin quercetin Kaempferol	Benefiting the liver and kidney, replenishing vital essence and improving eyesight	[3]
Hawthorn	0.1-2% wt/vol	rutin, hyperoside, Vitexin	Gastroprotective, stimulating Digestion, anti-microbial and anti-inflammatory activities	[4]
Ginkgo Biloba extract	240mg/g	Quercetin kaempferol Isorhamnetin	Improving peripheral blood flow, reducing cerebral insufficiency	[5]
Hippophae rhamnoides extract	10-439μg/g	Quercetin kaempferol Isorhamnetin	A cough relief, aiding digestion, invigorating blood circulation, and alleviating pain	[6]
Tea	4.9-136.3mg/g	Catechins theaflavins	Anti-oxidant activity, free radical scavengers	[7]
Soy bean	0.56-3.81mg/g	Daidzein genistein glycitein	Reduced risk of some diseases moderated by oestrogen (e.g.) breast cancer and osteoporosis	[8]

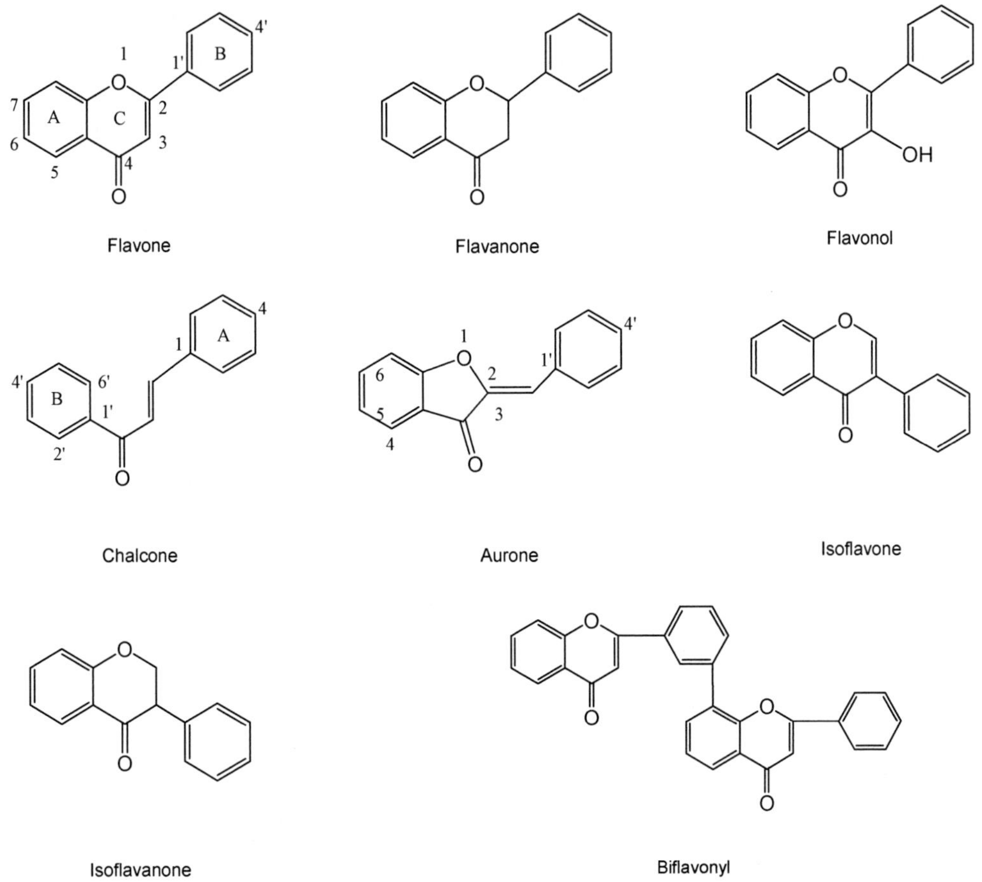

Figure 1. Basic structure of common subclasses of flavonoids.

The flavonoids are classified into at least 10 chemical groups. Figure 1 lists common subclasses of flavonoids and also demonstrates the chemical numbering system applied to both the atoms and rings (A, B and C) when comparing the structures of different flavonoids. Flavonoid compounds usually occur in plants as glycosides in which one or more of the phenolic hydroxyl groups are combined with sugar residues, forming an acid-labile glycoside O-C bond. There are also other forms of conjugated sugars (e.g. D-glucose, L-rhamnose) which contribute to the complex and diverse nature of the individual molecules that have been identified.

Analysis of Flavonoids – A Review

Due to the complex nature of the herbal remedies available (compared to usual pharmaceutical drugs which are composed mainly of a single active agent and formulation chemicals) the application of strict and stringent regulatory rules governing the "purity" of such a mixture is more complicated than those applied to drug moieties by the Food and Drug Administration Authority (FDA). Despite this, the World Health Organisation (WHO) have accepted that the "fingerprint" analysis of the levels of flavonoids and natural products in herbal remedies which claim the benefits of the presence of such compounds, is an acceptable methodology for monitoring the validity of any new or existing "natural product" [9]. This requirement was included in the European Economic Council guideline 75/318 "Quality of Herb Drugs" [10]. Taking *Gingko Biloba* extracts as an example, the flavonoids content is an important parameter in terms of quality control. The applied threshold for commercial standardized extracts of *Ginkgo* is that flavonoids constitute no less than 24% of the material and terpene lactones no less than 6% [11]. However in North America such extracts are considered to be a "dietary supplement" rather than a medicinal product and hence they do not attract the same level of scrutiny compared to Europe. The analysis of the levels of the flavonoids (considered to be – at least one of many – bioactive agents present in herbal extracts) is therefore useful in order to demonstrate that the individual taking the extract is obtaining the expected benefits from these herbal remedies. Furthermore, such analyses are also invaluable for the purpose of identifying any artificial fortification of extracts which are claimed to be "pure". Any such analysis can be used to study the entire flavonoid content of an extract and quantitate the levels of "active" flavonoids in a given sample (similar to any drug quality control assay). Alternatively "fingerprint" assays compare the entire profile of these compounds in a given sample to that of a "pure", unfortified extract in order to ensure that the extract has the properties associated with the herb. Such "fingerprint" analyses are however complicated due to the fact that the flavonoid composition of any herbal extract may be altered due to natural environmental or conditions in which the herb is grown prior to harvesting and so identifying an "ideal" flavonoid profile for comparison with commercial herbal extracts can be problematic. Despite these potential complications, these two major routes of bio-analysis of the flavonoid content of herbal extracts are commonly employed. Fingerprint analysis allows the evaluation of the quality of plant extracts and is able to provide comprehensive (including flavonoids and other components determination) and semi-quantitative information for complicated plant extract samples. More recently bioinformatic programs (e.g. fuzzy influence diagrams) have become available and may be applied in order to minimise subjective judgments when studying such data [12]. This development is a very important step when the active component is unknown in such complex biological extracts.

Fingerprint analysis of flavonoids can be achieved by using several chromatographic techniques including thin-layer chromatography (TLC) [13], high-performance liquid chromatography (HPLC) [14], gas chromatography (GC) [15] high-performance capillary electrophoresis (HPCE) [16] and high-speed counter-current chromatography (HSCCC) [17]. More recently, GC [18] and HPLC [19] in combination with mass spectrometry (MS) have become a popular alternative for fingerprint analysis as they have the advantage of providing more information compared to the previously applied techniques. Traditional quantitation of flavonoids has been achieved by spectrophotometry [20] and HPLC [21]. Both of these techniques require an acid hydrolysis step of the plant extract in order to convert the conjugated flavonoids into flavonoid aglycones. For spectrophotometry, rutin is normally chosen as the reference standard and only total flavonoid can be quantified as "rutin equivalent". HPLC is able to quantify individual flavonoids provided that their aglycone counterparts are available as standard reference compounds and flavonoids are quantified as aglycone equivalents in such assays. A 2-4 hours soxhlet extraction is required to convert the flavonoid glycosides to aglycones for the above two analytical methods. There are also reports of the quantitation of flavonoids in herbal remedies using GC/MS [22], offering better separation and specificity than spectrophotometry and HPLC. However, a time-consuming trimethylsilylate derivatisation step is required prior to GC/MS analysis.

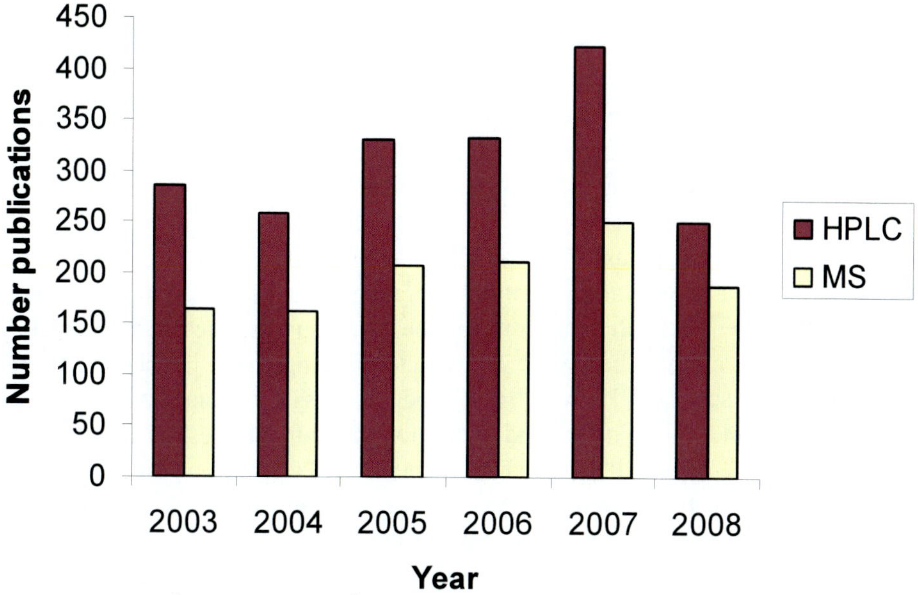

*Note 2008 data from 1st January until 31st October only.

Figure 2. Article title search results for flavonoid analysis by HPLC and MS between 2003 and 2008.

Capillary electrophoresis separation coupled with UV or ESI-MS detectors has also been applied to the study of flavonoids, offering an interesting alternative to HPLC separation [23]. In addition, UPLC is regarded as one way to achieve faster, more efficient separations with liquid chromatography by using smaller particle size stationary phase materials, and this separation technique has also applied to flavonoid analysis [24]. However, as a separation technique, HPLC is the more widely applicable and offers a larger range of choices (in terms of solid phases and column sizes) and when coupled to mass spectrometry detection it can provide structure-selective information concerning the analytes. This is very important in matrices as complicated as plant extracts. Hence, whilst HPLC-UV detection analysis remains well used for flavonoid analysis, mass spectrometry is becoming increasingly used also for such studies as can be seen Figure 2. Reports of the application of HPLC/MS for flavonoid analysis have more than doubled in the recent five years comparing to the previous five years. In this review therefore, we propose to focus on the mass spectrometric properties of flavonoids and mass spectrometric analysis of flavonoids in both plant extract and biological samples.

Mass Spectrometry and Its' Application to the Analysis of Flavonoids in Plant Extract and Metabolites *In Vivo*

Prior to mass spectrometry analysis, an extraction protocol is required in order to extract the flavonoids from the samples under study. This can be simply done by ultrasonic extraction or pressurised liquid extraction [25]. The sample is freeze-dried or crushed up (using a simple pestle and mortar) and methanol added to the resulting material. The solvent will solubilise the flavonoids whilst leaving other components of the sample undissolved and so either filtration or centrifugation can then be applied to the sample to remove this undissolved material and the "purified" flavonoid-methanol extract taken for analysis. Mass spectrometry allows the study of a mixture of compounds (with or without online separation by techniques such as HPLC) and analyses the flavonoids as ions generated from the neutral molecules. For a compound to be analysed by mass spectrometry, the first requirement is that the molecule must form such an ion- usually by formation of a proton adduct with a positive charge or the loss of a proton forming a negative ion. The most commonly utilised technique for forming ions from flavonoids to date is electrospray (ESI) which has been successfully applied to a large number of biological molecules ranging from small entities such as amino acids to peptides, proteins and oligonucleotides. The electrospray process requires that the ion is formed in solution and has the distinct advantage of being easily hyphenated to modern separation techniques such as HPLC. The ESI mode of mass spectrometry is often used for the analysis of flavonoids, since it is a kind of soft ionisation mode (i.e. the ionisation process does not fragment the compound being ionised). The ionised analytes are either protonated or depronated depnding on the solution chemistry. We have studied the flavonoids ability to form ions in an electrospray source and compared the ability of the technique to form both positive and negative ions. In ESI MS, the signal intensity of an individual flavonoid is much stronger (10^{2-3}) in negative mode than positive mode, and in positive mode, the pseudomolecular ion signal is very weak and sodium and potassium adducts are dominant, hence most flavonoid analysis is carried out in negative mode. In this mode, the deprotonated molecular ions will generally be the most abundant ion, and the agycone counterpart can be observed in all flavonoid glycoside mass spectra as an in-source derived fragment. The results, summarised in Figure 3, demonstrate that a negative ionisation approach is substantially more sensitive compared to the formation of positive ions when analysing flavonoids as the intensity of the ions formed is far greater. Given the structure of the flavonoids, this is a sensible conclusion as there are few atoms within the structure with the pre-requisite basic properties to attract a positive proton as would be required to form a positive adduct ion. Once formed, several different mass spectrometric experiments may be performed in order to gain information regarding the flavonoids present in a given sample. The first such method discussed here is accurate mass analysis.

Accurate mass analysis, analogous to modern "metabolomic" analyses, often utilises the direct infusion of the sample of interest. A large number of ions are generated as a result and catalogued. The mass of each ion is measured to a high degree of accuracy and the empirical formula of the compounds present is suggested from the *m/z* value of the ion. This technique requires high resolution mass spectrometers, usually fourier transform mass spectrometers, capable of generating the required degree of mass accuracy. An example spectrum of this type of analysis is indicated in Figure 4. The highlighted ions (indicated by an *) correspond to the flavonoids and in addition to these ions many terpene lactone ions are observed. The mass accuracy of the detected ions is presented in Table 2.

Such analysis allows the rapid analysis of complex samples with quick analysis times (Figure 4 analysis time was 1 minute), however there are a number of disadvantages related to the technique. Firstly, isobaric flavonoids cannot be distinguished as no separation of the compounds present is performed prior to their analysis. Hence, flavonoids with identical glycoside groups attached in a different orientation will give only one signal, for example, 3-*O*-[6-*O*- (α-L-rhamnosyl)-β-D-glucosyl] kaempferol and 3-*O*-[2-*O*-(β-D-glucosyl)-α-L-rhamnosyl] kaempferol, both of which exist in *Ginkgo biloba* extracts [26].

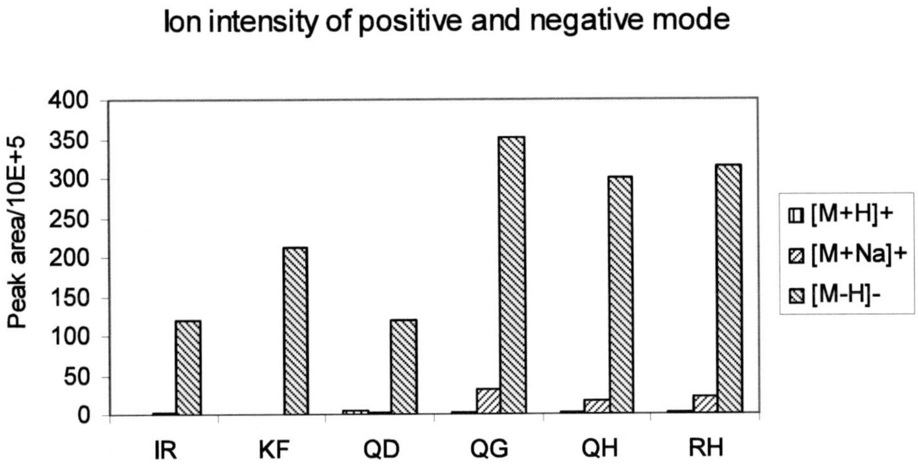

Figure 3. Comparison of ion intensity in positive and negative mode for some flavonoid components in *Ginkgo biloba.*

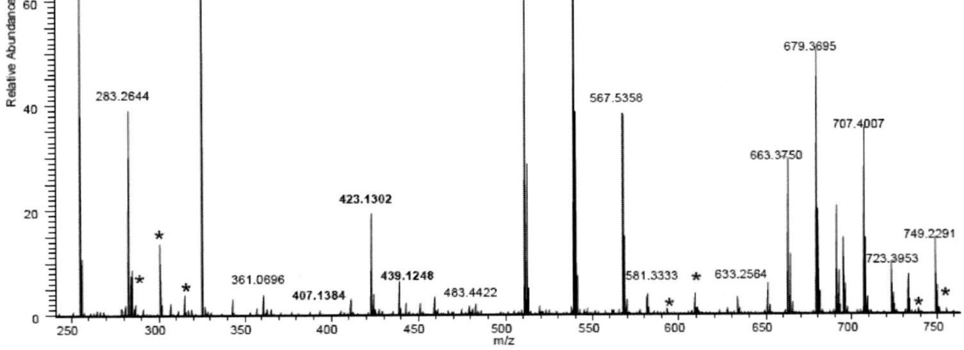

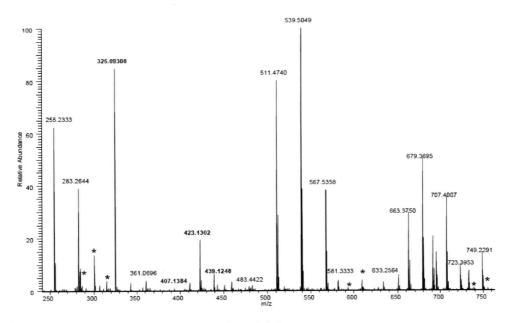

Figure 4. Mass spectrum of a direct infusion of a *G. biloba* extract on an accurate mass – mass spectrometer. (provided by Dr C. Williams, EPSRC National Mass Spectrometry Service Centre, Swansea University)

Table 2. Accurate mass analysis of a *Ginkgo biloba* extract

m/z	Theo. mass	Delta (ppm)	RDB equiv.	Formula	Identification
325.0930	325.0929	1.21	7.5	$C_{15}H_{17}O_8$	Bilobalide
423.1302	423.1297	1.25	9.5	$C_{20}H_{23}O_{10}$	Ginkgolide B/J
439.1248	439.1246	0.49	9.5	$C_{20}H_{23}O_{11}$	Ginkgolide C
407.1348	407.1348	0.11	9.5	$C_{20}H_{23}O_9$	Ginkgolide A
301.0355	301.0354	0.41	11.5	$C_{15}H_9O_7$	Quercetin
285.0406	285.0405	0.49	11.5	$C_{15}H_9O_6$	Kaempferol
315.0512	315.0510	0.55	11.5	$C_{16}H_{11}O_7$	Isorhametin
609.1461	609.1461	-0.01	13.5	$C_{27}H_{29}O_{16}$	Quercetin glycoside
593.1509	593.1512	-0.49	13.5	$C_{27}H_{29}O_{15}$	Kaempferol glycoside
739.1863	739.1880	-2.26	19.5	$C_{36}H_{35}O_{17}$	Kaempferol glycoside
755.1807	755.1829	-2.19	19.5	$C_{36}H_{35}O_{18}$	Quercetin glycoside

The *m/z* of both is 593Th as they exhibit identical empirical formulae, and hence these compounds cannot be distinguished by this method. As a result it is impossible to specify the exact nature of individual moieties as different arrangements of the sugars attached to the agylcone would generate identical data.

A further complication during accurate mass analysis arises due to the possibility of ion suppression. This occurs due to the fact that a specific amount of "charge" is available for the ionisation of the sample and hence the compounds present in the mixture "compete" for this charge. The presence of an easily ionised compound within the mixture may therefore limit the ionisation of others and hence the absence (or reduction in intensity) of a flavonoid ion may not represent an absence (or decrease in level) of the compound but may arise due to this factor. From this spectrum it can be noticed that *Ginkgo biloba* terpene lactone signals significantly suppressed the ionisation of flavonoids, despite the fact that the content of flavonoids is much higher than terpene lactones in the extract.

In order to address both of these issues, the application of a separation technique – preferably directly linked to the mass spectrometer – can be utilised. HPLC analysis is again applied with reverse phase (C18) stationary phases being the most commonly used. Recent developments in the miniaturisation of HPLC columns, and the systems used to run them, have led to lower mobile phase flow rates being applied in HPLC-MS analyses. This miniaturisation, due to the concentration sensitive nature of electrospray ionisation source of the mass spectrometer, leads to a significant increase in sensitivity. The reduction of the internal diameter of the HPLC from 4.6 mm to 0.3 mm (and reduction in required mobile phase flow rate from 1mL/min to 4μL/min) has been shown to result in a 80-100 fold increase in sensitivity of the HPLC-MS assay [27, 28]. The HPLC separation prior to analysis allows isobaric flavonoids to be separated and hence individually analysed and also removes the potential inaccuracy of the data obtained due to ion suppression effects. In order to further alleviate the problem of isobaric flavonoids in the extract, the combination of the HPLC separation of flavonoids with tandem mass spectrometry (MS/MS and MS^n analysis) - in which the ions are fragmented with an inert "collision" gas and the fragment ions determined – allows an information rich analysis to be performed without bias towards any particular flavonoid.

MS/MS requires the isolation of the ion of interest - the precursor ion- which is then fragmented to generate "product ions". These product ions can themselves be individually isolated and fragmented further in an MS^3 experiment. This type of analysis can be done in a "data dependent" fashion in which the mass spectrometer "decides" which ion to fragment (based on ion abundance and how often the ion is detected) and which of its product ions to fragment further. This type of analysis – most commonly applied to trypsin digests of proteins in proteomic analyses [29] – takes the most abundant ion in a given mass spectrum and fragments this ion, next the most abundant product ion is further fragmented generating further structural data.

As the flavonoids are eluted from the HPLC column, they each -for a given time window- become the most abundant such ion and so information on the majority of the flavonoids can be obtained in an automated fashion.

Under MS/MS conditions, flavonoids are fragmented into a series of product ions. For a flavonoid glycoside, the loss of the sugar moiety is commonly seen, producing the corresponding aglycone as the main fragment ion. This is a very important characteristic and can be used to facilitate the bioanalysis of individual flavonoid species in a mixture. For flavonoid aglycones, the diagnostic product ions produced by further fragmentation are illustrated in Figure 5.

Many of the modern mass spectrometers e.g. triple quadrupoles, Q-TOFs can carry out MS/MS analysis since there have two tandem analysers, however ion trap mass spectrometers have a unique capability in that it stores ions. Once an ion is stored, it can be manipulated in many different ways to perform multistage MS/MS experiments (MS^n), hence it is frequently used for the structural elucidation of unknown flavonoids.

The application of this fragmentation process to the identification of a flavonoid separated by the miniaturised HPLC separation and analysed by ESI-MS, MS/MS and MS^3 is shown in Figure 6 and Figure 7.

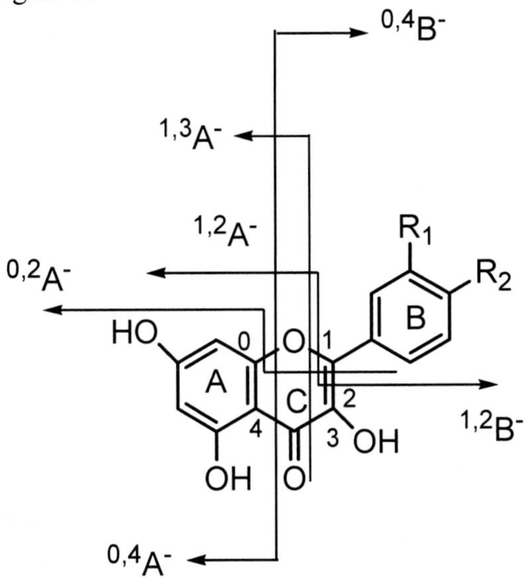

Figure 5. Nomenclature and diagnostic product ions of deprotonated flavonols formed by ESI-ion trap mass spectrometer, the symbols $^{i,j}A^+$ and $^{i,j}B^+$ are used to designate primary product ions containing intact A and B rings, respectively. The superscripts i and j refer to the bonds of the C-ring that have been broken [30].

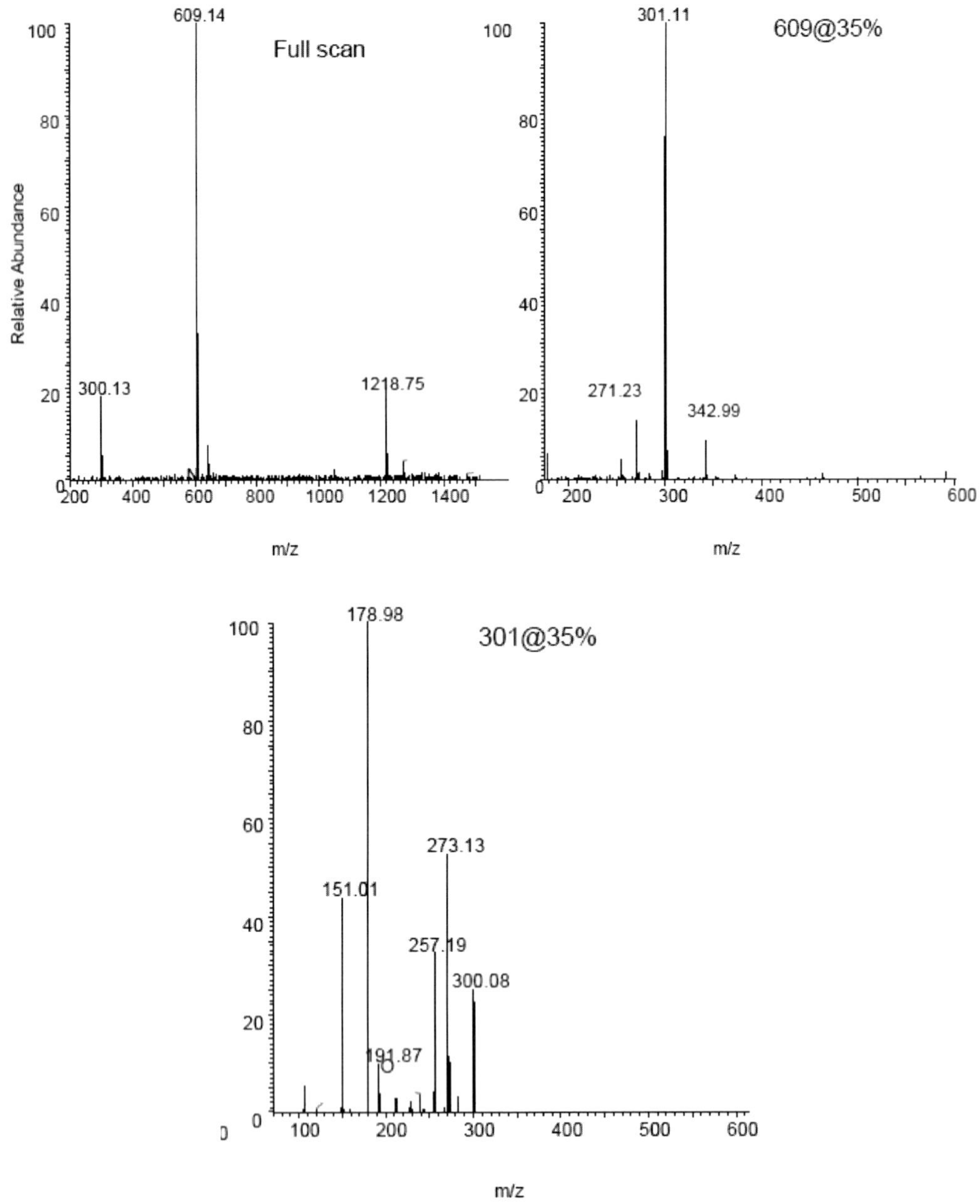

Figure 6. Data-dependent analysis rutin by HPLC-MS showing the full scan mass spectrum, the MS/MS spectrum of *m/z* 609 and the MS^3 spectrum of *m/z* 301 via m/z 609.

The information obtained from the data dependent fragmentation analysis can also be re-searched in order to study selectively specific types of flavonoid glycosides. This process is based on the knowledge that under MS/MS conditions, the loss of the sugar moiety is the first fragmentation event observed. The two most commonly bound sugars in these glycosides are a glucosyl group and a rhamnosyl group.

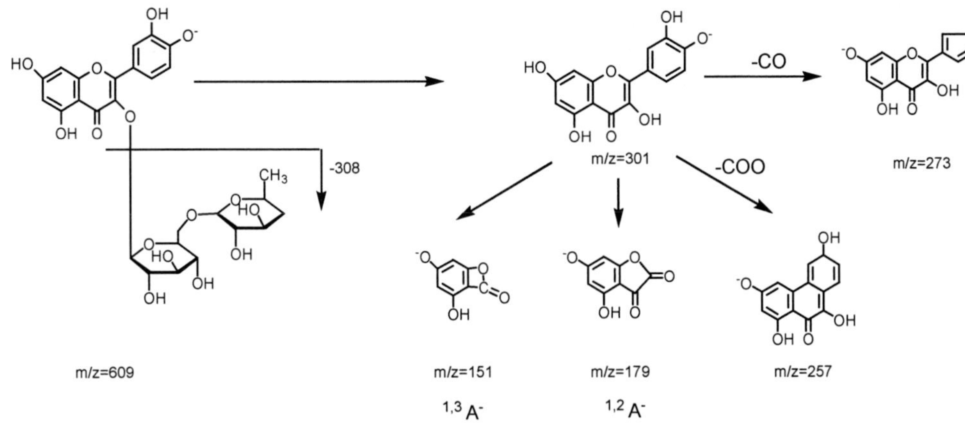

Figure 7. Illustration of the MS/MS and MS^3 fragmentation pathways observed during the fragmentation of rutin in an ion trap mass spectrometer (see Figure 6).

When these are lost in MS/MS experiments the product ion formed represents the loss of 162Da and 146Da respectively. Therefore a useful approach is to highlight in the complex dataset (obtained during the data dependent acquisition) all ions that exhibited these mass losses during fragmentation analysis. Figure 8 indicates the total ion chromatogram for a herbal extract indicating all ions monitored in the mass spectrometer compared to the selecting highlighting of those that lose 162 and 146Da.

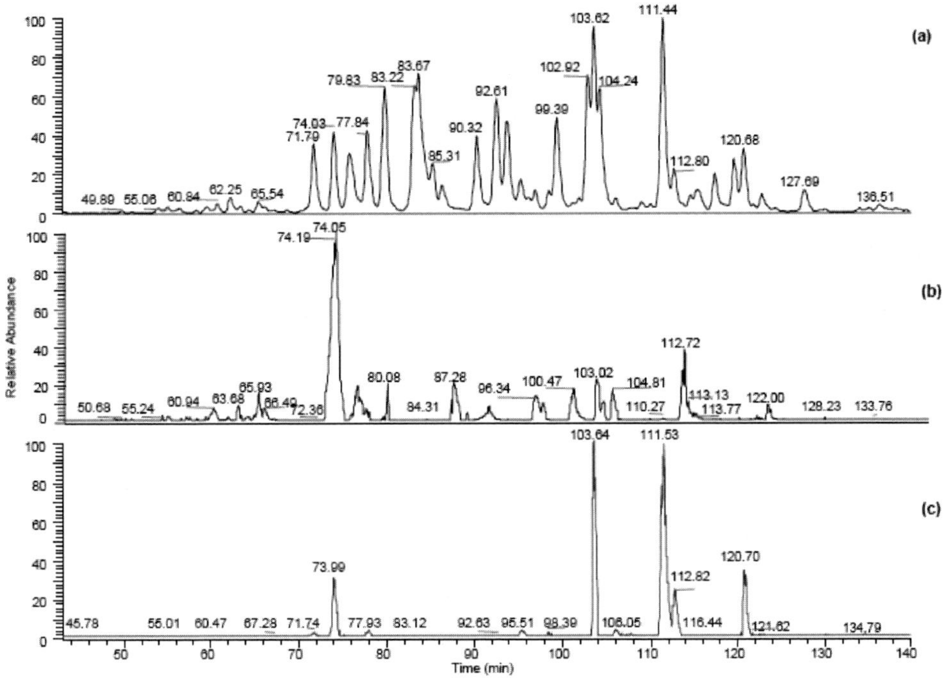

Figure 8. Capillary HPLC/MS total ion chromatogram (TIC) of *Gingko biloba* extract (a) base peak full scan (b) neutral loss of *m/z* 162 (c) neutral loss of *m/z* 146.

It can clearly be seen that this filtering process allows the specific study of such compounds and further study of these peaks confirmed their status as flavonoids.

Flavonoids show biological properties through their free radical-scavenging antioxidant activities and metal-ion-chelating abilities [31]. Despite the benefits of these components, their bioavailability after oral administration is considered to be a limiting factor [32]. Mass spectrometry has therefore also been more recently applied to the analysis of flavonoids in the urine of subjects who have taken herbal extracts in order to determine the time taken for the compounds to be eliminated from the body. After ingestion, flavonoid glycosides are thought to be first hydrolyzed by micro-organisms in the gastrointestinal tract to aglycones. The liberated aglycones can be absorbed through the intestinal wall and are eventually excreted in the urine and bile as glucuronides and sulphate conjugates [33]. The analysis of components excreted in urine is complicated due to their lower levels and the large number of other high abundant species also excreted. Therefore, the urine samples are generally incubated with the enzyme β-glucuronidase/sulfatase to convert flavonoids into their aglycones as a first step of the analysis. In doing so, aglycone concentrations are increased to a detectable level and the analysis is simplified. A number of analytical techniques have been utilized in order to evaluate the metabolism and bioavailability of flavonoids *in vitro* and *in vivo*. The methods utilised previously for the study of urinary and other biologically important flavonoids levels include HPLC [34-36] and mass spectrometry (GC/MS [37, 38] and HPLC/MS [39]). There are also reports of online solid phase extraction using a reverse phase trap column (the outline of such an experiment is shown in Figure 9 [40]) and this methodology was shown to allow the quick and efficient clean up of the injected urine sample.

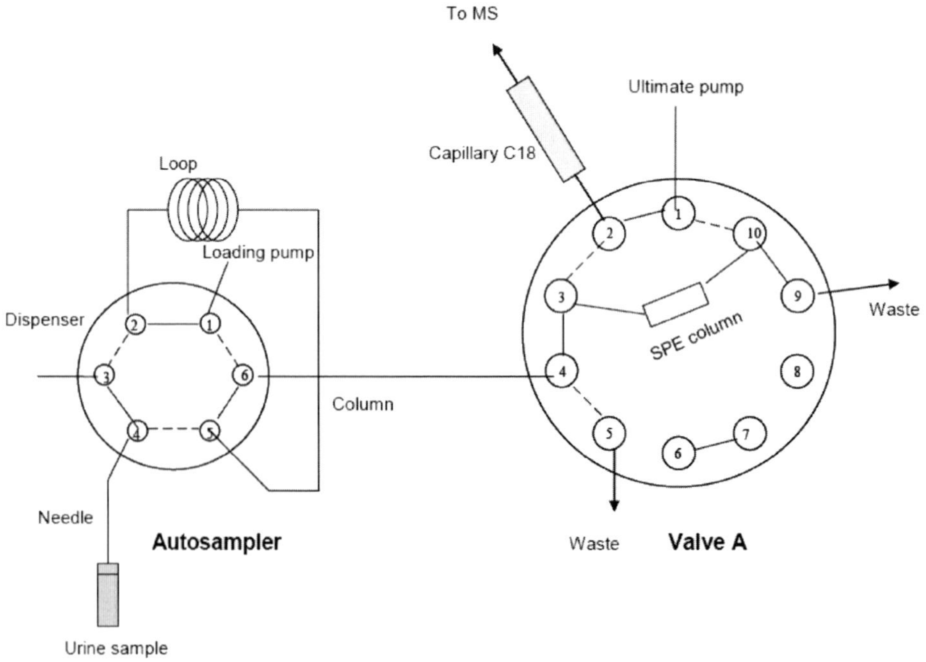

Figure 9. Illustration of a column-switching HPLC/MS system. The components to be analysed were retained on the C_{18}-Trap precolumn while the salt in the sample went to waste. After 3 minutes, Valve A was switched and components trapped on the precolumn were eluted to C_{18} analytical column and detected by mass spectrometry.

The comparison of the on-line clean-up method with off-line purification methodologies demonstrated that the on-line purification protocol does not suffer from any significant loss of analyte or interference from other matrix materials, and this method required minimal prior sample preparation and thereby facilitating higher throughput and greater automation.

CONCLUSION

Flavonoids are a diverse, yet important, group of chemical entities in many herbal extracts and their analysis in such materials is essential in order to gauge the appropriateness of different commercially available extracts. However, such an undertaking is complicated by the varied nature of these compounds. Fingerprint analysis – the comparison of the global metabolite profile of an extract compared to a "pure" standard - offers the ability to monitor such products and has been suggested as being beneficial by major regulatory organisations. Whilst many different techniques have been applied to such analyses in the past, the application of mass spectrometry offers an improvement in the quality of the data that can be obtained in an automated fashion. Furthermore, the ease by which the flavonoid-specific data can be extracted from the information (representing the total metabolite profile determined by such analyses) is improved by such experiments.

Mass spectrometry has a further application in the quantitation of flavonoid elimination via urinary excretion after the consumption of such herbal extracts and can therefore be of use in determining the longevity of the flavonoid. The application of the on-line clean-up and concentration of the flavonoids has been investigated and shown to allow accurate quantitation whilst minimising sample pre-treatment and work-up prior to analysis.

REFERENCES

[1] J.B.Harborne and C,A, Williams, *Phytochemistry*, 55 (2000) 481-504.

[2] F. Teillet, A. Boumendjel, J. Boutonnat and X. Ronot, *Med. Res. Rev.*, 28 (2008) 715-745.

[3] L. Kim, C. Francis and N. Ken, *Food Chemistry*,105 (2007) 353–363.

[4] V.M. Tadić, S. Dobrić and G.M. Marković , *et al. J Agric. Food Chem.*, 56 (2008) 700-7709.

[5] X. Mouren, P. Caillard, and F. Schwartz, *Angiology,* 45 (1994) 413-417.

[6] Q. Zhang and H. Cui, *J. Sep. Sci.,* 28 (2005) 1171–1178.

[7] M. Friedman, C.E. Levin, S.H. Choi, E. Kozukue and N. Kozukue, *Food Sci.*, 71 (2006) C328-C337.

[8] R.J. Fletcher, *British J. Nutrition,* (2003) S39-S43.

[9] World Health Organization, *Guidelines for the Assessment of Herbal Medcines*, Munich, 28.6.1991, WHO, Geneva, (1991).

[10] UNICEF/UNDP/World Bank/WHO, *Handbook of non-clinical safety testing*, (2004).

[11] T.A.van Beek, *J. Chromatogr. A*, 967 (2002) 21-55.

[12] H.Y.Kao, C.H. Huang, T.C.Kao and H.C. Kao, *International. J. Innovational Computing and Information Control*, 4 (2008) 2057-2067.

[13] C.D. Birk, G. Provensi, G. Gosmann, F.H. Reginatto and E.P. Schenkel, *J. Liq Chromatogr. Relat. Tech.*, 28 (2005) 2285-2291.
[14] C. Chen, H. Zhang, W. Xiao , Z.P.Yong and N. Bai, *J Chromatogr. A* , 1154 (2007) 250-259.
[15] P.Drasar and J. Moravcova, *J. Chromatogr. B*, 812 (2004) 3–21.
[16] C.B. Fang, X.C.Wan, C.J. Jiang, H.R. Tan, Y.H. Hu and H.Q. Cao, *J. Planar Chromatogr. Modern TLC*, 19 (2006) 348-354.
[17] M. Gu, Z.G. Su and O.Y. Fan, *J. Liq. Chromatogr. Relat. Tech.,* 29 (2006) 1503-1514.
[18] Y.P. Li, Z. Hu and L.C. He, *J. Pharmaceut. Biomed. Anal.*, 43 (2007) 1667-1672.
[19] S. Ding, E. Dudley, S. Plummer, J. Tang, R.P. Newton and A.G. Brenton, *Phytochemistry*, 69 (2008) 1555-1564.
[20] A. Rolim, C.P.M. Maciel, T.M. Kaneko, V.O. Consigilieri, I.M.N. Salgado- Santos and M.V.R. Velasco, *J. AOAC International*, 88 (2005)1015-1019.
[21] A.Kakasy, Z. Füzfai, L.Kursinszki, I. Molnár-Perl and E. Lemberkovics, *Chromatographia*, 63 (2006) S17-S22.
[22] Z. Füzfai and I. Molnár-Perl, , *J. Chromatogr. A*, 1149 (2007) 88-101.
[23] J.D. Henion, A.V. Mordehai, and J. Cai, *Anal. Chem.*, 66 (1994) 2103-2109.
[24] X.X. Ying, X.M. Lu, X.H. Sun, X.Q. Li and F.M. Li,Talanta, 72 (2007)1500-1506.
[25] X.J. Chen, B.L. Guo, S.P. Li, Q.W. Zhang, P.F. Tu and Y.T. Wang, *J. Chromatogr A*, 1163 (2007) 96-104.
[26] A. Hasler and O. Sticher, *J. Chromatogr.*, 605 (1992) 41-48.
[27] J. Liu, K.J. Volk, M.J. Mata, E.H. Kerns and M.S. Lee, *J. Pharm. Biomed. Anal.*, 15 (1997)1729.
[28] K. Lanckmans, A. Van Eeckhaut, S. Sarre, I. Smolders and Y.Michotte, *J. Chromatogr. A*, 1131 (2006) 166-175.
[29] B.R. Wenner and B.C. Lynn, *J. Am. Soc. Mass Spectrometry*, 15 (2004)150-157.
[30] Y.L. Ma, Q.M. Li, H. Van den Heuvel and M. Claeys, *Rapid Commun. Mass Spectrom.*, 11 (1997) 1357-1364.
[31] C.A. Rice-Evans, N.J. Miller and G. Paganga, *Trends Plant Sci.*, 2 (1997)152-159.
[32] F.V. DeFeudis and K. Drieu, *Current Drug Targets*, 1 (2000) 25-58.
[33] J.K. Prasain, C.C. Wang and S. Barnes, *Free Radical Biol. Med.*, 37 (2004) 1324 -1350.
[34] S.E. Nielsen and L.O. Dragsted, *J. Chromatogr. B*, 707 (1998) 81-89.
[35] I. Erlund, G. Alfthan, H. Siren, K. Ariniemi and A. Aro, *J. Chromatogr. B*, 727 (1999)179.
[36] F.M. Wang, , T.W. Yao and S. Zeng, *J. Pharm. Biomed. Anal.*, 33 (2003) 317-321.
[37] D.G. Watson and E.J. Oliveira, *J. Chromatogr. B*, 723 (1999) 203-210.
[38] D.G. Watson and A.R. Pitt, R*apid Commun. Mass Spectrom.*, 12 (1998) 153 -156.
[39] E.J. Oliveira and D.G. Watson, *FEBS letters*, 471 (2000) 1-6.
[40] S. Ding, E. Dudley, L. Chen, S. Plummer, J. Tang, R.P. Newton and A.G. Brenton, *Rapid Commun. Mass Spectrom.*, 20 (2006) 3619 – 3624.

In: Flavonoids: Biosynthesis, Biological Effects...
Editor: Raymond B. Keller
ISBN: 978-1-60741-622-7

Chapter 13

ANTIBACTERIAL EFFECTS OF THE FLAVONOIDS OF THE LEAVES OF *AFROFITTONIA SILVESTRIS*

Kola' K. Ajibesin
Department of Pharmacognosy,
Olabisi Onabanjo University, Ogun State

ABSTRACT

Afrofittonia silvestris Lindau, commonly known as the hunter's weed, is a procumbent herb trailing on moist ground. The leaves of the plant are used to heal sore feet, skin infections and as laxative. The leaves were macerated in 50 % ethanol and the liquid extract concentrated to dryness. The dry extract was evaluated for antibacterial activity by adopting agar diffusion method. The extract was partitioned between water, ethyl acetate and butanol successively and further subjected to antibacterial testing. The most active extract, ethyl acetate extract, was purified through various chromatographic methods to obtain pure compounds identified by spectroscopic methods as kaempferide 3–O–β–D–glucopyranoside and kaempferol 5,4'-dimethoxy-3,7-O- α-L-dirhamnoside. These compounds produced significant antibacterial effects, while the minimum inhibitory concentrations of the fractions and the pure compounds ranged between 25 and 250 μg/mL. These flavonoids are reported for the first time in this plant, while kaempferol 5,4'-dimethoxy-3,7-O- α-L-dirhamnoside is a new compound.

Keyword: *Afrofittonia silvestris*, antibacterial activity, kaempferide 3–O–β–D–glucopy ranoside, kaempferol 5,4'-dimethoxy-3,7-O- α-L-dirhamnoside.

INTRODUCTION

Afrofittonia silvestris is a procumbent herb trailing on moist ground and commonly known as the hunter's weed (Hutchinson and Dalziel, 1958). The plant grows throughout the year (Taylor, 1966). The leaves of the plant are employed in traditional medicine in the treatment of diseases such as digestive tract disorders, sores, skin diseases and constipation

(Burkill, 1985; Etukudo, 2003; Ajibesin et al., 2008). Although no chemical report of this plant is in literature, its nutritional values have been established (Odoemena et al., 2002).

This study was designed to isolate and identify the antibacterial principles of *Afrofittonia silvestris*.

MATERIALS AND METHODS

General Experimental Procedures

The NMR spectra were recorded on a Brucker DR – 500 MHz (^{1}H 1) and 50 MHz (^{13}C), in CD_3OD using TMS as internal standard. Mass spectroscopy was determined using Electro spray ionization (ESI) Full MS and Finnigan LCQ Deca-MS, Agilent series 1100-LC. UV spectroscopy was determined by Dionex, UVD 340 S Dionex. Melting points were determined on a Kofler hot-stage microscope (uncorrected). TLC was carried out on silica gel 60 F_{254} (Merck). Solvent systems such as EtOAc-CH_3OH; 8:2 (A), CH_2Cl_2-MeOH; 9:1 (B), CH_2Cl_2-MeOH; 4:1 (C), CH_2Cl_2-MeOH; 7:3 (D), CH_2Cl_2-MeOH-H_2O; (7:3:1) were employed. UV light (λ max 254 nm and 366 nm), $FeCl_3$ spray, vanillin/H_2SO_4 and conc. H_2SO_4 sprays followed by activating at 100°C for 5 min., were used for detection of spots.

Plant Material

The leaves (6 kg) of *Afrofittonia silvestris* were collected in July, 2000, at Ikot Ekpene in Akwa Ibom State, Nigeria. The plant was identified and authenticated by Dr. U. Essiett of the Department of Botany, University of Uyo, Uyo, Nigeria. Voucher specimen (KKA 2) was deposited in the Department of Pharmacognosy and Natural Medicine herbarium, Faculty of Pharmacy, University of Uyo, Uyo, Nigeria.

Extraction of *A. Silvestris* Leaves

The dried leaf powder (4 kg) of *A. silvestris* was extracted by maceration using 50 % EtOH (10 L). It was filtered and the marc re-extracted with the fresh solvent mixture for 12 h (x2) and filtered. The filtrates were pooled together and concentrated to dryness *in vacuo* at 40°C.

Antibacterial Test

The extracts and the fractions were reconstituted in MeOH-H_2O (1:1) to obtain a stock solution of 20 mg/mL. 50 µl of this solution was introduced into each of the equidistant wells (8 mm) bored on the agar plate surface previously inoculated with each of the test organisms. A control well containing Gentamicin (5 µg/mL) was placed in each of the plates seeded with bacteria. The bacteria were incubated at 37 °C for 24 h (Alade and Irobi, 1993). Antibacterial activity was expressed as average diameter of the zones of inhibition calculated as a difference in diameter of the observed zones and those of the wells.

Minimum Inhibitory Concentration

The minimum inhibitory concentration (MIC)was determined by incorporating various amounts (250 – 6.25 μg/mL) of the solution of extracts and fractions into sets of test tubes containing the culture media.50 μl of the standard test bacterial broth cultures were added into each of the test tubes. The set of tubes containing a mixture of bacteria and the sample (extracts and fractions) were incubated at 37 ^{O}C for 24 h (Cos et al., 2006).

A positive control tube containing only the growth medium of each of the organisms was also set up. The MIC was regarded as the lowest concentration of the extract or fraction that did not permit any visible growth when compared with that of the control tubes.

Activity-Guided Fractionation of A. *Silvestris*

The dry extract was dissolved in water and successively shaken with EtOAc (6x300 mL) and BuOH (6x300 mL) to afford ethylacetate (20 g), butanol (25 g) and aqueous extracts (35 g) respectively.

The resultant 3 fractions were evaluated against the test organisms at 20 mg/mL in aqueous methanol ($MeOH:H_2O$; table 2). The antibacterial principles were partitioned more largely into ethyl acetate fraction followed by butanol and aqueous fractions respectively.

Isolation and Characterization

The EtOAc, butanol and aqueous fractions of the plant species were subjected to TLC analysis, using solvent systems A, D and E respectively, visualized under the UV light (λ 254 nm) before using 100 % H_2SO_4 and $FeCl_3$ solution as detecting spray reagents. The most active EtOAc fraction (16 g) showed flavonoid components and was chromatographed on silica (Merck, 0.040-0.063 mm particle size) by accelerated gradient chromatography (AGC) column and eluted with C_6H_{14} containing increasing amount of CH_2Cl_2, followed by increasing amount of CH_3OH (4:1, 9:1). Four flavonoid fractions coded A, B, C, D were obtained, two (B, C) of which showed significant antibacterial effects. The more active (C) of the two flavonoid fractions was further fractionated on silica by vacuum liquid chromatography (VLC), using EtOAc in gradient with CH_3OH and H_2O (7:2:1). Final purification was carried out on silica by preparative thin layer chromatography (prep. TLC), using EtOAc-CH_3OH (4:1) as mobile phase to give **1** (30 mg). The less active flavonoid fraction was purified by repeated AGC (silica) to yield **2** (21 mg). The two compounds along with the fractions were subjected to antibacterial test.

kaempferol 5,4'-dimethoxy-3,7-O- α-L-dirhamnoside **1**. Yellow powder, mp 220 ^{0}C (MeOH), UV CH_3OH λ max nm: 272, 334, ESI Full MS – m/z (rel. int.): 607 $[M+H]^+$ (100), 461 $[M+H\text{-}Rham.]^+$ (25), 299 $[M+H\text{-}2Rham.]^+$ (5). ^{1}HNMR (CD_3OD): δ 6.70 (1h, d, J= 2.2 Hz, H-6), 6.77 (1H, d, J= 2.2 Hz, H-8), 7.10 (1H, d, J= 8.8 Hz, H-3', 5'), 7.98 (1H, dd, J= 8.8

Hz, H-2', 6'), 5.48 (1h, d, J= 1.4 Hz, H-1'''), 5.24 (1H, d, J= 1.4 Hz, H-1'''), 0.72 (3H, d, J= 6.2 Hz, H-6'''), 0.64 (3H, d, J= 6.2 Hz, H-6''), 3.29 (3H, s, -OMe), 3.95 (3H, s, -OMe), 2.40-4.92 (8H, sugar protons).

^{13}CNMR: see table 1.

Table 1. ^{13}CNMR spectral data for compounds 1 and kaempferol 3,7- dirhamnoside

Aglycone			sugar moiety		
C	1	K	C	1	K
2(C)	157.0	156.4	1″(CH)	102.3	102.2
3(C)	134.8	134.8	1‴(CH)	100.0	99.8
4(C)	180.0	178.2	2″(CH)	70.5	70.5
5(C)	163.5	161.2	2‴(CH)	70.4	70.4
6(CH)	93.5	98.7	3″(CH)	71.7	71.0
7(C)	164.0	162.0	3‴(CH)	71.1	70.6
8(CH)	93.0	94.9	4″(CH)	72.0	71.9
9(C)	157.1	157.1	4‴(CH)	71.5	71.4
10(C)	106.0	106.0	5″(CH)	70.4	70.4
1′(C)	122.0	120.6	5‴(CH)	70.1	70.1
2′,6′ (C)	131.2	131.0	6″(CH3)	18.0	18.2
3′,5′ (C)	112.3	115.8	6‴(CH3)	17.9	17.8
4′(C)	163.2	160.5			
MeO	57.8				
	58.0				

K= kaempferol 3,7- dirhamnoside.

Known compound **2** was identified by comparing its spectroscopic data with those in literature (Lahtinen et al., 2005).

RESULTS AND DISCUSSION

Two flavonoids were isolated from the leaves of *A. silvestris*. Kaempferol-5,4′-dimethoxy–3,7–O–α–L–dirhamnoside 1, a yellow powder, was isolated with the aid of accelerated gradient chromatography (AGC), vacuum liquid chromatography (VLC) and preparative thin layer chromatography (prep. TLC), while kaempferide 3–O–β–D–glucopyranoside 2 was separated with AGC alone. Compound 1 gave a UV spectrum which showed absorption maxima at 271 (band II) and 335 nm (band I) which indicated a flavonoid structure skeleton (Toker et al., 2004). The ESI Full mass spectrum showed a $[M+H]^+$ peak at m/z 607 consistent with the molecular formula $C_{29}H_{34}O_{14}$. The peak at m/z 461 was due to the loss of one rhamnose unit. The fragment ion corresponding to m/z 299 indicated the successive loss of two rhamnose units.

In the ^{1}HNMR spectrum, the meta-coupled protons of H-6 and H-8 appeared separately as doublets at δ6.70 and δ6.77 (J = 4.9Hz) respectively. In the B ring, the protons at C-3′/5′ showed a doublet at δ7.10 (1H, J = 8.8 Hz), while their coupled protons at ortho position C-2′/6′ occurred as two doublets at δ7.98 (1H, J = 8.8 Hz). Two singlets at δ3.29 and δ3.95 integrating for 3H respectively represented two methoxy groups. The signals at δ0.64 and δ0.72 (d, J = 6.2 Hz), each integrated for 3-protons, assigned rhamnose-CH_3 protons (Mabry et al., 1970). In addition, two anomeric protons assigned to H-1 of the two rhamnose moieties were observed at δ5.24 and δ5.48 as narrow doublets for α configuration of the glycosidic linkage (Toker et al., 2004).

The structure indicated by the ^{1}HNMR was supported by ^{13}CNMR spectrum. The two methoxy groups attached at positions 5 and 4′ were indicated by the signals at 57.8 and 58.0 ppm respectively. The ^{13}C NMR spectra gave many similarities with kaempferol 3,7-O- α-dirhamnoside (Gohar and Elmazar, 1997) in the benzopyrone ring and sugar moiety. However, the position of the 1st methoxy group of 1 was indicated by the downfield shift of C-4′ by 2.7 ppm and the upfield shift of the ortho carbons (C-3′/5′) by 3.5 ppm with respect to the same signals in the ^{13}C NMR spectra of kaempferol 3, 7-O- α-dirhamnoside. Furthermore, the position of the other methoxy group on C-5 was shown by the downfield shift of C-5 by 2.3 ppm when compared with the ^{13}C NMR signal of the same kaempferol 3,7-O- α- dirhamnoside, while the ortho carbon C-6 shifted much upfield by 5.2 ppm. Thus, the main distinction between kaempferol 3,7-O- α- dirhamnoside and 1 appears to be the methoxy groups present in the latter, which was further confirmed by its larger molar mass. Similar distinctions were made when 1 was compared with another kaempferol 3,7- O-α-L-dirhamnoside isolated from *Tilia argentea* (Toker et al., 2004). Also, 1 shared some resonance characteristics when compared with the aglycone of kaempferide 3 rhamnoside where only one methoxy was attached at C-4′ to form kaempferide (Bilia et al. 1993). The glycosylation at C-3 and C-7 was shown by their ^{13}CNMR signals at 134.8 ppm (s) and 164.0 ppm (s) respectively. The MS fragmentation of 1 also suggested O-glycosilation at C-3 and C-7. The sugar region gave eight sugar carbon signals at ca. 70.1-72.0 ppm, with the anomeric carbons resonating at 102.3 ppm (s, C-1″) and 100.0 ppm (s, C-1‴) respectively. The presence of two characteristic rhamnose methyl signals at 17.9 and 18.0 ppm further confirmed the presence of two rhamnose residues (Agrawal, 1989; Neeru et al., 1990). Consequently, the data for compound 1 are uniquely consistent with the structure of kaempferol -5,4′-dimethoxy-3,7-O- α-L-dirhamnoside, a compound hitherto not reported in literature. The data showed that 1 is different from kaempferol-3,7- O- α-L-dirhamnoside earlier isolated from *Chenopodium* species and *Tilia argentea* in that it has two extra methoxyl groups (Gohar and Elmazar, 1997; Toker et al., 2004).

Kaempferide 3-O-β-glucoside 2, earlier detected in the larval faeces of sawfly species (Lahtinen et al., 2005), was also present in the plant.

The antibacterial effects of A. silvestris have been determined to be due mainly to kaempferol -5,4′-dimethoxy-3,7-O- α-L-dirhamnoside, while Kaempferide 3-O-β-glucoside was also isolated as antibacterial principle showing less inhibitory activity. It is noteworthy that kaempferol -5,4′-dimethoxy-3,7-O- α-L-dirhamnoside elicited better antibacterial effect than Gentamicin, the standard drug used. Antimicrobial activity of phenolics has been similarly established in Acalypha species (Adesina et al., 2000).

CONCLUSION

No previous report of the antibacterial effects of kaempferol -5,4′-dimethoxy-3,7-O- α-L-dirhamnoside and Kaempferide 3-O-β-glucoside was found in literature. The two conpounds are responsible for the antibacterial effects of the plant, and this validates its uses in traditional medicine for treating infections.

Table 2. Antibacterial activity of the extracts of *A. silvestris*

Zone of inhibition of organisms(mm)[a]						
Microorganism	L	E	B	Aq	Gen	MeOH:H2O
E. coli NCIB 86	9±1.00*	7±1.41*	4±0.00	3±0.00	12±1.58*	0
B. cereus						
NCIB 6349	10±1.00 *	7±1.73*	5±2.12	4±2.20	13±1.41*	0
S. aureus						
NCIB 8588	12±1.41*	10±1.58*	7±1.00*	4±0.00	13±1.00*	0
Ps. aeruginosa						
NCIB 950	10±2.20*	8±0.00*	5±1.00	3±1.00	15±2.12*	0

L: leaf extract, E: ethyl acetate extract, B: butanol extract, Aq: aqueous extract, Gen: gentamicin, values are mean±SD(n=4), *: p<0.01 with respect to control.

Table 3. Antibacterial activity of fractions and flavonoids isolated from *A. silvestris*

Microorganism	A	B	C	D	1	2	Gen	MeOH: H2O (1:1)
E.coli NCIB 86	5±0.00	8±1.40*	9±1.00*	4±2.12	15±2.20*	13±1.00*	12±1.58*	0
B. cereus								
NCIB 6349	6±0.00	9±1.00*	11±1.00*	5±0.00	16±2.12*	13±1.41*	13±1.41*	0
S. aureus								
NCIB 8588	6±2.45	8±1.41*	12±2.82*	5±1.00	18±1.41*	14±2.82*	13±1.00*	0
Ps. aeruginosa								
NCIB 950	5±1.00	7±2.45	11±1.41*	4±0.00	20±1.00*	15±2.45*	15±2.12*	0

Values are mean±SD (n=4), *: p<0.01 with respect to control, Gen: gentamicin.

Table 4. MIC of the fractions and flavonoids isolated from *A. silvestris* (μg/mL)

Microorganism	A	B	C	D	1	2	Gen
E.coli NCIB 86	>250	250	200	>250	50	100	200
B. cereus							
NCIB 6349	>250	200	100	>250	25	100	100
S. aureus							
NCIB 8588	>250	250	100	>250	25	50	50
Ps. aeruginosa							
NCIB 950	>250	250	100	>250	25	50	50

Gen: gentamicin.

REFERENCES

Adesina, S K, Idowu, O, Ogundaini, A O, Oladimeji, H, Olugbade, T A, Onawunmi, G O and Pais, M (2000). Antimicrobial constituents of the leaves of *Acalypha wilkesiana* and *Acalypha hispida*. *Phytother. Res.* 14: 371-374.

Agrawal, P K (1989). Carbon-13 NMR of Flavonoids. Armsterdam, Elsevier.

Ajibesin, K K, Ekpo, B A, Bala, D N, Essien, E E and Adesanya, S A (2008). Ethnobotanical survey of Akwa Ibom State of Nigeria. *J. Ethnopharmacol.* 115(3): 387-408.

Alade, P I and Irobi, O N (1993). Antimicrobial activities of crude leaf extracts of *Acalypha wilkesiana*. *J. Ethnopharmacol.* 39: 171-174.

Bilia, A R, Palmae, E, Marsili, A, Pistelli, I and Morelli, I (1993) A flavonol glycoside from *Agrimonia eupatoria*. *Phytochemistry.* 32 (4): 1078-1079.

Burkill, H M (1985). The Useful Plants of West Tropical Africa (Edition 2), Vol. 1, Families A-D. Kew: Royal Botanic Gardens.

Cos, P, Vlietnick, A J, Berghe, D V and Maes, L (2006). Anti-infective potential of natural products: How to develop a stronger in vitro 'proof-of-concept'. *J. Ethnopharmacol.* 106: 290-302.

Etukudo, I (2003). Ethnobotany: convention and traditional uses of plants. Nigeria: Verdict press.

Gohar, A A and Elmazar, M M A (1997). Isolation of hypotensive flavonoids from *Chenopodium* species growing in Egypt. *Phytother. Res.* 11: 564-567.

Hutchinson, J and Dalziel, J M (1958). Flora of West Tropical Africa, Vol. 1, part II, Vol. II. London: Crown Agents for Overseas Government.

Lahtinen, M, Kapari, L, Ossipov, V, Salminen, J, Haukioja, E and Pihlaja, K (2005). Biochemical transformation of birch leaf phenolics in larvae of six species of sawflies. *Chemoecology.* 15 (3): 153-159.

Neeru, J, Sarwar, Alam M, Kamil, M, Ilyas, M, Niwa, M and Sakae, A (1990). Two flavonoid glycosides from *Chenopodium ambrosoides*. *Phytochemistry.* 29 (12): 3988-3991.

Odoemena, C S, Sampson, E A, Bala, D N and Ajibesin, K K (2002). Phytochemical study and nutritive potential of *Afrofritomia sylevestris* leaf. *Nig. J. Nat. Prod. and Med.* 6: 42-43.

Taylor, S R (1966). Investigation on plants of West Africa III, phytochemical studies of some plants of Sierra Leone. Africa Noire 28: 5.

Toker, G, Memisoglu, M, Yesilada, E and Aslan, M (2004). Main flavonoids of *Tilia argentea* DESF. ex DC. Leaves. *Turk. J. Chem.* 28: 745-749.

In: Flavonoids: Biosynthesis, Biological Effects...
Editor: Raymond B. Keller
ISBN: 978-1-60741-622-7

Chapter 14

WHY IS BIOAVAILABILITY OF ANTHOCYANINS SO LOW?

Sabina Passamonti*
Department of Life Sciences, University of Trieste
Via L. Giorgieri 1, 34127 Trieste

1. CHEMISTRY, DIETARY INTAKE AND BIOAVAILABILITY OF ANTHOCYANINS

Following ingestion, anthocyanins are detected intact in blood [5, 6] in a time lapse considerably shorter than that observed with other dietary flavonoids [7]. However, the anthocyanins concentrations in plasma barely exceed 10^{-7} M, which translates into less than 0.1% absorption, including anthocyanin metabolites [8]. These features are indicative of various biochemical issues underlying the quite limited bioavailability of anthocyanins in mammalian organisms.

2. GENERAL MECHANISTIC ASPECTS OF LIMITED ANTHOCYANIN BIOAVAILABILITY

2.1. Transporter-Mediated Absorption at the Cellular Level

Being found in plasma as intact glycosylated compounds, anthocyanins must have diffused across the gastro-intestinal barrier via membrane transporters catalysing their specific, sequential translocation from the gastro-intestinal lumen into the epithelial cells and from the cells into the blood. Molecules as polar as dietary anthocyanins cannot permeate epithelial barriers without the involvement of specific membrane transporters [9], unless epithelial barriers are disrupted, in which case para-cellular transport can occur [10].

---

* Email: spassamonti@units.it

2.1.1. Consequences of Transporter-Mediated Absorption: Rapidity

In turn, transporter-mediated absorption of anthocyanin provides the kinetic mechanism for their rapid absorption. Similarly to enzymes that are powerful enhancers of the rate of chemical transformations, membrane transporters are powerful enhancers of the rate of transport of solute molecules across membrane-bordered compartments [11].

2.1.2. Consequences of Transporter-Mediated Absorption: Saturability

Transporter-mediated absorption of anthocyanin implies that the rate of their absorption must display saturation with respect to their concentration. Similarly to enzymes, transporters kinetics obeys the Michaelis-Menten law, which is based on the existence of a transporter-substrate complex, featured by a Michaelis-Menten constant, Km, and a maximal velocity of transport, Vmax. Transport kinetics may deviate from the Michaeli-Menten law, yielding a sigmoidal dependence of transport rate as a function of the substrate concentration; also in such case Vmax is predicted to occur at infinite substrate concentrations. High-affinity transporters are quite efficient at transporting solutes at low solute concentrations, but are also inevitably saturated at relatively low solute concentrations. As a consequence, a high-affinity transporter specific for anthocyanins and expressed in the gastro-intestinal epithelium will also be a low-capacity transporter and therefore will enable low absorption.

2.1.3. Bilitranslocase: An Anthocyanin-Specific Membrane Transporter

Bilitranslocase is a membrane transporter originally identified in the liver [12] and extensively characterised for its transport function [13]. It is assayed in vitro using rat liver plasma membrane vesicles, which contain bilitranslocase, and the phthalein dye bromosulfophthalein as the transport substrate [14, 15]. This synthetic dye displays pH-dependent tautomerism, shifting between the phenolic, colourless species and the quinoidal, purple one. In this respect, BSP and anthocyanins are quite similar and this provided the rationale for the investigation of the interaction of these pigments with bilitranslocase. It was found that all six aglycones, their mono- as well as their di-glucosides behaved as competitive inhibitors of bilitranslocase transport activity [16]. Subtle changes in the glycosyl moiety were found to be associated with decreased affinity or with a change of the inhibition modality, i.e. from competitive to non-competitive inhibition [16]. The transporter seems to be quite selectively specific for anthocyanins, since related flavonols with the same pattern of glycosylation do not interact with bilitranslocase [17], presumably because they are not able to fit to the transport site, that accepts only planar molecules [17, 18]. The affinity of bilitranslocase for anthocyanins is described by their inhibition constants, ranging 2-22 μM. For these values, bilitranslocase should reasonably play a role in the uptake of anthocyanins from plasma, where they occur at very low concentrations, into the liver. Indeed, transport of anthocyanins into human hepatic cells is bilitranslocase-mediated, as shown by the strong inhibition of uptake caused by specific anti-bilitranslocase antibodies [19]. No other anthocyanin-specific membrane transporter has yet been identified, but certainly will be discovered, since membrane transport is rarely determined by just a single type of carrier.

2.2. Environment-Dependent Absorption at the Supra-Cellular Level

At the level of supra-cellular structures, like the gastro-intestinal tract, more complex factors combine to yield profound impacts on both the rate and extent of absorption of anthocyanins.

2.2.1. Distribution and Density of Anthocyanin-Specific Transporters

The first factor to be considered is the distribution and density of anthocyanin-specific transporters along the cranio-caudal axis of the gastro-intestinal tract. Consequently, the more upstream the transporter localisation, the fastest will be the absorption of anthocyanins, and vice-versa. Furthermore, critical is the sub-cellular localisation of transporters in absorptive epithelia, made by polarised cells that are distinctively equipped with influx and efflux transporters, so to favour the unidirectional trans-cellular passage of nutrients and other solutes.

2.2.2. Occurrence of Bilitranslocase in the Gastro-Intestinal Epithelium

This carrier is found in the gastric epithelium [20], more specifically at the level of two of the four main cell types lining the gastric glands, i.e. the mucus-secreting cells that are found at the luminal surface of the mucosa and the acid-secreting parietal cells, that are located more deeply in the columnar setting of the glands [21]. Moreover, it has recently been found also in the intestinal epithelium at the level of the apical (luminal) plasma membrane domain (unpublished data).

This localisation seems to adequately justify both the prediction that anthocyanins might be absorbed form the stomach [22] and its subsequent demonstration [22, 23]. A deeper mechanistic demonstration is difficult to be obtained with gastric epithelial cells, that are heterogeneous both morphologically and functionally [24].

2.2.3. Absorption of Anthocyanins into Intestinal Cell Monolayers: A Unique Role for Bilitranslocase?

The occurrence of bilitranslocase on the apical domain of intestinal cells offers an interpretation of data obtained testing anthocyanins absorption by human intestinal cell (Caco-2) monolayers [25]. The data show a striking correspondence between the extent of absorption of various anthocyanins and the affinity of anthocyanins for bilitranslocase [16]. Delphinidin 3-glucoside, the poorest anthocyanidin monoglucoside inhibitor of bilitranslocase (Ki=8.6 μM), was the least absorbed compound; the most absorbed ones, peonidin 3-glucoside and malvidin 3-glucoside, are also the best bilitranslocase ligands (Ki=1.8 and 1.4 μM, respectively). The correspondence also recurs with the glycosylated derivatives of cyanidin: cyanidin 3-glucoside is better absorbed than cyanidin 3-galactoside and the former is a better bilitranslocase ligand (Ki=5.8 μM) than the latter (Ki=35 μM).

The possible role of glucose transporters in anthocyanin translocation from the lumen into intestinal cells has been ruled out on the basis that glucose fails to decrease cyanidin 3-glucoside absorption both *in vivo* [26] and in *in vitro* intestinal models [27]. No experimental data is currently available to put forward speculations about the possible involvement of other apical transporters in anthocyanin absorption.

2.2.4. Retention of Anthocyanins into the Intestinal Epithelium: Absence of Efflux Transporters?

In the above-mentioned study, only <4% of the dose applied in the luminal compartment appeared in the serosal one [25]. In another study [28], appearance of anthocyanins in the serosal compartment could not even be detected. However, in both investigations, retention of anthocyanins into the cell monolayer was rather extensive, up to 60%. Thus, anthocyanins might enter into Caco-2 cells via bilitranslocase, but would find a barrier for their diffusion across the basolateral (serosal) side of the cell membrane, where bilitranslocase is absent and the various other nutrient efflux transporters (e.g. the facilitative glucose transporter isoforms 2 GLUT2 [29], various aminoacid transporters [30]), seem to play no significant role in the cellular efflux of anthocyanins.

Even more surprisingly, primary active transporters, such as the Multidrug Resistance Associated Protein MRP1, MRP3, MRP4 and MRP5 [31], also seem not to promote anthocyanin efflux from intestinal cells, though their role as flavonoid transporters has been demonstrated [31].

Alternative mechanisms for the escape of intracellular anthocyanins from the enteric epithelium into the blood should be taken in consideration. A very attractive one is that already highlighted for quercetin, which is not transported directly into the mesenteric portal capillaries, but rather into the lymphatic system [32], likely in association with lipoproteins.

2.3. Anthocyanin Instability in the Intestinal Tract and in Plasma: Chemistry or Biochemistry?

Anthocyanins are said to be unstable in the intestine, because of pH conditions favouring their degradation. However, their loss in simulated intraluminal conditions is limited (<10%) and certainly not enough to account for their poor bioavailability [33, 34]; rather, when in contact with the colonic microflora, they are rapidly deglycosylated and the aglycones are then easily converted to phenolic metabolites [35, 36]. In plasma, anthocyanins are also said to be easily lost, due to their very low concentration and to their association with plasma proteins. However, further mechanisms of anthocyanin "instability" might be envisaged. In particular, the question if anthocyanins are degraded in the gut, in cells or in plasma by enzyme-catalysed mechanisms has never been addressed. This possibility is not unreasonable. In the gut, microbial flora might cause flavonoid C-ring fission by secreting a chalcone isomerase, as the latter has been shown to be a specific enzyme of the faecal anaerobe *Eubacterium ramulus* [37]. Its N-terminal amino-acid sequence does not align with any protein sequence in data bases [37], suggesting that genomic analysis is not fully predictive of phenotypes.

CONCLUSIONS

In conclusion, the poor bioavailability of anthocyanis seems to stem from the fact that they are transported into intestinal cells by a carrier-mediated mechanism, that displays high affinity though low capacity of transport. Contrary to many other organic anions, these pigments are apparently not transported by other intestinal membrane carriers besides bilitranslocase, though this issue needs to be further investigated. Surprisingly, anthocyanins are retained into the intestinal cells, being unable to be transported across the basolateral domain of the enterocyte plasma membrane. The high intracellular concentration is certainly a factor limiting sustained uptake of anthocyanin from the lumen. In the colon, anthocyanins undergo de-glycosylation and rapid C-ring fission, perhaps catalysed by bacterial chalcone isomerase. Enzyme-based degradation of anthocyanins in biological fluids is an issue that deserves investigation, in order to assess all aspects of the limited anthocyanin bioavailability in mammalian organisms.

REFERENCES

[1] Andersen MØ, Jordheim M. The Anthocyanins. In: Andersen MØ, Markham KR, Ed. Flavonoids. Boca Raton, Florida, USA, CRC Press 2006; 471-551.

[2] Mazza G, Miniati, E. Anthocyanins in fruits, vegetables and grains. Boca Raton, Florida, CRC Press 1993; 379.

[3] Wu X, Beecher GR, Holden JM, Haytowitz DB, Gebhardt SE, Prior RL. Concentrations of anthocyanins in common foods in the United States and estimation of normal consumption. *J. Agric Food Chem.* 2006; 54: 4069-75.

[4] Kuhnau J. The flavonoids. A class of semi-essential food components: their role in human nutrition. *World Rev. Nutr. Diet* 1976; 24: 117-91.

[5] McGhie TK, Walton MC. The bioavailability and absorption of anthocyanins: towards a better understanding. *Mol. Nutr. Food Res.* 2007; 51: 702-13.

[6] Prior RL, Wu X. Anthocyanins: structural characteristics that result in unique metabolic patterns and biological activities. *Free Radic. Res.* 2006; 40: 1014-28.

[7] Manach C, Williamson G, Morand C, Scalbert A, Remesy C. Bioavailability and bioefficacy of polyphenols in humans. I. Review of 97 bioavailability studies. *Am. J. Clin. Nutr.* 2005; 81: 230S-42S.

[8] Mazza GJ. Anthocyanins and heart health. *Ann. Ist. Super Sanita* 2007; 43: 369-74.

[9] Lipinski CA, Lombardo F, Dominy BW, Feeney PJ. Experimental and computational approaches to estimate solubility and permeability in drug discovery and development settings. *Adv. Drug Deliv. Rev.* 2001; 46: 3-26.

[10] Turner JR. Molecular basis of epithelial barrier regulation: from basic mechanisms to clinical application. *Am. J. Pathol.* 2006; 169: 1901-9.

[11] Stein WD. Kinetics of transport: analyzing, testing, and characterizing models using kinetic approaches. *Methods Enzymol.* 1989; 171: 23-62.

[12] Sottocasa GL, Lunazzi GC, Tiribelli C. Isolation of bilitranslocase, the anion transporter from liver plasma membrane for bilirubin and other organic anions. *Methods Enzymol.* 1989; 174: 50-7.

[13] Sottocasa GL, Passamonti S, Battiston L, Pascolo L, Tiribelli C. Molecular aspects of organic anion uptake in liver. *J. Hepatol.* 1996; 24: 36-41.

[14] Passamonti, S., Sottocasa, G.L. Bilitranslocase: structural and functional aspects of an organic anion carrier. In: G.S.Pandalai, Ed. Recent Research Developments in Biochemistry. Kerala, Research Signpost, Kerala, India 2002.

[15] Baldini G, Passamonti S, Lunazzi GC, Tiribelli C, Sottocasa GL. Cellular localization of sulfobromophthalein transport activity in rat liver. *Biochim Biophys Acta* 1986; 856: 1-10.

[16] Passamonti S, Vrhovsek U, Mattivi F. The interaction of anthocyanins with bilitranslocase. *Biochem. Biophys. Res. Commun.* 2002; 296: 631-6.

[17] Karawajczyk A, Drgan V, Medic N, Oboh G, Passamonti S, Novic M. Properties of flavonoids influencing the binding to bilitranslocase investigated by neural network modelling. *Biochem. Pharmacol.* 2007; 73: 308-20.

[18] Passamonti S, Sottocasa GL. The quinoid structure is the molecular requirement for recognition of phthaleins by the organic anion carrier at the sinusoidal plasma membrane level in the liver. *Biochim. Biophys. Acta.* 1988; 943: 119-25.

[19] Passamonti S, Vanzo A, Vrhovsek U, Terdoslavich M, Cocolo A, Decorti G, et al. Hepatic uptake of grape anthocyanins and the role of bilitranslocase. *Food Res. Int.* 2005; 38: 953-60.

[20] Battiston L, Macagno A, Passamonti S, Micali F, Sottocasa GL. Specific sequence-directed anti-bilitranslocase antibodies as a tool to detect potentially bilirubin-binding proteins in different tissues of the rat. *FEBS Lett.* 1999; 453: 351-5.

[21] Nicolin V, Grill V, Micali F, Narducci P, Passamonti S. Immunolocalisation of bilitranslocase in mucosecretory and parietal cells of the rat gastric mucosa. *J. Mol. Histol.* 2005; 36: 45-50.

[22] Passamonti S, Vrhovsek U, Vanzo A, Mattivi F. The stomach as a site for anthocyanins absorption from food. *FEBS Letters* 2003; 544: 210-3.

[23] Talavera S, Felgines C, Texier O, Besson C, Lamaison JL, Remesy C. Anthocyanins Are Efficiently Absorbed from the Stomach in Anesthetized Rats. *J. Nutr.* 2003; 133: 4178-82.

[24] Karam SM, Leblond CP. Identifying and counting epithelial cell types in the "corpus" of the mouse stomach. *Anat Rec* 1992; 232: 231-46.

[25] Yi W, Akoh CC, Fischer J, Krewer G. Absorption of anthocyanins from blueberry extracts by caco-2 human intestinal cell monolayers. *J. Agric. Food Chem.* 2006; 54: 5651-8.

[26] Felgines C, Texier O, Besson C, Vitaglione P, Lamaison JL, Fogliano V, et al. Influence of glucose on cyanidin 3-glucoside absorption in rats. *Mol. Nutr. Food Res.* 2008; 52: 959-64.

[27] Walton MC, McGhie TK, Reynolds GW, Hendriks WH. The flavonol quercetin-3-glucoside inhibits cyanidin-3-glucoside absorption in vitro. *J. Agric. Food Chem.* 2006; 54: 4913-20.

[28] Steinert RE, Ditscheid B, Netzel M, Jahreis G. Absorption of black currant anthocyanins by monolayers of human intestinal epithelial Caco-2 cells mounted in ussing type chambers. *J. Agric. Food Chem.* 2008; 56: 4995-5001.

[29] Kwon O, Eck P, Chen S, Corpe CP, Lee JH, Kruhlak M, et al. Inhibition of the intestinal glucose transporter GLUT2 by flavonoids. *Faseb. J.* 2007; 21: 366-77.

[30] Broer S. Amino acid transport across mammalian intestinal and renal epithelia. *Physiol. Rev.* 2008; 88: 249-86.

[31] Brand W, Schutte ME, Williamson G, van Zanden JJ, Cnubben NH, Groten JP, et al. Flavonoid-mediated inhibition of intestinal ABC transporters may affect the oral

bioavailability of drugs, food-borne toxic compounds and bioactive ingredients. *Biomed. Pharmacother.* 2006; 60: 508-19.

[32] Murota K, Terao J. Quercetin appears in the lymph of unanesthetized rats as its phase II metabolites after administered into the stomach. *FEBS. Lett.* 2005; 579: 5343-6.

[33] Talavera S, Felgines C, Texier O, Besson C, Manach C, Lamaison JL, et al. Anthocyanins are efficiently absorbed from the small intestine in rats. *J. Nutr.* 2004; 134: 2275-9.

[34] Uzunovic A, Vranic E. Stability of anthocyanins from commercial black currant juice under simulated gastrointestinal digestion. *Bosn. J. Basic. Med. Sci.* 2008; 8: 254-8.

[35] Keppler K, Humpf HU. Metabolism of anthocyanins and their phenolic degradation products by the intestinal microflora. *Bioorg Med. Chem.* 2005; 13: 5195-205.

[36] Fleschhut J, Kratzer F, Rechkemmer G, Kulling SE. Stability and biotransformation of various dietary anthocyanins in vitro. *Eur. J. Nutr.* 2006; 45: 7-18.

[37] Herles C, Braune A, Blaut M. First bacterial chalcone isomerase isolated from Eubacterium ramulus. *Arch. Microbiol.* 2004; 181: 428-34.

INDEX

A

B

I

J

K

L

M

N

O

P

Q

R

S

T

U

V

W

X

Y